Horizons in Medicine

number 16

Edited by

Jayne Franklyn

Professor of Medicine, Institute of Biomedical Research, The Medical School, Edgbaston, Birmingham

Royal College of Physicians of London

Acknowledgement

The Royal College of Physicians acknowledges the contribution of The Lavenham Press towards the cost of printing this book.

Front cover photograph:
LAWRENCE LIVERMORE LABORATORY/SCIENCE PHOTO LIBRARY
False-colour scanning tunnelling micrograph of DNA

Royal College of Physicians of London
11 St Andrews Place, London NW1 4LE

Registered Charity No. 210508

ISBN 1 86016 233 9

Typeset by Dan-Set Graphics, Telford, Shropshire
Printed in Great Britain by The Lavenham Press Ltd, Sudbury, Suffolk

British Library Cataloguing in Publication Data
A catalogue record of this book is available from the British Library

Editor's introduction

This volume in the Horizons in Medicine series represents an update of a wide-ranging group of subjects reaching across all areas of medicine. As organiser of the 2004 Advanced Medicine Conference, I was allowed the luxury of seeking out UK leaders of national and international repute working at the cutting edge in their field and inviting them to contribute. This publication reflects their input to one of the most important, topical and popular conferences organised by the Royal College of Physicians.

The trend of increasing specialisation, and even subspecialisation, within medicine determines that it is increasingly difficult to keep abreast of new developments in fields other than our own. The vast array of information available, especially electronically, sometimes hinders rather than helps, emphasising the need for those at the forefront of their field to put such information into context and to give pragmatic advice based on their practical experience.

The chapters reflect many aspects of medicine. Topics covered include the importance of preventive medicine and the potential impact of better management of highly prevalent risk factors such as obesity and hypertension; information about novel therapies and interventions in common medical diagnoses such as gastrointestinal bleeding, lung cancer and chronic liver disease; best practice in areas of medicine such as coronary artery disease and osteoporosis where a sometimes bewildering array of options is available; and also the role of 'super-specialist' input in complex areas such as the medicine of pregnancy, hepatology and nephrology. In addition, this volume reflects the conference highlights: the Lumleian lecture, which illustrates to perfection the translation of molecular biology to disease management and risk prediction, and the Croonian lecture, which so elegantly displays the genetic and biological unravelling of multiple sclerosis, an all too common disease.

In these times of change for the physician, both in training and in consultant practice, it is easy to lose sight of the clinical excellence which exists within the UK. Academic medicine is perceived as being under threat. It remains critical to protect professional flexibility and time, within both the NHS and university sectors, to allow the fostering and development of talents and innovations, which could all too readily be swamped by increasing constraints.

This volume illustrates some of those talents and, in so doing, provides a practical guide to best practice in medicine in 2004.

JAYNE FRANKLYN

August 2004

Contributors

JOHN C ATHERTON *Professor of Gastroenterology and MRC Senior Clinical Fellow, Wolfson Digestive Diseases Centre and Institute of Infection, Immunity and Inflammation, University of Nottingham, C Floor, South Block, University Hospital, Nottingham NG7 2UH*

NIGEL J BRUNSKILL *Senior Lecturer/Honorary Consultant Nephrologist, Department of Nephrology, Leicester General Hospital, Gwendolen Road, Leicester LE5 4PW*

ALASTAIR COMPSTON *Professor of Neurology, Department of Clinical Neurosciences, University of Cambridge, Addenbrooke's Hospital, Hills Road, Cambridge CB2 2QQ*

PAUL A CORRIS *Professor of Thoracic Medicine, University of Newcastle and Regional Cardiothoracic Centre, Freeman Hospital, Newcastle upon Tyne NE7 7DN*

JOHN S DUNCAN *Professor of Neurology, Department of Clinical and Experimental Epilepsy, Institute of Neurology, UCL, National Hospital for Neurology and Neurosurgery, Queen Square, London WC1N 3BG*

RICHARD EASTELL *Professor of Bone Metabolism, Academic Unit of Bone Metabolism, Section of Human Metabolism, Division of Clinical Sciences, University of Sheffield Clinical Sciences Centre, Northern General Hospital, Herries Road, Sheffield S5 7AU*

I SADAF FAROOQI *Wellcome Clinician Scientist Fellow, University Departments of Medicine and Clinical Biochemistry, Box 232, Addenbrooke's Hospital, Cambridge CB2 2QQ*

JAYNE FRANKLYN *Professor of Medicine, Associate Dean for Graduate School, Institute of Biomedical Research, Wolfson Drive, The Medical School, Edgbaston, Birmingham B15 2TT*

MICHAEL D GAMMAGE *Reader in Cardiovascular Medicine, Department of Cardiovascular Medicine, Centre for Cardiovascular Studies, Queen Elizabeth Hospital, University of Birmingham, Birmingham B15 2TH*

LORRAINE HARPER *Senior Lecturer (Medicine) and Honorary Renal Consultant, Renal Immunobiology, The Medical School, University of Birmingham, Edgbaston, Birmingham B15 2TT*

CHRIS J HAWKEY *Professor of Gastroenterology, Co-Director – Institute of Clinical Research, Wolfson Digestive Diseases Centre, University Hospital, Nottingham NG7 2UH*

ANTHONY HEAGERTY *Professor of Medicine, Department of Medicine, Manchester Royal Infirmary, Oxford Road, Manchester M13 9WL*

NICHOLAS A HOENICH *Lecturer, School of Clinical Medical Sciences, University of Newcastle; Honorary Clinical Scientist, Newcastle upon Tyne Hospitals NHS Trust, Framlington Place, Newcastle upon Tyne NE2 4HH*

HOWARD S JACOBS *Emeritus Professor of Reproductive Endocrinology, Royal Free and UCL Medical School; London Diabetes and Lipid Centre, 14 Wimpole Street, London W1G 9SX*

OLIVER F W JAMES *Head of School, Clinical Medical Sciences, University of Newcastle, Framlington Place, Newcastle upon Tyne NE2 4HH*

LIZ LIGHTSTONE *Senior Lecturer and Honorary Consultant Renal Physician, Renal Section, Division of Medicine, Faculty of Medicine, Imperial College London, Hammersmith Campus, Du Cane Road, London W12 0NN*

IAIN C MACDOUGALL *Consultant Nephrologist and Honorary Senior Lecturer, Department of Renal Medicine, King's College Hospital, East Dulwich Grove, London SE22 8PT*

VIAS MARKIDES *Consultant Cardiologist, Cardiology Department, St Mary's Hospital and Imperial College, Praed Street, London W2 1NY*

JANET M McCOMB *Consultant Cardiologist, Freeman Hospital, Newcastle upon Tyne NE7 7DN*

KEVIN MOORE *Senior Lecturer in Medicine, Centre for Hepatology, Department of Medicine, Royal Free Campus, University College London, Rowland Hill Street, London NW3 2PF*

KAREN E MORRISON *Professor of Neurology, Head of Department of Clinical Neurosciences, Honorary Consultant Neurologist, 2nd Floor, Institute of Biomedical Research, The Medical School, University of Birmingham, Edgbaston, Birmingham B15 2TT*

DAVID MUTIMER *Consultant Hepatologist, The Liver and Hepatology Unit, 3rd Floor, Nuffield House, Queen Elizabeth Hospital, Edgbaston, Birmingham B15 2TH*

KELVIN PALMER *Consultant Gastroenterologist, Western General Hospital, Crew Road, Edinburgh EH4 2XU*

DAVID PATCH *Consultant Hepatologist, Department of Surgery, 9th Floor, Royal Free Hospital, Pond Street, London NW3 2QG*

NICHOLAS S PETERS *Professor of Cardiology, Head of Cardiac Electrophysiology, Imperial College at St Mary's Hospital, Praed Street, London W2 1NY*

RICHARD POULSOM *Histopathology Unit, Cancer Research UK, London Research Institute, 44 Lincoln's Inn Fields, London WC2A 3PX; Bart's and the London, Queen Mary's School of Medicine and Dentistry, London*

PETER M ROTHWELL *Professor of Clinical Neurology, University of Oxford; Stroke Prevention Research Unit, University Department of Clinical Neurology, Radcliffe Infirmary, Woodstock Road, Oxford OX2 6HE*

PETER SELBY *Consultant Physician, Manchester Royal Infirmary; Honorary Senior Lecturer, University of Manchester, Department of Medicine, Manchester Royal Infirmary, Oxford Road, Manchester M13 9WL*

MICHAEL C SHEPPARD *William Withering Professor of Medicine and Vice Dean, Medical School, University of Birmingham, Edgbaston, Birmingham B15 2TT*

STEPHEN G SPIRO *Head, Department of Respiratory Medicine, University College London Hospital, The Middlesex Hospital, Mortimer Street, London W1T 3AA*

ROBERT A STOCKLEY *Professor in Medicine, Department of Medicine, Queen Elizabeth Hospital, Edgbaston, Birmingham B15 2TH*

IAN D SWAIN *Consultant Biomedical Engineer, Department of Medical Physics and Biomedical Engineering, Salisbury District Hospital, Salisbury SP2 8BJ; Academic Biomedical Engineering Research Group, Bournemouth University*

PAUL N TAYLOR *Principal Clinical Engineer, Department of Medical Physics and Biomedical Engineering, Salisbury District Hospital, Salisbury; Academic Biomedical Engineering Research Group, Bournemouth University*

DOUGLAS THORBURN *Consultant Hepatologist, The Liver and Hepatology Unit, 3rd Floor, Nuffield House, Queen Elizabeth Hospital, Birmingham B15 2TH*

SARA THORNE *Consultant Cardiologist, University Hospital Birmingham, Birmingham B15 2TH*

TZYNG-HAI YEN *Histopathology Unit, Cancer Research UK, London Research Institute, 44 Lincoln's Inn Fields, London WC2A 3PX; Bart's and the London, Queen Mary's School of Medicine and Dentistry, London; Department of Nephrology, Chang Gung Memorial Hospital, Taipei, Taiwan*

MARK VANDERPUMP *Consultant Physician and Honorary Senior Lecturer in Endocrinology and Diabetes, Department of Endocrinology, Royal Free Hospital Trust, Pond Street, London NW3 2QG*

ALASTAIR J M WATSON *Professor of Medicine, Department of Medicine, University of Liverpool Medical School, Daulby Street, Liverpool L69 3GA*

PETER N T WELLS *Emeritus Professor of Physics and Engineering in Medicine, University of Bristol, Bristol General Hospital, Bristol BS1 6SY*

DAVID C WHEELER *Senior Lecturer in Nephrology, Centre for Nephrology, Royal Free and University College Medical School, Rowland Hill Street, London NW3 2PF*

TOM WONG *Research Fellow, Cardiology Department, St Mary's Hospital and Imperial College, Praed Street, London W2 1NY*

MARK WOODHEAD *Consultant in General and Respiratory Medicine, Manchester Royal Infirmary, Oxford Road, Manchester M13 9WL*

NICHOLAS A WRIGHT *Histopathology Unit, Cancer Research UK, London Research Institute, 44 Lincoln's Inn Fields, London WC2A 3PX; Bart's and The London, Queen Mary's School of Medicine and Dentistry, Warden's Office, Turner Street, Whitechapel, London E1 2AD*

Contents

NEUROLOGY

RENAL

RESPIRATORY

GASTROENTEROLOGY

HEPATOLOGY

TRANSPLANTATION

MEDICINE IN PREGNANCY

Oncology

Should we be more aggressive in the management of lung cancer?

Stephen Spiro

□ INTRODUCTION

Lung cancer kills more men than any other common cancer and is close to breast cancer in women for annual mortality. The death rates for men and women from lung cancer exceed those of colorectal, breast, pancreatic and prostate cancer combined. In 2003, there were 172,000 and 38,000 new cases in the USA and the UK, respectively, with 157,000 and 36,000 deaths. The five-year survival in 1975 from all presentations of lung cancer was 12%; it has barely improved since 1998 when it was 15%. This lack of improved survival for lung cancer, with no substantial progress in treatments, compares relatively unfavourably with the advances seen in colorectal, breast and prostate cancers. Surgical management has improved over the last two decades in case selection, postoperative care and a reduced peri-operative death rate. The effect of radiotherapy as a radical treatment for locally advanced disease is disappointing (0–17% five-year survival). Radical radiotherapy in medically inoperable but technically resectable patients achieves a five-year survival rate well below that for resection. Chemotherapy has provided only modest benefit in non-small-cell lung cancer (NSCLC), improving the median survival for patients with advanced metastatic disease from approximately four months with best supportive care to 8–9 months with modern platin-containing chemotherapy.

□ AGGRESSIVE MANAGEMENT

Current areas of more aggressive management include:

- the potential of low-dose spiral computed tomography (LDCT) as a screening tool for earlier stage lung cancer
- the value of positron emission tomography (PET) in reducing the futile thoracotomy rate
- a possible role for chemotherapy either before (neo-adjuvant) or after (adjuvant) surgery, and
- similarly, the potential for adding chemotherapy to radical radiotherapy.

At present, the role of chemotherapy in advanced disease seems limited and unsatisfactory. The attempt to consider biological growth modifying agents is therefore a current 'hot topic' for patients with advanced disease.

☐ SMALL-CELL LUNG CANCER

There was real progress in the management of small-cell lung cancer (SCLC) in the 1970s and 1980s. This involved refining the intensity and duration of chemotherapy and confirmation of the value of adding mediastinal irradiation to patients whose tumours responded well to chemotherapy. The role of prophylactic cranial irradiation has also shown a small survival advantage and better control of the incidence of cerebral relapse in patients who had responded to chemotherapy or chemotherapy-radiotherapy to the primary tumour site. However, many attempts to increase survival further with early or late intensification of chemotherapy doses, using alternating non-cross-resistant regimens and gentler chemotherapy in the elderly all failed. The current interest in biological growth modifying agents does not seem to be as valuable in SCLC although anti-angiogenic agents are being evaluated in large multicentre trials in this cell type.

☐ SCREENING FOR PRIMARY TUMOURS

Half way through the life of a solid tumour, the mass is 1 mm in diameter. Lung cancer is diagnosed on routine chest X-ray at approximately 3–4 cm in diameter which represents approximately 37 of the total 40 volume doubling times comprising the life of a cancer. Although chest X-ray *may* identify a 1 cm tumour, it may be missed in up to 85% of cases when reviewed retrospectively. The use of LDCT as a screening tool to identify smaller primary tumours has been the subject of several recent hypothesis generating studies, mainly in Japan and the USA where adenocarcinoma is the commonest cell type. In western Europe, squamous cell cancers predominate, a cell type that tends to occur centrally, cause symptoms of breathlessness, cough, wheeze, infection and haemoptysis, and usually diagnosed via the bronchoscope. Adenocarcinomas generally arise peripherally within the lung and are silent, and therefore seem an attractive proposition for earlier detection by LDCT. However, any potential screening study would require a control group and have to take into account the biases of lead time, length time and overdiagnosis. Ultimately, screening for lung cancer will be effective only if it is shown to reduce mortality.

To date, the published studies have focused on high risk populations, mainly men over the age of 50 years at entry, and smokers of at least 20 pack-years (Table 1).[1–4] The pick up of primary lung cancers on prevalence screens has ranged from 0.27–2.8%, depending on the risk status of the chosen population. Up to 80% of tumours identified have been of the most favourable tumour-nodal status (metastases) stage (ie stage Ia). Conventionally, this stage has a five-year survival of approximately 65% after resection. Most stage Ia tumours found on initial screens have been resectable, but the cure rate for these individuals is not yet known. In addition to prevalence screening, incidence screening (usually one year after the prevalence screen) has shown a continuing pick up of cancers, but at a much lower rate than on the prevalence screen, with a smaller proportion (ca 65%) of incidence cancers stage Ia.

Table 1 Spiral computed tomography screening studies.

Study	Patients				False-positive scans (%)
	No.	Data	Primary cancers	Stage Ia	
Kaneko[1]	1,369	>50 years >20 pack-years 82% men	15	14	11.4
Henschke[3]	1,000	>60 years 45 pack-years	27	23	19
Svensen[4]	1,520	>50 years >20 pack-years	22	15	51

Confounding factors

A major confounding factor in all screening studies has been the high incidence of benign non-calcified nodules (11% in Japanese studies, 20% in the USA). In midwestern USA, where fungal infection with histoplasmosis and coccidioido-mycosis is particularly common, the incidence of false-positive findings on LDCT is up to 98%! Screening is a subject of great interest, but so far all studies published are hypothesis generating, and the average size of tumours detected is 16 mm which is larger than anticipated. It is still debatable whether there is a relationship between tumour size and survival. The high false-positive rate has led to patients having biopsies or resections for benign disease, with many being submitted to regular follow-up with high-resolution CT, causing an accumulating exposure to irradiation.

It is difficult to know which population should be studied, and the whole question of LDCT screening will not be settled until large randomised controlled trials (RCTs) have been performed. Such a study has already started in the USA; it aims for 50,000 entrants, but it will be 10 years before any effect on mortality is seen – assuming the study is positive.

□ STAGING TESTS

Positron emission tomography

The five-year survival for the most favourable (Ia) and poorest resectable (IIIa) stage NSCLC is 65% and 12%, respectively. Clinical examination, CT scanning, bone isotope scans and abdominal ultrasound often fail to identify metastatic disease. PET scanning is likely to improve this. Several studies comparing PET and CT for lymph node status in potentially operable NSCLC show that the sensitivity, specificity and accuracy of PET are 89%, 92% and 90%, respectively, and 65%, 80% and 75% with CT. The best results are obtained with both techniques combined (CT/PET).

A recent Dutch randomised study in patients with potentially operable NSCLC compared conventional work-up (96 patients) with conventional work-up plus

PET (92). Eighteen patients in the conventional work-up group and 32 in the PET group did not have a thoracotomy. In the conventional group, 39 patients had a futile thoracotomy compared with only 19 in the PET group. PET, therefore, saved unnecessary surgery in 20% of patients.[5] PET scanning outside the thorax is also likely to prove valuable.

PET scanners in the UK are scarce compared with more than 700 in the USA (at present, fewer than 10 PET scanners are available in the NHS), but the government has recently promised a small number of new scanners.

Current recommendations for scanning

The current recommendation is that a biopsy should be performed if CT of the thorax reveals enlarged lymph nodes in the mediastinum or an enlarged mass outside the thorax (eg adrenal gland, liver mass). If, however, a patient staged for surgery is operable on CT staging, a PET scan should be carried out to ascertain that normal sized or borderline (10 mm) lymph nodes do not contain metastatic disease. PET scanning is likely to be accurate, with a high negative predictive value (95%) in nodes as small as 8 mm in diameter.

□ NON-SMALL-CELL LUNG CANCER

Neo-adjuvant chemotherapy

In 1994, two small studies (60 patients with 30 randomised to each arm) reported that neo-adjuvant chemotherapy in resectable patients had a highly significant survival advantage compared with surgery alone.

In 2002, a European study of 355 patients was reported in which primary surgery alone in clinically staged resectable patients was compared with primary surgery preceded by two courses of mitomycin, ifosfamide and cisplatin chemotherapy followed by two further postoperative courses to responding patients.[6] The pre-operative response to chemotherapy in the neo-adjuvant arm was 64%. Postoperative mortality was acceptable (neo-adjuvant 6.7%, surgery alone 4.5%); median survival was 37 months for neo-adjuvant chemotherapy and 26 months for surgery alone ($p = 0.15$).

This large study was negative, suggesting that all patients seriously considered for neo-adjuvant chemotherapy should still participate in a clinical trial as more comparative trials are needed. In fact, several large clinical trials are in progress to see whether this more aggressive approach to operable patients will improve the five-year survival. It is hoped that the answer will be found within the next few years.

Adjuvant therapy

Chemotherapy

A meta-analysis in 1995 showed that the addition of chemotherapy following surgery gave a non-statistically significant 5% five-year survival advantage for adjuvant chemotherapy.[7] Several studies are re-examining this and are now beginning to report. One study comparing three courses of mitomycin, vindesine and platinum following surgery with surgery alone in 1,209 patients was negative, with no survival advantage for postoperative chemotherapy. Another study of similar design from France in 1,800 patients comparing 3–4 cycles of platin-based chemotherapy following surgery with surgery alone showed a five-year survival advantage of 5% for the adjuvant arm. Four other studies will soon complete. It is then likely that the important question will be answered whether patients should receive chemotherapy following successful surgery. The survival advantage may be small, but in a common disease would benefit thousands of patients undergoing successful resection.

Radiotherapy

The role of adjuvant radiotherapy with surgery has been clarified to some extent in a meta-analysis of nine RCTs; following successful surgery, patients were randomised to two groups, one of which received postoperative radiotherapy. A statistically significant disadvantage was found for patients who received postoperative radiotherapy, and it was therefore no longer recommended.[8] This study has been criticised because the radiation fractionations were different from those currently in use, less aggressive, and given by older, out-of-date equipment. Nevertheless, current evidence suggests no advantage for postoperative irradiation.

Locally advanced disease

It is increasingly accepted that radical radiotherapy fails primarily because of the emergence of distant metastases despite reasonable local control of the treated area. During the last 15 years several studies have added chemotherapy to radical radiotherapy as either neo- or adjuvant treatment. Others have adopted this approach, but have also attempted to improve the effects of radiotherapy by escalating the radical dose or giving it as a hyperfractionated regimen (usually twice daily). A few studies have shown a small survival advantage for the more aggressive treatment arm, more related to the addition of chemotherapy than to a change in the radiotherapy schedule.

There is current interest in giving chemotherapy concurrently with radiotherapy rather than sequentially, but only one published study has compared this approach in locally advanced disease.[9] In the concurrent arm (156 patients), radiotherapy was started on day 2 with 28 Gy given in 14 daily fractions. The same radiotherapy schedule was repeated after a 10-day rest period, making a total of 56 Gy given to the tumour. On day 1, prior to commencing radiotherapy, chemotherapy was started (cisplatin, vindesine and mitomycin) and repeated for four courses. In the sequential arm (158 patients), chemotherapy was given for four courses, with radiotherapy (56 Gy in daily fractions) on completion of the chemotherapy. The median survival for concurrent and sequential treatment was 16.5 months and 13.3 months, respectively, with a statistically significant survival advantage for concurrent treatment ($p < 0.04$). Further studies are in progress to confirm these data; a large study in the UK will begin in June 2004.

Advanced metastatic disease

The role of cytotoxic chemotherapy in advanced metastatic disease has shown no specific chemotherapy regimen to be superior. Most regimens in the UK now contain two rather than three cytotoxic agents. The commonest schedules include carboplatin and gemcitabine or carboplatin and vinorelbine. In the USA, paclitaxel is used more commonly with carboplatin or cisplatin than in the UK where the expense of paclitaxel is considered excessive. All the studies of these regimens show median survival figures of 7-9 months, with isolated studies reporting medians of 11 months (Table 2).[10] The one-year survival without chemotherapy (ie best supportive care) in advanced NSCLC is 28%, increasing to 30–40% with chemotherapy.

Table 2 Chemotherapy in advanced non-small-cell lung cancer.[10]

				Survival	
Chemotherapy	**Cycle frequency (days)**	**No. of patients**	**Stage III/IV**	**Mean (months)**	**One-year (%)**
Cisplatin 75 mg/m^2 Paclitaxel 135 mg/m^2 over 24 hours	21	288	11/89	7.8	31
versus Cisplatin 100 mg/m^2 Gemcitabine 1,000 mg/m^2 (days 1, 8, 21)	28	288	14/86	8.1	36
versus Cisplatin 75 mg/m^2 Docetaxel 75 mg/m^2	21	289	14/86	7.4	31
versus Carboplatin, AUC 6 Paclitaxel 225 mg/m^2 over 3 hours	21	290	14/86	8.1	34

Many recent studies do not contain quality of life (QoL) data. This appears to be an essential requirement when considering palliative chemotherapy in advanced NSCLC. A recent British study comparing chemotherapy versus best supportive care in 273 patients with advanced disease showed no significant advantage in global health score for the addition of chemotherapy compared with best supportive care alone. The side effects of chemotherapy seem to counterbalance the improvement achieved by chemotherapy for the systemic symptoms associated with advanced lung cancer. However, there seems to be no *disadvantage* in terms of overall QoL, so it is reasonable to offer chemotherapy to suitable patients – in general, those with a good performance status. There is no recommended age cut-off. Elderly patients (>70 years) respond as well as younger patients, with a similar progression free interval, but toxicity and the need for dose reductions of the chemotherapy are greater.

Docetaxel is recommended for second-line chemotherapy. The response rate is about 15%; approximately 20% of patients who relapse after an initial response to first-line chemotherapy are still considered fit enough to receive docetaxel.

□ BIOLOGICAL GROWTH MODIFYING AGENTS

Gefitinib (Iressa), an epidermal growth factor receptor antagonist, has been studied as a second-, third- or fourth-line agent in relapsed advanced NSCLC. It has also been given as initial treatment in addition to chemotherapy compared with chemotherapy alone. Two studies in relapsed disease after 1–3 previous chemotherapy regimens have shown a 10–18% response rate with gefitinib, a prolonged survival and substantial improvement in QoL scores in up to 40% of patients. Response rates, median survivals and QoL improvements are more frequent in patients who enter a gefitinib study having relapsed after one regimen of cytotoxic chemotherapy than in those who have received three or four different regimens.[11] The two other large studies comparing different doses of gefitinib given at the start of chemotherapy compared with chemotherapy alone have been negative.

Several agents in this class are being evaluated in lung cancer. It is too early to know if these well tolerated agents will find an important therapeutic role. Clinical trials in advanced disease are in progress with erlotinib (Tarceva). The place of the anti-angiogenic agent, thalidomide, is also being actively investigated in studies in both SCLC and advanced NSCLC.

□ SMOKING AND LUNG CANCER

The outlook for lung cancer remains tough. It is hard to get away from the fact that smoking is the cause of more than 80% of all lung tumours. There is a dose response and a dose duration effect with smoking and all four cell types are associated with tobacco consumption. A recent study has shown that the incidence is independent of the tar content of cigarette smoke.[12] It is no longer tenable to believe that low tar-containing tobacco is less likely to cause lung cancer. Women have twice the risk of acquiring lung cancer and its incidence is rising in women in the UK. It is rising even more rapidly – and alarmingly – in France and the Mediterranean countries where smoking amongst women is high. Attempts to reduce smoking within the population must remain an important primary aim. Smoking prevalence reduced by 50% in the UK between 1950 and 1990, but current smokers in 1990 were more likely to be lifelong smokers. Nevertheless, the earlier individuals stop smoking, the lower their risk of acquiring this almost always fatal disease.

REFERENCES

1 Kaneko M, Eguchi K, Ohmatsu H, Kakinuma R *et al.* Peripheral lung cancer: screening and detection with low-dose spiral CT versus radiography. *Radiology* 1996;**201**:798–802.

2 Sone S, Takashima S, Li F, Yang Z *et al.* Mass screening for lung cancer with mobile spiral computed tomography scanner. *Lancet* 1998;**351**:1242–5.

3 Henschke CI, McCauley DI, Yankelevitz DF, Naidich DP *et al.* Early Lung Cancer Action Project: overall design and findings from baseline screening. *Lancet* 1999;**354**:99–105.

4 Swensen SJ, Jett JR, Sloan JA, Midthun DE *et al.* Screening for lung cancer with low-dose spiral computed tomography. *Am J Respir Crit Care Med* 2002;**165**:508–13.

5 van Tinteren H, Hoekstra OS, Smit EF, van den Bergh JH *et al.* Effectiveness of positron emission tomography in the preoperative assessment of patients with suspected non-small-cell lung cancer: the PLUS multicentre randomised trial. *Lancet* 2002;**359**:1388–93.

6 Depierre A, Milleron B, Moro-Sibilot D, Chevret S *et al.* Preoperative chemotherapy followed by surgery compared with primary surgery in resectable stage I (except T1N0), II, and IIIa non-small-cell lung cancer. *J Clin Oncol* 2002;**20**:247–53.

7 Chemotherapy in non-small cell lung cancer: a meta-analysis using updated data on individual patients from 52 randomised clinical trials. Non-small Cell Lung Cancer Collaborative Group. *BMJ* 1995;**311**:899–909.

8 Postoperative radiotherapy in non-small-cell lung cancer: systematic review and meta-analysis of individual patient data from nine randomised controlled trials. PORT Meta-analysis Trialists Group. *Lancet* 1998;**352**:257–63.

9 Furuse K, Fukuoka M, Kawahara M, Nishikawa H *et al.* Phase III study of concurrent versus sequential thoracic radiotherapy in combination with mitomycin, vindesine, and cisplatin in unresectable stage III non-small-cell lung cancer. *J Clin Oncol* 1999;**17**:2692–9.

10 Schiller JH, Harrington D, Belani CP, Langer C *et al.* Comparison of four chemotherapy regimens for advanced non-small-cell lung cancer. *N Engl J Med* 2002;**346**:92–8.

11 Fukuoka M, Yano S, Giaccone G, Tamura T *et al.* Multi-institutional randomized phase II trial of gefitinib for previously treated patients with advanced non-small-cell lung cancer. *J Clin Oncol* 2003;**21**:2237–46.

12 Harris JE, Thun MJ, Mondul AM, Calle EE. Cigarette tar yields in relation to mortality from lung cancer in the cancer prevention study II prospective cohort, 1982-8. *BMJ* 2004;**328**:72.

Who should be screened for colorectal cancer?

Alastair Watson

☐ INTRODUCTION

Screening is a healthcare strategy that can bring great benefits by preventing disease in an entire population. The decision to start a screening programme can be momentous, particularly if it is to be on a national scale, because the costs can be considerable as new services frequently have to be established. Screening also carries the potential of doing serious harm if the test procedures are dangerous. Also, few screening programmes are 100% sensitive or specific; this can cause distress through the raising of false expectations. Some people who consider themselves healthy object to having their lives interrupted by being contacted by health services. For these reasons, it is essential to have clear criteria for deciding whether screening for a particular disease is justified.

It is now accepted that the criteria for screening (Table 1) laid down by Wilson and Jünger form a good framework for guiding thought about the merits of a screening programme.[1] The case for screening for colorectal cancer will be considered in this chapter according to those criteria.

Table 1 The Wilson and Jünger criteria for screening.[1]

- Is the disease an important health problem?
- Is there an early or latent stage?
- Is the natural history of the condition known?
- Is there a suitable screening test?
- Are there agreed criteria for who should be treated?
- Are diagnostic and treatment facilities available?
- Is the programme economically viable?

☐ IS COLORECTAL CANCER AN IMPORTANT HEALTH PROBLEM?

In 1999, 35,579 new cases of colorectal cancer were diagnosed, and in 2001 it caused the death of 16,152 people in the UK.[2] Colorectal cancer is the second commonest cause of cancer death, accounting for 16% of all cancer deaths and 3% of deaths from all causes (Figs 1 and 2).[3]

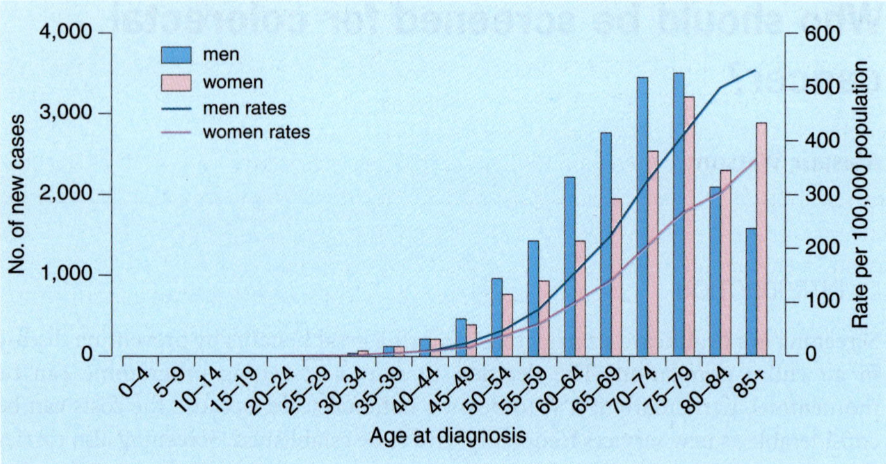

Fig 1 Number of new cases of colorectal cancer diagnosed and age-specific rates per 100,000 population, by sex, UK 1999.[3]

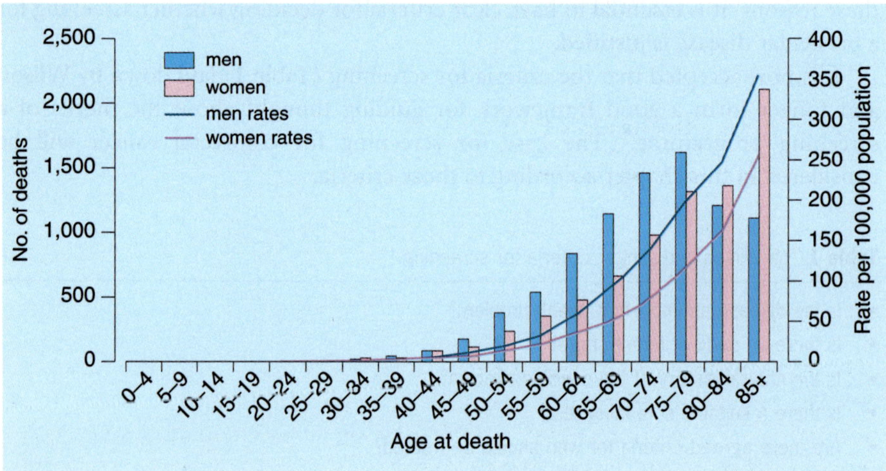

Fig 2 Number of deaths from colorectal cancer and age-specific mortality rates per 100,000 population, by sex, UK 1999.[3]

Colorectal cancer can be cured if treated early in its natural history. Patients with cancer limited to the bowel wall (Duke's A) have a five-year survival of over 95%. The problem is that only about 10% of patients present with Duke's A histology, most presenting with more advanced disease that carries a far worse prognosis. A significant minority of patients present as emergencies through the casualty department with bowel obstruction or perforation secondary to their cancer, significantly worsening their prognosis. The challenge for the clinician is that Duke's A cancer is often asymptomatic and therefore requires measures to be taken with the general population who consider themselves to be healthy.

☐ IS THERE AN EARLY LATENT STAGE AND IS THE NATURAL HISTORY KNOWN?

It is now accepted that most colorectal cancers arise from pre-existing adenomas. Evidence in support is that adenomas and carcinomas share some risk factors and genetic alterations. Colorectal cancer and adenomas often coexist, and some adenomas contain a focus of malignant change. However, the average age of adenoma diagnosis is 10 years younger than that of colorectal cancer.[4,5] Moreover, only one in six adenomas develops into cancer, with risk factors being size (>1 cm), multiplicity (>3) and villous histology. Such high risk adenomas have a prevalence of about 6% in 55 year olds. The progression of adenoma to carcinoma is slow and estimated to take 10–15 years. Thus, there is a large window of opportunity to identify and remove adenomas before they transform into potentially lethal carcinomas. Removal of pedunculated and sessile polyps fails to prevent about 25% of cancer; it is possible that these cancers arise from flat or depressed adenomas.

☐ IS THERE A SUITABLE SCREENING TEST?

One of the complexities of planning colorectal cancer screening is the large number of tests and procedures that could potentially be used.

Established tests

There are several well established tests:

- ☐ faecal occult blood (FOB)
- ☐ barium enema
- ☐ flexible sigmoidoscopy, and
- ☐ colonoscopy.

The gold standard for testing the efficacy of a screening tool is a randomised controlled trial (RCT) demonstrating a reduction in population mortality from colorectal cancer in a screened population compared with an unscreened population. Only screening with FOB has been tested against this stringent criterion. A reduction of population mortality from colorectal cancer of 15–20% has been demonstrated.[6–8] A trial of flexible sigmoidoscopy is underway in the UK, but it has not yet reported. Any further RCTs of screening tools are unlikely because it is becoming impossible to recruit a control group that will not undergo some sort of screening test during the trial. Policy makers have to rely more on case-control and cohort studies to inform their decisions than in many other areas of medicine.

Newer screening tests

There are also much newer tests based on computed tomography (CT) and magnetic resonance (MR) scanning and tests for the detection of cancer products in the stool. Both CT virtual colonoscopy and MR colonography are undergoing continuous development.[9,10] The latest scanning protocols achieve similar sensitivity and specificity to colonoscopy. The detection of DNA cancer markers in the stools of patients is an attractive strategy as it is minimally invasive and does not require capital expenditure on an endoscopy, CT or MR unit. Methods for the detection of microsatellite instability, mutations of APC, p53, BAT-26 or K-ras, or the detection of high molecular weight DNA from non-apoptotic cells all show promise, but require more work to establish their sensitivity and specificity in average risk populations.[11]

☐ ARE THERE AGREED CRITERIA FOR WHO SHOULD BE SCREENED?

In broad terms, there are agreed criteria about who should be screened. There is substantial international agreement between gastroenterologists on screening criteria for individual patients who consult them about colorectal cancer,[4,12,13] but little agreement on the details of patient selection or what test should be used. This is important as apparently minor differences in screening protocols can have huge cost implications. At a government level, there is little international consensus.

Screening stages

Colorectal cancer screening should be thought of as a three-stage procedure:

1. Formal assessment of the patient's risk for developing colorectal cancer.
2. A screening test to eliminate patients with no disease.
3. A definitive diagnostic and treatment stage.

Colonoscopy has the advantage of combining stages 2 and 3.

Risk stratification

Risk stratification should establish answers to the following questions:

1. Has the patient ever had colorectal cancer or an adenomatous polyp?
2. Does the patient have inflammatory bowel disease (IBD)?
3. Has the patient had a previous adenomatous polyp?
4. Has a family member had colorectal cancer? If so, were they a first-degree relative and how old were they at diagnosis?

If the answer to these questions is 'no', the patient is defined as being of average risk. This will account for about 70% of patients. Those who answer 'yes' have a higher risk and require a different screening or surveillance strategy.

☐ SCREENING PEOPLE OF AVERAGE RISK

Faecal occult blood testing

Testing of faecal blood has a low sensitivity (ca 50%) and specificity for the detection of colorectal cancer, but with repeated annual use can detect as many as 92% of cancers.

Three statistically powerful RCTs have been undertaken.[6–8] Over a follow-up of at least 10 years, colorectal mortality in the screened population was reduced by 18–21%.

The US Multisociety Task Force on Colorectal Cancer recommends an annual test with a guaic-based test without rehydration following a three-day abstention from red meat.[14] The NHS National Screening Committee is still formulating its recommendations on FOB screening but has recently completed pilot studies demonstrating the feasibility of FOB testing in the NHS. About a third of screenees will have a positive FOB and require colonoscopy and polypectomy if a polyp is detected or surgery if a cancer is found.

Flexible sigmoidoscopy

Flexible sigmoidoscopy examines the left side of the colon to a variable extent. It has the advantage over colonoscopy in that the patient does not require a full three-day bowel preparation but only an enema immediately prior to the procedure. It is also frequently acceptable to the patient to omit sedation.

Dr Wendy Atkin has proposed, and is now testing with a large RCT, that a single flexible sigmoidoscopic examination at age 55 is sufficient substantially to reduce the lifetime risk of colorectal cancer if the finding of significant adenoma (>1 cm in diameter, multiple adenomas or villous histology) is used as an indication for full colonoscopy.[15] This will identify about 50% of advanced right-sided neoplasms.[16] A Scandinavian study has reported that colorectal cancer incidence in individuals with polyps was reduced by 80% with screening sigmoidoscopy followed by colonoscopy.[17] This strategy is attractive because it considerably reduces the number of colonoscopies that need to be performed, thereby increasing patient acceptability and safety, and substantially reducing cost.

Colonoscopy

Unlike FOB testing and flexible sigmoidoscopy, colonoscopy will probably never be evaluated as a screening tool by RCT, but two cohort studies have shown that colonoscopy and polypectomy substantially reduce (by 60–80%) the incidence of colorectal cancer.[18,19] The US Multisociety Task Force on Colorectal Cancer recommends colonoscopy every 10 years starting at age 50.[14] A recent study found that individuals whose initial colonoscopy was negative had a less than 1% chance of an adenomatous polyp being found at a second colonoscopy five years later. Flat adenomas can be difficult to identify by routine colonoscopy so some authorities recommend highlighting either by dyes such as indigo carmen or by magnifying colonoscopy.

☐ SCREENING PEOPLE OF INCREASED RISK

Previous colorectal cancer

Patients with colorectal cancer are at a sixfold increased risk of developing a second cancer compared with patients with benign adenomatous polyps. If a patient has undergone surgery with curative intent there is a strong case for screening for second metachronous cancers. It is important to ensure that the patient has only one cancer at the time of initial surgery and that all adenomas are removed. If a patient is obstructed at initial surgery, colonoscopy can be undertaken in the subsequent six months to ensure the bowel is cleared of polyps. Second cancers develop from polyps at the same rate as other colorectal cancers (anastomotic recurrence of colorectal cancer is rare). There is a broad consensus on both sides of the Atlantic that a second screening colonoscopy is not needed for 3–5 years, but should be performed five yearly thereafter.

Previous adenoma

Risk stratification based on the findings of initial colonoscopy when the first polyp was removed is central to deciding on an appropriate surveillance protocol. The evidence suggests that the greatest benefit is accrued from the first colonoscopy and polypectomy. Patients with more than five adenomas of any size or three of which one is larger than 1 cm in diameter are at greatest risk (villous histology is another risk factor, but difficult to define with accuracy).

British Society of Gastroenterology (BSG) guidelines state that such high risk patients should have a further colonoscopy at one year to ensure complete clearance, then every 3–5 years depending on the result of the second colonoscopy (Table 2).[5] Patients with low risk polyps (defined as 1–2 polyps both <1 cm in diameter) should have five-yearly colonoscopy until no polyps are found, at which time surveillance should stop. Similar, though not identical, guidelines are in place in the USA. The evidence underpinning this guidance is still evolving and it is likely that recommendations will change in the future.

Inflammatory bowel disease

The risk of colon cancer is increased approximately fivefold in patients with ulcerative colitis or colonic Crohn's disease compared with age-matched controls. The risk is higher in patients who were young at the onset of IBD, who have disease of long duration and in whom there is extensive colonic involvement. There is a wide consensus that surveillance by colonoscopy should start after eight years of disease, then repeated three yearly.[4] Biopsies should be taken every 10 cm in all four quadrants.

There is also agreement that the finding of high-grade dysplasia or 'dysplasia associated mass lesion', confirmed by two independent pathologists, is an indication for colectomy or mucosal resection as there is a 42% chance of a coexisting cancer. There is little agreement on the correct management of low-grade dysplasia because of low interobserver agreement between pathologists. A sensible course of action might be to increase the frequency of surveillance until the dysplasia either resolves or becomes high-grade. There are never likely to be RCTs in the area so recommendations are inevitably based on case-control studies and expert opinion. It is suggested in the literature that the risk of colon cancer in IBD may be falling, so surveillance protocols may change in the future.

Table 2 British Society for Gastroenterology and Association of Coloproctology guidelines for colorectal screening of high risk groups.[5]

Family groups	Lifetime risk of death from CRC	Screening procedure	Age at initial screen	Interval	No. of procedures/ 300,000 population
FAP	1 in 2.5	Genetic testing/ Flexible sigmoidoscopy + OGD	Puberty	12-monthly colectomy if +ve	6
Juvenile polyposis and Peutz-Jeghers syndrome	1 in 3	Genetic testing/ Colonoscopy + OGD	Puberty	12-monthly colectomy if +ve	6
HNPCC	1 in 2	Colonoscopy + OGD	Age 25	2-yearly colonoscopy	48
2 FDR with CRC	1 in 6	Colonoscopy	Age 35–40	If first colonoscopy clear, next aged 55	23
1 FDR <45 years with CRC	1 in 10	Colonoscopy	Age 35–40	If first colonoscopy clear, next aged 55	12

CRC = colorectal cancer; FAP = familial adenomatous polyposis; FDR = first-degree relative; HNPCC = hereditary non-polyposis colorectal cancer; OGD = gastroscopy.

Patients with a family history

Patients with one first-degree relative with colorectal cancer aged below 45 years or two first-degree relatives of any age have a lifetime risk of colorectal cancer of one in six and one in 10, respectively. The BSG recommends a full colonoscopy at age 35–40 followed by a second examination at age 55.[5] The primary purpose of the first colonoscopy is to reassure, as there is only a one in 3,618 chance of preventing a colorectal cancer death at that time. By contrast, the second colonoscopy has a one in 213 chance of preventing death and is the main preventive intervention.[13]

Hereditary non-polyposis colorectal cancer

Patients with a clinical diagnosis of hereditary non-polyposis colorectal cancer have a 50% lifetime risk of colorectal cancer. In this syndrome, characterised by a defect repair of mismatch errors in DNA, cancer develops from a polyp but both faster and at a younger age than from sporadic polyps. Surveillance should be by colonoscopy starting at age 25 and then every two years.[20] X-rays should be avoided as these patients are at an increased theoretical risk of radiation-induced malignancy. They should also undergo surveillance of the stomach by gastroscopy and, in the case of women, the uterus by ultrasound.

Familial adenomatous polyposis

Patients at risk of familial adenomatous polyposis should undergo genetic testing after counselling. Surveillance by annual sigmoidoscopy should start at puberty until polyps develop, then the timing of colectomy should be considered.

□ ARE SCREENING FACILITIES AVAILABLE?

The only screening protocol whose implementation in the NHS has been studied in detail is for FOB, followed by colonoscopy and polypectomy for FOB-positive individuals. This screening programme was piloted in North-East Scotland and the Coventry area in 1999–2003.[21] It was accompanied by an exhaustive research programme evaluating patient acceptability, outcomes, health economics and impact on workload and other routine services. Both sites were able to complete the screening programme, though often with disruption of diagnostic services for symptomatic patients. Colonoscopy workload was increased by 80%, with consequent knock-on effects on pathology, radiology and surgery. It was concluded that implementation of such a screening programme in the NHS would be possible if both the capacity and quality of endoscopic and other services were increased.

□ IS SCREENING FOR COLORECTAL CANCER ECONOMICALLY VIABLE?

The cost-effectiveness of FOB screening was calculated in this pilot study. The gain in life-days saved was only modest (14 days), but this was offset by low costs such that the net cost per quality-adjusted life-year (QALY) gained was £2,000–3,000.[21]

This is well within the limit of £30,000 per QALY gained set by the National Institute for Clinical Excellence. FOB screening compares favourably with prevention schemes such as statins in secondary prevention of heart disease and screening for breast or cervical cancer. Studies in the USA, where there is greater provision of colonoscopy services, show that colonoscopy can also be highly cost-effective.

□ CONCLUSIONS

Colorectal cancer fulfils the Wilson and Jünger criteria for screening,[1] particularly in the case of high risk individuals. The principal challenge for the implementation of a national screening programme in the UK is the provision of adequate colonoscopy capacity and skills. In any case, this issue needs to be addressed urgently for the benefit of symptomatic patients. Introduction of a screening programme is likely to highlight current shortcomings and drive up colonoscopy standards and capacity, with consequent benefit for all patients undergoing colonoscopy.

Appropriate communication with screenees will be essential as no screening strategy can completely prevent colon cancer. It will be vital to emphasise that the purpose of screening is to reduce risk but that it does not eliminate it.

Acknowledgements

I am grateful to Professor Jon Rhodes for his critical reading of the manuscript and for helpful discussions with Professor Tony Morris and all other members of the National Endoscopy Training Centre at the Mersey School of Endoscopy.

REFERENCES

1 Wilson JM, Jünger JJ. *Principles and Practice of Screening for Disease.* Geneva: World Health Organization, Geneva, 1968:34.
2 http://www.cancerresearchuk.org
3 www.statistics.gov.uk
4 Winawer S, Fletcher R, Rex D, Bond J *et al.* Colorectal cancer screening and surveillance: clinical guidelines and rationale – update based on new evidence. *Gastroenterology* 2003;**124**: 544–60.
5 Atkin WS, Saunders BP; British Society for Gastroenterology; Association of Coloproctology for Great Britain and Ireland. Surveillance guidelines after removal of colorectal adenomatous polyps. *Gut* 2002;**51**(Suppl 5):V6–9.
6 Hardcastle JD, Chamberlain JO, Robinson MH, Moss SM *et al.* Randomised controlled trial of faecal-occult-blood screening for colorectal cancer. *Lancet* 1996;**348**:1472–7.
7 Mandel JS, Church TR, Ederer F, Bond JH. Colorectal cancer mortality: effectiveness of biennial screening for fecal occult blood. *J Natl Cancer Inst* 1999;**91**:434–7.
8 Kronborg O, Fenger C, Olsen J, Jorgensen OD, Sondergaard O. Randomised study of screening for colorectal cancer with faecal-occult-blood test. *Lancet* 1996;**348**:1467–71.
9 Pickhardt PJ, Choi JR, Hwang I, Butler JA *et al.* Computed tomographic virtual colonoscopy to screen for colorectal neoplasia in asymptomatic adults. *N Engl J Med* 2003;**349**:2191–200.
10 Ajaj W, Pelster G, Treichel U, Vogt FM *et al.* Dark lumen magnetic resonance colonography: comparison with conventional colonoscopy for the detection of colorectal pathology. *Gut* 2003;**52**:738–43.

11 Boynton KA, Summerhayes IC, Ahlquist DA, Shuber AP. DNA integrity as a potential marker for stool-based detection of colorectal cancer. *Clin Chem* 2003;**49**:1058–65.

12 Atkin WS, Cuzick J, Northover JM, Whynes DK. Prevention of colorectal cancer by once-only sigmoidoscopy. *Lancet* 1993;**341**:736–40.

13 Dunlop MG; British Society for Gastroenterology; Association of Coloproctology for Great Britain and Ireland. Guidance on large bowel surveillance for people with two first degree relatives with colorectal cancer or one first degree relative diagnosed with colorectal cancer under 45 years. *Gut* 2002;**51**(Suppl 5):V17–20.

14 US Preventive Services Task Force. Screening for colorectal cancer: recommendation and rationale. *Ann Intern Med* 2002;**137**:129–31.

15 UK Flexible Sigmoidoscopy Screening Trial Investigators. Single flexible sigmoidoscopy screening to prevent colorectal cancer: baseline findings of a UK multicentre randomised trial. *Lancet* 2002;**359**:1291–300.

16 Watson AJ. Are proximal colorectal cancers always associated with distal adenomas? *Gut* 2003;**52**:317–8.

17 Thiis-Evensen E, Hoff GS, Sauar J, Langmark F *et al.* Population-based surveillance by colonoscopy: effect on the incidence of colorectal cancer. Telemark Polyp Study I. *Scand J Gastroenterol* 1999;**34**:414–20.

18 Winawer SJ, Zauber AG, Ho MN, O'Brien MJ *et al.* Prevention of colorectal cancer by colonoscopic polypectomy. The National Polyp Study Workgroup. *N Engl J Med* 1993;**329**: 1977–81.

19 Citarda F, Tomaselli G, Capocaccia R, Barcherini S, Crespi M; Italian Multicentre Study Group. Efficacy in standard clinical practice of colonoscopic polypectomy in reducing colorectal cancer incidence. *Gut* 2001;**48**:812–5.

20 Dunlop MG; British Society for Gastroenterology; Association of Coloproctology for Great Britain and Ireland. Guidance on gastrointestinal surveillance for hereditary non-polyposis colorectal cancer, familial adenomatous polyposis, juvenile polyposis, and Peutz-Jeghers syndrome. *Gut* 2002;**51**(Suppl 5):V21–7.

21 Alexander F, Weller D. *Evaluation of the UK Colorectal Cancer Screening Pilot.* London: National Health Service, 2003.

☐ ONCOLOGY SELF ASSESSMENT QUESTIONS

Should we be more aggressive in the management of lung cancer?

1 Positron emission tomography scanning in lung cancer staging:
(a) Saves futile thoracotomies
(b) Has a high positive predictive value
(c) Identifies malignant lesions smaller than 6 mm diameter
(d) Saves the need for computed tomography (CT) scanning
(e) Distinguishes inflammatory from malignant lesions

2 Low-dose spiral CT scanning:
(a) Identifies mainly stage I cancers
(b) Is good at identifying central tumours
(c) Identifies more prevalence than incidence lesions
(d) Identifies a high incidence of benign disease
(e) Improves resection rates and mortality

3 Surgical outcomes for lung cancer:
(a) Can be improved by neo-adjuvant chemotherapy
(b) May be improved by adjuvant chemotherapy
(c) Is improved by postoperative thoracic irradiation
(d) Five-year survival for stage I tumours is as high as 90%
(e) Five-year survival is the same for medically unfit, resectable patients treated by radical radiotherapy

4 The treatment of advanced non-metastatic non-small-cell lung cancer with chemotherapy:
(a) Should be limited to patients with performance status 0 and 1
(b) Provides better results in younger patients
(c) Should be withheld in patients over 70 years
(d) Has a definite benefit on global quality of life
(e) Is better if given together with an epidermal growth factor receptor antagonist

Who should be screened for colorectal cancer?

1 Colorectal cancer:
(a) Duke's A cancer can be cured
(b) Emergency presentation has no influence on the prognosis of colorectal cancer
(c) Adenomas rapidly progress to carcinomas
(d) Villous histology is a risk factor for progression to cancer
(e) Colorectal cancer can develop from flat adenomas

2 Screening tests:
(a) Faecal occult blood (FOB) testing reduces population mortality from colorectal cancer

(b) CT tomography scanning cannot detect colorectal cancer
(c) Barium enema is the most popular screening test in the USA
(d) Flexible sigmoidoscopy based screening cannot detect casual cancers
(e) Molecular cancer markers in the stools of patients have been evaluated by randomised controlled trial

3 General issues:
(a) Risk stratification is not part of screening
(b) Previous colorectal cancer increases the risk of subsequent adenomas
(c) FOB testing reduces mortality by 20%
(d) 50% of right-sided advanced colonic neoplasms are accompanied by left-sided polyps
(e) Patients with a relative under the age of 45 with colorectal cancer have an increased risk of its development

Cardiology

Contemporary treatment for atrial fibrillation

Tom Wong, Nicholas Peters and Vias Markides

☐ INTRODUCTION

Atrial fibrillation (AF) is the commonest sustained cardiac arrhythmia in humans, affecting approximately 1% of the population. In the UK alone more than half a million people suffer from this arrhythmia.[1] The prevalence of AF is constantly rising, even after adjusting for age and presence of structural heart disease. It is associated with significant morbidity and mortality: the risk of stroke increases sixfold and mortality doubles,[2,3] while up to two-thirds of patients report that the arrhythmia is disruptive to their lives.[4]

This chapter will review, first, the classification and pathophysiology of AF and, secondly, the treatment of the arrhythmia, both pharmacological and non-pharmacological, including anticoagulation for the prevention of thrombo-embolism as well as surgery.

☐ CLASSIFICATION

The classification of AF has traditionally been based on aetiology. Most patients with AF have structural heart disease secondary to conditions such as hypertension, valvular and ischaemic heart disease but 15% of AF have no identifiable aetiology: so-called 'lone AF'.

More recently, a classification system based on the temporal pattern of the arrhythmia has been recommended as follows:[5]

- A patient may present to medical attention with a *first detected episode* of AF or, if previous episodes have been documented, *recurrent* arrhythmia.
- Episodes themselves may be *paroxysmal* if they terminate spontaneously, usually within seven days, or *persistent* if the arrhythmia continues and requires electrical or pharmacological cardioversion to terminate.
- AF is termed *permanent* if it does not respond to cardioversion or is of long duration (>1 year) and cardioversion has not been attempted.

☐ PATHOPHYSIOLOGY

The pathogenesis of AF is now thought to involve a fundamental interaction between triggers responsible for initiation of the arrhythmia and the atrial substrate that is largely responsible for its perpetuation.

Focal triggers of atrial fibrillation

Foci capable of producing rapid ectopic activity, often located in muscular sleeves that extend from the left atrium into the proximal parts of thoracic veins (most frequently the pulmonary veins), are now known to play a pivotal role in the initiation of AF in humans.[6] Initiation of AF by rapid focal activity has been demonstrated not only in patients with paroxysmal AF but also during the process of reinitiation of persistent AF after electrical cardioversion, both in the presence and absence of associated structural heart disease.[7] In some patients, continuous activity from focal triggers may also contribute towards maintenance of the arrhythmia.

Tissue substrate capable of maintaining atrial fibrillation

Both experimental and human mapping studies have demonstrated that persistent AF is often characterised by the presence of multiple re-entrant wavelets of excitation that propagate around the atrial myocardium. More recent work has suggested that electrical rotors, most frequently present in the left atrium, may also have a pivotal role in perpetuation of the arrhythmia. Perpetuation is facilitated by the existence or development of an abnormal atrial tissue substrate.[8] Re-entry within the atrial myocardium is encouraged by conduction slowing and shortening of the refractory period, both of which have been demonstrated in animal models and patients with AF. AF in itself can cause progressive changes in atrial electrophysiology (as described above), further facilitating perpetuation of the arrhythmia ('AF begets AF').[9] Reduced expression of L-type calcium channels, increased expression of repolarising potassium channels, connexin changes[10] and microfibrosis of the atrial myocardium have all been demonstrated to contribute towards this process.

□ TREATMENT

In patients with short paroxysms of AF, therapeutic strategies should generally concentrate on controlling the arrhythmia itself. In patients with persistent AF, however, the clinician has the choice of two strategies:

- □ to aim for restoration and maintenance of sinus rhythm (rhythm control), or
- □ to accept the arrhythmia and aim to control the ventricular rate (rate control); in fact, rate control is often the only meaningful strategy for patients with permanent AF.

Anticoagulation

Regardless of the arrhythmia pattern (paroxysmal, persistent or permanent) or the therapeutic strategy chosen (rhythm or rate control), all patients with AF and risk factors for thromboembolism should be considered for anticoagulation. When warfarin is contraindicated or associated with unacceptable risk of bleeding, antiplatelet therapy such as aspirin may be of benefit – a strategy that may also be used in patients at intermediate risk of thromboembolism.

AF increases the risk of stroke sixfold and is the attributable cause in 15% of all strokes. The efficacy (in terms of prevention of stroke and peripheral embolism) and safety (risk of bleeding events) of warfarin and aspirin in patients with AF have been extensively studied.[11-14] Both warfarin and aspirin have been shown to be more efficacious than placebo in the setting of primary and secondary prevention. A comparison of warfarin and aspirin strongly favours warfarin for stroke prevention. Full anticoagulation (target international normalised ratio 2.0–3.0) has also been shown to be more efficacious than the combination of low-dose warfarin and aspirin or low-dose warfarin alone. Younger patients, for whom the risk of thromboembolism without warfarin is similar to the risk of major bleeding with warfarin, may not benefit from anticoagulation. The current joint American College of Cardiology/American Heart Association/European Society of Cardiology task force recommendation for anticoagulation therapy for the prevention of stroke in patients with AF is largely based upon the presence or absence of other risk factors for stroke (Table 1).[5]

□ RESTORATION OF SINUS RHYTHM

Restoration of sinus rhythm in patients with AF may improve symptoms and cardiac haemodynamics. It is associated with improvements in exercise capacity and peak oxygen consumption both in patients with structural heart disease and those with normal hearts.[15]

Table 1 American College of Cardiology/American Heart Association/European Society of Cardiology treatment guidelines for antithrombotic therapy in patients with atrial fibrillation (AF).[5]

Risk category	Patient features	Antithrombotic therapy
Lowest	Age <60 years, no heart disease (lone AF)	Aspirin 325 mg/day or no therapy
Low	Age <60 years, heart disease but no risk factors for thromboembolism (including heart failure, LV ejection fraction ≤0.35, history of hypertension) Age ≥60 years, no risk factors for thromboembolism	Aspirin 325 mg/day
High	Age ≥60 years with diabetes mellitus or coronary artery disease	Oral anticoagulation (INR 2.0–3.0); optional addition of aspirin 81–162 mg/day
	Age ≥75 years, especially women	Oral anticoagulation (INR .2.0)
	Heart failure (LV ejection fraction ≤0.35) Thyrotoxicosis Hypertension	Oral anticoagulation (INR 2.0–3.0)
Highest	Rheumatic heart disease (mitral stenosis) Prosthetic heart valves Prior thromboembolism Persistent atrial thrombus on transoesophageal echocardiography	Oral anticoagulation (INR target of at least 2.0–3.0; INR 2.5–3.5 or higher may be appropriate)

INR = international normalised ratio; LV = left ventricular.

There is an important inverse association between duration of AF and likelihood of successful cardioversion or recurrence of the arrhythmia, so it is important that attempts to restore sinus rhythm are made as soon as possible and safe. Most guidelines suggest that cardioversion, whether pharmacological or electrical, performed within 48 hours of arrhythmia onset has a low risk of thromboembolism even without anticoagulation but, pragmatically, anticoagulation early after clinical presentation of AF is often advisable – particularly as this allows considerably more freedom for patient management.

For patients whose duration of AF is longer or in whom the duration of the arrhythmia is not clear, a minimum period of anticoagulation of three weeks is recommended prior to cardioversion.[5] An alternative approach, particularly useful if there is clinical urgency to restore sinus rhythm, is to perform transoesophageal echocardiography in an attempt to exclude the presence of left atrial thrombus prior to cardioversion. However, even if this is achieved, patients should be anticoagulated for at least one month after cardioversion since mechanical atrial function may be slow to return after cardioversion.

Pharmacological cardioversion

Conversion pharmacologically is often possible for patients presenting within 48 hours of AF onset. Intravenous flecainide in patients with AF of recent onset has been shown to restore sinus rhythm in 72–95% of patients, with the greatest success rates in patients receiving therapy within 24 hours of AF onset. Flecainide also appears to be superior to both propafenone and amiodarone in this setting.

Pharmacological cardioversion is much less likely to be effective when AF has persisted for more than 48 hours. Administration of dofetilide to patients with persistent AF of more than two weeks' duration restored sinus rhythm in 22–42% within three days. There is a significant risk of pro-arrhythmia so therapy must be initiated in hospital with continuous monitoring. Amiodarone appears to be the most effective agent for restoring sinus rhythm in patients with persistent AF; one small study demonstrated sinus rhythm restoration in up to 68% of patients.[16]

Atrial defibrillators

Although implantable atrial defibrillators are effective at terminating AF episodes (96% success),[17] they are often poorly tolerated because of significant discomfort associated with shocks and are thus not in routine clinical use.

Sinus rhythm maintenance

Flecainide and propafenone have been shown to be similarly effective at suppressing symptomatic paroxysms of AF and, in the absence of structural heart disease, neither drug appears to cause significant pro-arrhythmia. In general, these class Ic agents tend to be better tolerated and more effective than class Ia agents such as quinidine and disopyramide.

Beta-adrenoceptor antagonists

Pure beta-adrenoceptor antagonists have a small beneficial effect in maintaining sinus rhythm in patients who have been cardioverted from AF. One study demonstrated no difference between pure beta1-antagonists and sotalol in either reduction of AF burden in patients with paroxysmal AF or the likelihood of AF relapse after cardioversion.[18] Sotalol may be better than propafenone at preventing AF paroxysms.

Amiodarone

The efficacy of amiodarone in maintaining sinus rhythm has been shown both in patients with paroxysmal AF and in those cardioverted from persistent AF refractory to other drugs, with a probability of arrhythmia suppression of 50–80% at 1–3 years. In a direct comparison, amiodarone has more recently been found superior to both propafenone and sotalol at maintaining sinus rhythm.[19] However, the side effect profile of amiodarone makes its routine use undesirable, especially long-term.

Ultimately, the choice of pharmacological agent for sinus rhythm maintenance needs to be tailored to the individual patient. Beta-adrenoceptor antagonists may be preferred in patients with relatively normal hearts, with class Ic agents as an alternative, reserving amiodarone for patients unresponsive to other drugs or those with poor ventricular function.

□ VENTRICULAR RATE CONTROL

Digoxin

Digoxin is widely used for ventricular rate control during AF. It is generally safe even in patients with poor ventricular function, but it appears to be less effective than other agents at controlling ventricular rate, particularly during acute paroxysmal AF, exercise or critical illnesses. Digoxin may also prolong the duration of paroxysms.[20]

Diltiazem

Diltiazem is effective at controlling ventricular rate in patients with AF and fast ventricular rates. Both diltiazem and verapamil are superior to digoxin at controlling ventricular rates during exercise, and allow modest improvements in exercise capacity without causing resting bradycardia or pauses.

The benefits of both calcium-channel blockers and beta-blockers over digoxin are particularly marked in patients with impaired diastolic filling, such as those with mitral stenosis or left ventricular hypertrophy. Combinations of digoxin with calcium-channel blockers or beta-blockers may not only improve ventricular rate control, both at rest and during exercise, but also improve exercise capacity even in patients with underlying ventricular dysfunction.

Atrioventricular node ablation and pacemaker insertion

In a minority of patients in whom the ventricular rate cannot be adequately controlled by pharmacological therapy, atrioventricular (AV) node ablation and insertion of permanent pacemaker can be used as a last resort. Creating a permanent AV block with ablation allows total control of the ventricular rate and restores regular ventricular contraction from ventricular pacing, both of which might help to improve cardiac haemodynamics. However, as AF continues, the atria cannot actively contribute to ventricular filling and the risk of stroke persists.[21] In patients with paroxysmal AF, the procedure increases the likelihood of progression to permanent AF,[22] and there are reports of the development of late ventricular dysfunction after the procedure as a result of chronic right ventricular pacing.[23,24]

Percutaneous catheter ablation

The recent recognition of the role of myocardial sleeves within the pulmonary veins as important contributors to the initiation and possibly perpetuation of AF has led to the development of percutaneous catheter ablation techniques for the treatment of AF.

Elimination or isolation of the triggers that initiate AF, commonly located in the pulmonary veins, has been shown to be effective at maintaining sinus rhythm, particularly in patients who have paroxysmal AF. More recently, atrial substrate modification, involving linear ablation in the left atrium around the pulmonary vein ostia, has been shown to be at least as effective, allowing AF to be cured in up to 88% of patients with paroxysmal arrhythmia at baseline.[25]

As the various techniques for AF ablation and the technology behind them continue to evolve rapidly, especially with increasing evidence of their superiority, ablation procedures – usually reserved for patients with highly symptomatic arrhythmia refractory to medical therapy – may be offered to an increasing number of patients.[26]

□ ARRHYTHMIA SURGERY

The surgical Maze procedure, first described more than a decade ago by Cox,[27] consists of multiple 'cut-and-sew' lesions in both atria. The aim is to produce electrical compartmentalisation of the atria, such that re-entry of multiple wavelets cannot be sustained. Various modifications of the original lesion set have subsequently been developed and proven effective at restoring and maintaining sinus rhythm. More recently, surgeons have replaced the surgical blade with linear cryoablation, radiofrequency or microwave ablation probes with ablated areas acting as lines of conduction block. The early results in terms of restoration and maintenance of sinus rhythm are promising, but surgery remains associated with substantial morbidity and mortality. Such procedures are thus predominantly performed in patients undergoing cardiac surgery for other concomitant cardiac conductions such as mitral valve repair or replacement.

□ RATE VERSUS RHYTHM CONTROL

Rhythm control, which aims to restore sinus rhythm and thus synchronised AV contraction, should theoretically help slow or prevent the progression to permanent

AF and reduce the risk of thromboembolism. However, the findings from clinical studies are not conclusive.

Four recent randomised control trials (RCTs) [28–31] found that in selected groups of patients (mainly elderly patients who could symptomatically tolerate the AF at baseline) sole ventricular rate control was at least similar to – if not better than – continued treatment for rhythm control in terms of morbidity and mortality.

The Atrial Fibrillation Follow-up Investigation of Rhythm Management (AFFIRM) trial[28] was the largest trial. More than 4,000 patients (mean age 70 years) were enrolled, with mainly persistent AF, at least one risk factor for stroke or death accompanying AF and able symptomatically to tolerate the arrhythmia at baseline. Patients randomised to rate control received digoxin, beta-blockers or calcium antagonists, whereas those randomised to rhythm control received amiodarone, sotalol or propafenone and, if necessary, DC cardioversion. At follow-up, sinus rhythm was achieved in 60% of patients in the rhythm arm whereas satisfactory rate control was achieved in 80% of those in the rate control arm. The primary end-point of the study, namely all-cause mortality, was not significantly different between the two groups, although there was a trend towards lower mortality with rate control.

There were no differences in secondary end-point components, including stroke rate, quality of life or functional status, although there was again a trend favouring rate control. However, anticoagulation was discontinued in more patients in the rhythm group – particularly relevant since the majority of strokes in both groups occurred in patients who were either not anticoagulated at the time or had subtherapeutic levels of anticoagulation. Moreover, in the predefined group of patients in the study below 65 years (ca 25%) there was a trend favouring rhythm control.

The other three RCTs,[29-31] which included similar patient populations (predominantly elderly patients with persistent AF), produced similar findings. It is important to note that these trials did not include highly symptomatic or young patients for whom a rate control strategy may not be suitable. Not uncommonly a rhythm control strategy may prove necessary on symptomatic grounds alone.

In a more recent, non-randomised prospective study by Pappone *et al*,[26] over 1,000 patients with paroxysmal or persistent AF were treated either medically or with left atrial radiofrequency ablation around the pulmonary vein ostia, aiming for rhythm control. Ablation was not only much more effective at maintaining sinus rhythm than medical therapy (>80% vs <40% at 3-year follow-up) but was also associated with a 50% reduction in all-cause mortality and major cardiovascular events including ischaemic stroke and heart failure and also with normalisation of quality of life.

□ CONCLUSIONS

AF is a common and increasingly prevalent arrhythmia associated with substantial morbidity and mortality. Pharmacological therapy is the mainstay of treatment for most patients but catheter-based treatment is used increasingly frequently as experience and technological improvements allow for continuously increasing efficacy. In the light of recent findings from randomised trials rate control may be the preferred treatment strategy for elderly patients with persistent AF who do not have disabling symptoms from arrhythmia. Rhythm control should be offered to patients with paroxysmal AF and to symptomatic or relatively young patients with persistent AF.

Regardless of the arrhythmia management strategy, antithrombotic therapy for stroke prevention forms an integral part of the treatment for patients with AF and risk factors for thromboembolism.

The predominant focus of recent developments in pharmacological therapy for AF has been the development of novel class III anti-arrhythmic agents, each with characteristic effects on potassium channels. In general, they have proven moderately efficacious but carry a significant risk of pro-arrhythmia. Novel agents with specific action on the atrial myocardium are currently being developed.

The advancement in catheter ablation techniques may greatly facilitate safe isolation of multiple pulmonary veins for patients with predominantly paroxysmal AF, whereas further development of catheters that will enhance safe linear ablation in the left atrium accompanied by 3-dimensional atrial mapping and catheter navigation may facilitate the creation of complete left atrial linear lesions, thus improving the success in treating patients with persistent AF.

REFERENCES

1 Stewart S, Murphy N, Walker A, McGuire A, McMurray JJ. Cost of an emerging epidemic: an economic analysis of atrial fibrillation in the UK. *Heart* 2004;**90**:286–92.

2 Benjamin EJ, Wolf PA, D'Agostino RB, Silbershatz H, Kannel WB. Impact of atrial fibrillation on the risk of death: the Framingham heart study. *Circulation* 1998;**98**:946–52.

3 Wolf PA, Abbott RD, Kannel WB. Atrial fibrillation as an independent risk factor for stroke: the Framingham study. *Stroke* 1991;**22**:983–8.

4 Hamer ME, Blumenthal JA, McCarthy EA, Phillips BG, Pritchett EL. Quality-of-life assessment in patients with paroxysmal atrial fibrillation or paroxysmal supraventricular tachycardia. *Am J Cardiol* 1994;**74**:826–9.

5 Fuster V, Ryden LE, Asinger RW, Cannon DS *et al.* ACC/AHA/ESC Guidelines for the Management of Patients With Atrial Fibrillation: Executive Summary. A Report of the American College of Cardiology/American Heart Association Task Force on Practice Guidelines and the European Society of Cardiology Committee for Practice Guidelines and Policy Conferences (Committee to Develop Guidelines for the Management of Patients With Atrial Fibrillation) Developed in Collaboration With the North American Society of Pacing and Electrophysiology. *Circulation* 2001;**104**:2118–50.

6 Haissaguerre M, Jais P, Shah DC, Takahashi A *et al.* Spontaneous initiation of atrial fibrillation by ectopic beats originating in the pulmonary veins. *N Engl J Med* 1998;**339**:659–66.

7 Lau CP, Tse HF, Ayers GM. Defibrillation-guided radiofrequency ablation of atrial fibrillation secondary to an atrial focus. *J Am Coll Cardiol* 1999;**33**:1217–26.

8 Allessie MA, Lammers WJ, Smeets JL, Bonke F, Hollen J. Total mapping of atrial excitation during acetylcholine-induced atrial flutter and fibrillation in the isolated canine heart. In: Kulbertus HE, Olsson SB, Schlepper M (eds). *Atrial fibrillation.* Mölndal, Sweden: Lindgren and Soner, 1982:44–52.

9 Wijffels MC, Kirchhof CJ, Dorland R, Allessie MA. Atrial fibrillation begets atrial fibrillation. A study in awake chronically instrumented goats. *Circulation* 1995;**92**:1954–68.

10 Kanagaratnam P, Cherian A, Stanbridge RD, Glenville B *et al.* Relationship between connexins and atrial activation during human atrial fibrillation. *J Cardiovasc Electrophysiol* 2004;**15**:206–16.

11 The effect of low-dose warfarin on the risk of stroke in patients with nonrheumatic atrial fibrillation. The Boston Area Anticoagulation Trial for Atrial Fibrillation Investigators. *N Engl J Med* 1990;**323**:1505–11.

12 Secondary prevention in non-rheumatic atrial fibrillation after transient ischaemic attack or minor stroke. EAFT (European Atrial Fibrillation Trial) Study Group. *Lancet* 1993;**342**:1255–62.

13 Adjusted-dose warfarin versus low-intensity, fixed-dose warfarin plus aspirin for high-risk patients with atrial fibrillation: Stroke Prevention in Atrial Fibrillation III randomised clinical trial. *Lancet* 1996;**348**:633–8.

14 Ezekowitz MD, Bridgers SL, James KE, Carliner NH *et al.* Warfarin in the prevention of stroke associated with nonrheumatic atrial fibrillation. Veterans Affairs Stroke Prevention in Nonrheumatic Atrial Fibrillation Investigators. *N Engl J Med* 1992;**327**:1406–12.

15 Gosselink AT, Crijns HJ, van den Berg MP, van den Broek SA *et al.* Functional capacity before and after cardioversion of atrial fibrillation: a controlled study. *Br Heart J* 1994;**72**:161–6.

16 Kerin NZ, Faitel K, Naini M. The efficacy of intravenous amiodarone for the conversion of chronic atrial fibrillation. Amiodarone vs quinidine for conversion of atrial fibrillation. *Arch Intern Med* 1996;**156**:49–53.

17 Wellens HJ, Lau CP, Luderitz B, Akhtar M *et al.* Atrioverter: an implantable device for the treatment of atrial fibrillation. *Circulation* 1998;**98**:1651–6.

18 Steeds RP, Birchall AS, Smith M, Channer KS *et al.* An open label, randomised, crossover study comparing sotalol and atenolol in the treatment of symptomatic paroxysmal atrial fibrillation. *Heart* 1999;**82**:170–5.

19 Roy D, Talajic M, Dorian P, Connolly S *et al.* Amiodarone to prevent recurrence of atrial fibrillation. Canadian Trial of Atrial Fibrillation Investigators. *N Engl J Med* 2000;**342**:913–20.

20 Rawles JM, Metcalfe MJ, Jennings K. Time of occurrence, duration, and ventricular rate of paroxysmal atrial fibrillation: the effect of digoxin. *Br Heart J* 1990;**63**:225–7.

21 Takahashi Y, Yoshito I, Takahashi A, Harada T *et al.* AV nodal ablation and pacemaker implantation improves hemodynamic function in atrial fibrillation. *Pacing Clin Electrophysiol* 2003;**26**:1212–7.

22 Marshall HJ, Harris ZI, Griffith MJ, Holder RL, Gammage MD. Prospective randomized study of ablation and pacing versus medical therapy for paroxysmal atrial fibrillation: effects of pacing mode and mode-switch algorithm. *Circulation* 1999;**99**:1587–92.

23 Vanderheyden M, Goethals M, Anguera I, Nellens P *et al.* Hemodynamic deterioration following radiofrequency ablation of the atrioventricular conduction system. *Pacing Clin Electrophysiol* 1997;**20**:2422–8.

24 Zile MR, Blaustein AS, Shimizu G, Gaasch WH. Right ventricular pacing reduces the rate of left ventricular relaxation and filling. *J Am Coll Cardiol* 1987;**10**:702–9.

25 Oral H, Scharf C, Chugh A, Hall B *et al.* Catheter ablation for paroxysmal atrial fibrillation: segmental pulmonary vein ostial ablation versus left atrial ablation. *Circulation* 2003;**108**: 2355–60.

26 Pappone C, Rosanio S, Augello G, Gallus G *et al.* Mortality, morbidity, and quality of life after circumferential pulmonary vein ablation for atrial fibrillation: outcomes from a controlled nonrandomized long-term study. *J Am Coll Cardiol* 2003;**42**:185–97.

27 Cox JL. The surgical treatment of atrial fibrillation. IV. Surgical technique. *J Thorac Cardiovasc Surg* 1991;**101**:584–92.

28 Wyse DG, Waldo AL, DiMarco JP, Domanski MJ *et al*; Atrial Fibrillation Follow-up Investigation of Rhythm Management (AFFIRM) Investigators. A comparison of rate control and rhythm control in patients with atrial fibrillation. *N Engl J Med* 2002;**347**:1825–33.

29 Van Gelder IC, Hagens VE, Bosker HA, Kingma JH *et al.* A comparison of rate control and rhythm control in patients with recurrent persistent atrial fibrillation. *N Engl J Med* 2002;**347**:1834–40.

30 Hohnloser SH, Kuck KH, Lilienthal J. Rhythm or rate control in atrial fibrillation – Pharmacological Intervention in Atrial Fibrillation (PIAF): a randomised trial. *Lancet* 2000;**356**:1789–94.

31 Carlsson JO, Miketic S, Windeler J, Cuneo A *et al.* Randomized trial of rate-control versus rhythm-control in persistent atrial fibrillation: the Strategies of Treatment of Atrial Fibrillation (STAF) study. *J Am Coll Cardiol* 2003;**41**:1690–6.

Risk stratification post-myocardial infarction

Janet McComb

□ INTRODUCTION

There have been several major changes in the management of patients with acute myocardial infarction (AMI) in the past 25 years leading to a marked reduction in mortality.[1] As new therapies have been developed, risk stratification has become important to ensure that those patients most likely to benefit from the many therapies now available can be identified and treated.

Three important complications of AMI cause death and major morbidity:

- recurrent ischaemia
- heart failure
- sustained ventricular arrhythmias and sudden cardiac death.

These are not independent risk factors:

- recurrent ischaemia can cause further infarction predisposing to heart failure
- ischaemia can precipitate sudden death
- heart failure is associated with excess sudden death and ventricular arrhythmias etc.

□ RECURRENT ISCHAEMIA

Recurrent ischaemia occurs prior to hospital discharge in up to half of those with AMI who have either reinfarction or, more frequently, chest pain at rest or on minimal exertion. These patients are at high risk of recurrent events and should undergo angiography with a view to revascularisation by either percutaneous coronary intervention or bypass graft surgery. Other clinical indicators of high risk include increasing age, previous infarction and the presence of multiple clinical risk factors, including hypertension, hypercholesterolaemia etc. These patients should also undergo angiography.

Patients not identified at high risk using simple clinical criteria should undergo risk stratification by exercise testing and assessment of left ventricular function. Exercise testing should be carried out within six weeks of the index infarction, symptom limited unless performed in the first week when it should be submaximal.[2,3] Angiography is indicated if significant ischaemia is identified on stress testing. This approach is summarised in Fig 1.

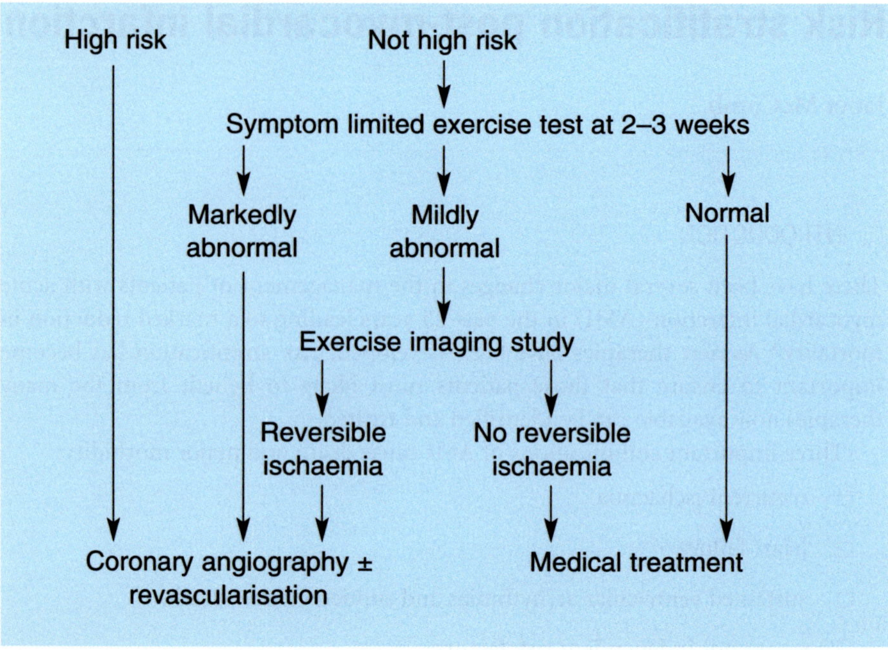

Fig 1 Algorithm for identifying patients at high risk following myocardial infarction using exercise stress testing.

Figure 2 shows the relationship between exercise testing and outcome in the Gruppo Italiano per lo Studio della Sopravvivenza Nell'Infarto (GISSI 2) trial, confirming that low risk patients can be identified by stress testing.[4] A comparison of the outcome of invasive and non-invasive strategies after MI, based on identification of ischaemia by exercise testing, found a significant reduction in mortality and major adverse cardiac events with the former strategy (Fig 3).[5]

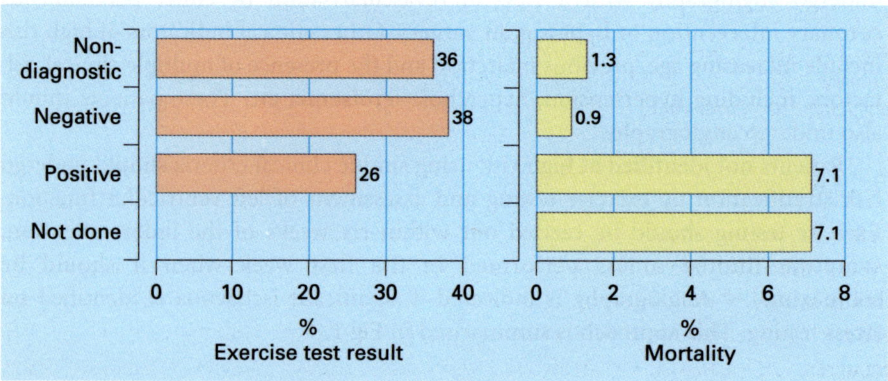

Fig 2 Exercise test results in relation to mortality in the Gruppo Italiano per lo Studio della Sopravvivenza Nell'Infarto trial (GISSI 2).[4]

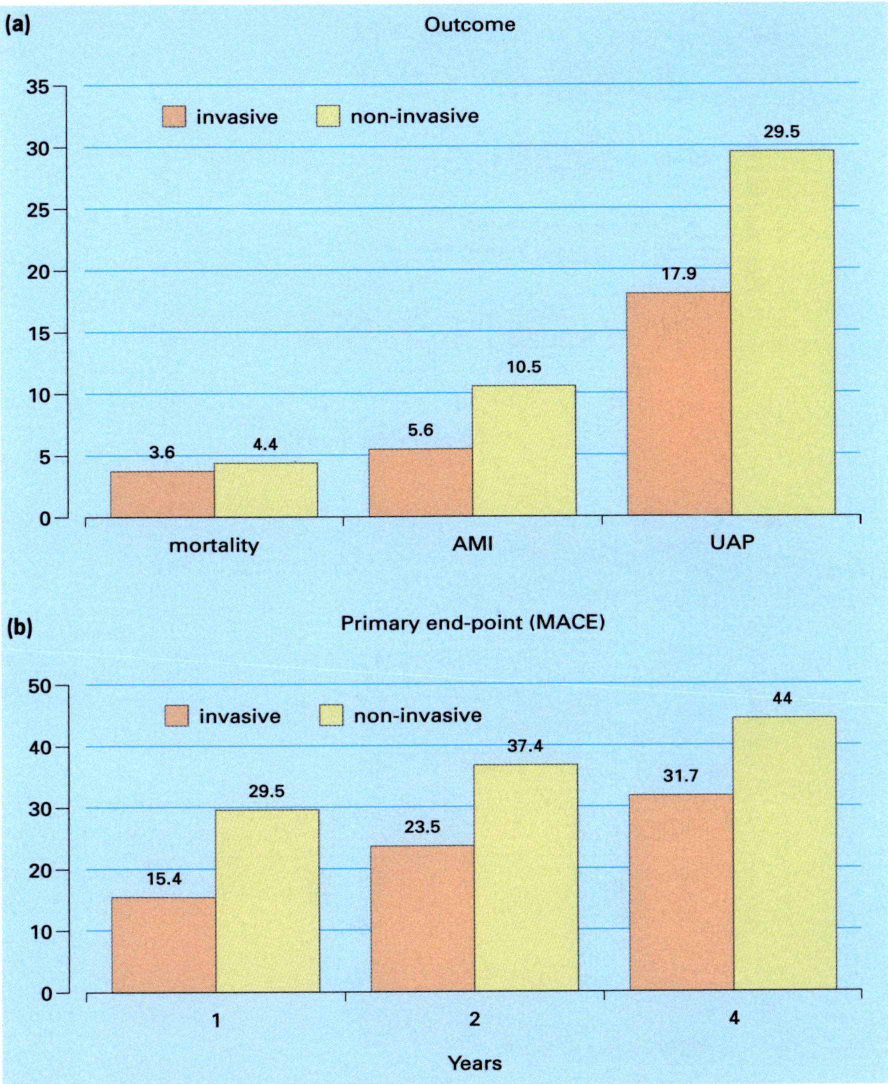

Fig 3 The Danish Multicenter Study of Acute Myocardial Infarction (DANAMI):[5] **(a)** outcome and **(b)** primary end-point in relation to treatment strategy (invasive versus conservative) (AMI = acute myocardial infarction; MACE = major adverse cardiac event; UAP = unstable angina pectoris).

□ HEART FAILURE

Left ventricular ejection fraction is one of the most accurate predictors of adverse events after MI.[6] Preservation of myocardial function is therefore most important; this is achieved by identifying and treating patients at high risk in order to try to reduce both infarct size and reinfarction. Heart failure may be associated with recurrent ischaemia; if so, an invasive approach (as above) is recommended. Both beta-blockers[7] and angiotensin-converting enzyme inhibitors (ACEIs)[8] should be given to reduce mortality and heart failure readmissions after AMI.

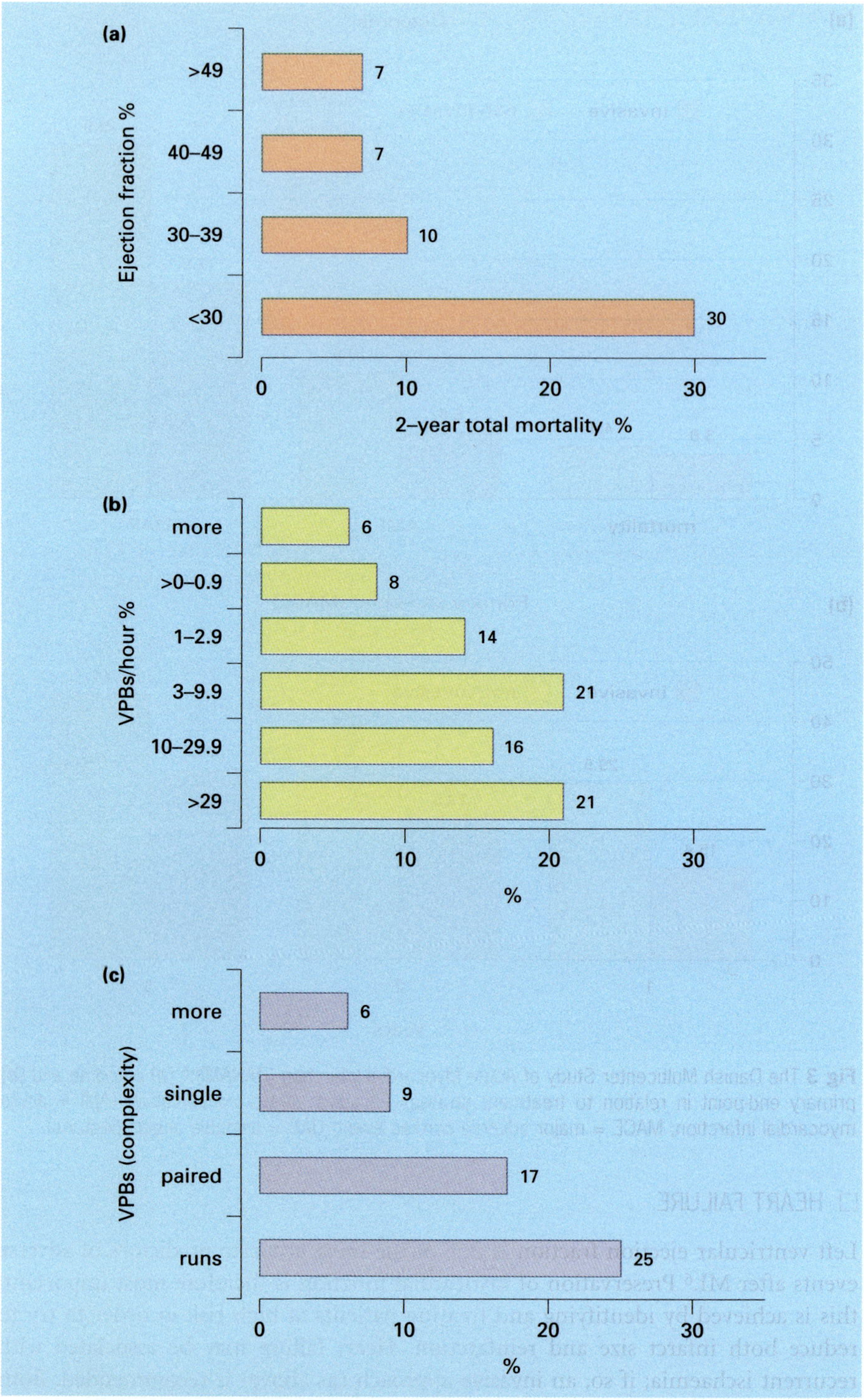

Fig 4 Mortality post-myocardial infarction in relation to **(a)** ejection fraction, **(b)** ventricular premature beats (VPBs) per hour and **(c)** complexity of VPBs.[6]

☐ ARRHYTHMIAS AND SUDDEN CARDIAC DEATH

Sustained ventricular tachycardia or ventricular tachycardia more than 24 hours after an AMI are associated with a high risk of death. Coronary angiography is indicated as ventricular arrhythmias may be a marker of continuing ischaemia. In the absence, or after treatment, of ischaemia consideration of antiarrhythmic therapy, including beta-blockade, amiodarone and an implantable cardioverter defibrillator, is appropriate.

Implantable cardioverter defibrillator

It has been known for 20 years that ejection fraction and ventricular ectopy (both the number and complexity of ectopics) can be used to identify patients at high risk of death after MI.[6] The influence of these risk factors on mortality after MI is shown in Fig 4. Antiarrhythmic drugs do not confer any benefit, despite suppressing ectopy, and may cause harm.[9]

The implantable cardioverter defibrillator (ICD) has however been shown to reduce total and sudden mortality in postinfarction patients shown to be at high risk.[10] The National Institute for Clinical Excellence[11] recommends that patients undergo risk stratification according to the screening cascade employed in the Multicenter Automatic Defibrillator Implantation Trial (MADIT) (Fig 5). This trial demonstrated benefit of the ICD in post-MI patients with reduced ejection fractions (≤35%), non-sustained ventricular tachycardia on 24-hour ECG monitoring and inducible ventricular tachycardia on electrophysiological testing.

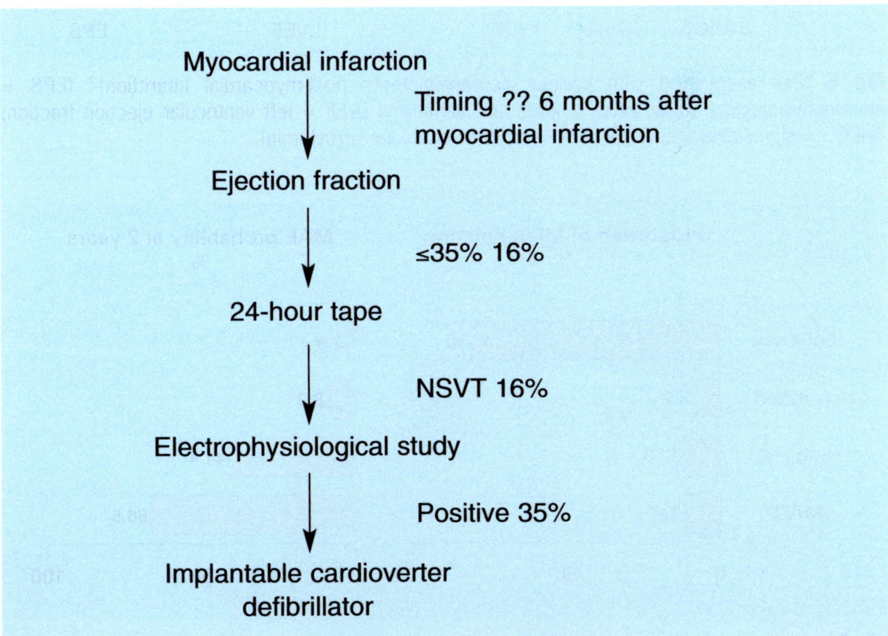

Fig 5 The screening cascade used in the Multicenter Automatic Defibrillator Implantation Trial[10] (NSVT =non-sustained ventricular arrhythmia).

Other known risk stratifiers (eg heart rate variability, signal averaged ECG) have also been tested in this population (Fig 6) in an attempt to target ICD therapy. However, various combinations of tests used in complex screening cascades have less predictive accuracy than the MADIT screening approach (Fig 7).[12]

□ CONCLUSIONS

It has been clearly shown that thrombolysis, ACEIs, beta-blockade, aspirin and statins may all improve outcomes after MI. There is increasing evidence that an aggressive invasive approach in those at high risk will also improve outcome. This strategy

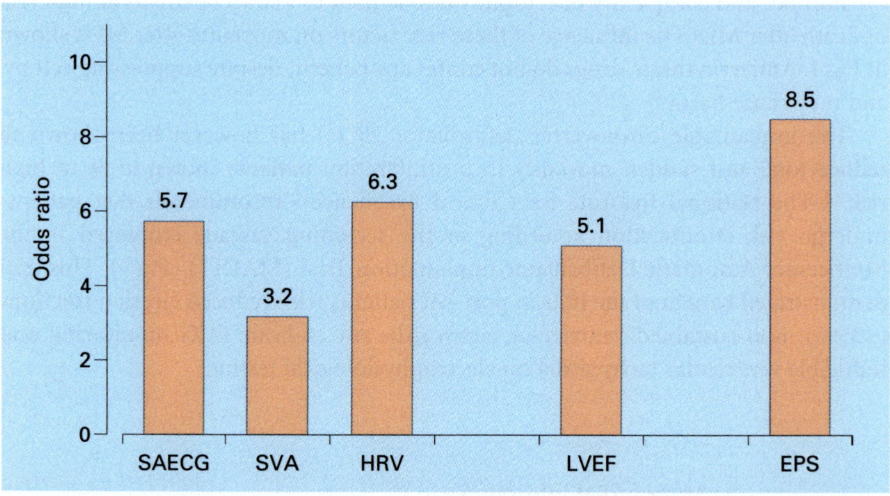

Fig 6 Risk associated with various screening tests post-myocardial infarction[12] (EPS = electrophysiological study; HRV = heart rate variability; LVEF = left ventricular ejection fraction; SAECG = signal averaged ECG; SVA = serious ventricular arrhythmia).

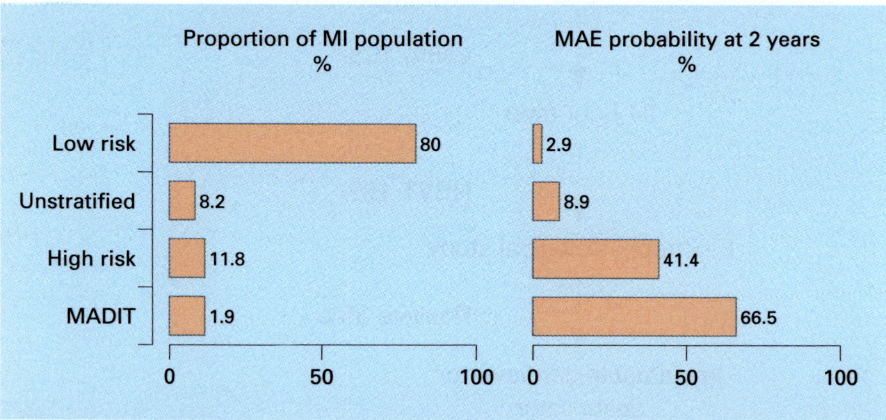

Fig 7 Risk stratification using several risk stratifiers and outcome in comparison with the Multicenter Automatic Defibrillator Implantation Trial (MADIT) screening cascade[12] (MAE = major adverse event; MI = myocardial infarction).

includes an invasive approach with a view to revascularisation in those identified as having spontaneous or inducible ischaemia and the implantation of the ICD in those deemed at high risk of sudden cardiac death. Risk stratification is therefore important, so that these invasive (and expensive) therapies can be targeted appropriately.

REFERENCES

1 Hasdai D, Behar S, Wallentin L, Danchin N *et al.* A prospective survey of the characteristics, treatments and outcomes of patients with acute coronary syndromes in Europe and the Mediterranean basin; the Euro Heart Survey of Acute Coronary Syndromes (Euro Heart Survey ACS). *Eur Heart J* 2002;**15**:1190–201.

2 Van de Werf F, Ardissino D, Betriu A, Cokkinos DV *et al.* Management of acute myocardial infarction in patients presenting with ST-segment elevation. The Task Force on the Management of Acute Myocardial Infarction of the European Society of Cardiology. *Eur Heart J* 2003;**24**:28–66.

3 Ryan TJ, Antman EM, Brooks NH, Califf RM *et al.* 1999 update: ACC/AHA guidelines for the management of patients with acute myocardial infarction. A report of the American College of Cardiology/American Heart Association Task Force on Practice Guidelines (Committee on Management of Acute Myocardial Infarction). *J Am Coll Cardiol* 1999;**34**:890–911.

4 Villella A, Maggioni AP, Villella M, Giordano A *et al.* Prognostic significance of maximal exercise testing after myocardial infarction treated with thrombolytic agents: the GISSI-2 data-base. Gruppo Italiano per lo Studio della Sopravvivenza Nell'Infarto. *Lancet* 1995;**346**:523–9.

5 Madsen JK, Grande P, Saunamaki K, Thayssen P *et al.* Danish multicenter randomized study of invasive versus conservative treatment in patients with inducible ischemia after thrombolysis in acute myocardial infarction (DANAMI). DANish trial in Acute Myocardial Infarction. *Circulation* 1997;**96**:748–55.

6 Bigger J, Fleiss JL, Kleiger R, Miller JP, Rolnitzky LM. The relationships among ventricular arrhythmias, left ventricular dysfunction, and mortality in the 2 years after myocardial infarction. *Circulation* 1984;**69**:250–8.

7 Lechat P, Packer M, Chalon S, Cucherat M *et al.* Clinical effects of beta-adrenergic blockade in chronic heart failure: a meta-analysis of double-blind, placebo-controlled, randomized trials. *Circulation* 1998;**98**:1184–91.

8 Flather M, Yusuf S, Kober L, Pfeffer M *et al.* Long-term ACE-inhibitor therapy in patients with heart failure or left-ventricular dysfunction: a systematic overview of data from individual patients. ACE-Inhibitor Myocardial Infarction Collaborative Group. *Lancet* 2000;**355**: 1575–81.

9 Echt DS, Liebson PR, Mitchell LB, Peters RW *et al.* Mortality and morbidity in patients receiving encainide, flecainide, or placebo. The Cardiac Arrhythmia Suppression Trial. *N Engl J Med* 1991;**324**:781–8.

10 Moss AJ, Hall WJ, Cannom DS, Daubert JP *et al.* Improved survival with an implanted defibrillator in patients with coronary disease at high risk for ventricular arrhythmia. Multicenter Automatic Defibrillator Implantation Trial Investigators. *N Engl J Med* 1996;**335**:1933–40.

11 National Institute for Clinical Excellence. *Guidance on the use of implantable cardioverter defibrillators for arrhythmias.* Technology Appraisal Guidance no 11. London: NICE, 2000.

12 Bailey JJ, Berson AS, Handelsman H, Hodges M. Utility of current risk stratification tests for predicting major arrhythmic events after myocardial infarction. *J Am Coll Cardiol* 2001;**38**:1902–11.

Cardiovascular funny turns

Michael Gammage

☐ INTRODUCTION

Those who suffer from frequent and severe fainting often die suddenly
Hippocrates, 1000 BC

Only if one knows the causes of syncope will he be able to recognise its onset and combat the cause
Maimonides, 1135–1204

Funny turns of cardiovascular origin have been recognised for centuries and are generally the result of intermittent impairment of cerebral perfusion. This transient reduction in cerebral perfusion will not always result in syncope, but this is the classic symptom with which patients present. This chapter will address the recommended approach to the investigation and management of the patient presenting with syncope.

☐ SYNCOPE

Syncope is a symptom, the characteristics of which are a transient, self-limited loss of consciousness, usually leading to falling. Onset of syncope is relatively rapid, subsequent recovery is spontaneous, complete and usually prompt, and the underlying mechanism is relatively abrupt cerebral hypoperfusion.[1]

The Framingham study found an incidence of 7.2 per 1,000 person-years in a broad population sample. Assuming a constant incidence rate over time, a 6% 10-year cumulative incidence can be calculated from the study.[2] In selected populations such as the elderly the annual incidence may be as high as 6%, with a recurrence rate of 30%.

The prognosis of patients with syncope depends highly on the underlying cause: those suffering syncope with underlying cardiac disease are at the highest risk, while vasovagal syncope carries a relatively benign prognosis.[2] For this reason, an understanding of the causes, together with investigation and management of syncope, may have a major impact on outcome.

Is it syncope?

No branch of medicine illustrates the maxim that the history is 90% of the diagnosis more clearly than syncope. A careful and thorough history, preferably including observations made by family and/or friends, will allow many patients to receive a diagnosis, appropriate advice/therapy and reassurance. The history requires information about:

- the circumstances in which the attack(s) occurred
- details relating to the onset of the attack
- duration of the event, and
- events associated with termination/recovery from the attack.

In addition, a careful assessment of risk factors for syncope should be undertaken; in particular, previous stroke or transient ischaemic attack (TIA), presence of cardiac medication, hypertension and diabetes have been shown to be predictive of syncope.[3]

Many patients with cardiovascular syncope are inappropriately labelled as having seizures. This has a significant impact on lifestyle, especially in the younger patient, as it will influence career opportunities, driving and leisure activities. For this reason alone, it is important to examine the symptoms and signs associated with episodes in order to direct further investigation and avoid incorrect diagnosis and the associated problems. A brief and simple approach to differentiating between seizures and syncope is shown in Table 1.[4]

Table 1 Differentiation between seizures and syncope (from Ref 4).

Observation	Seizures	Syncope/hypotension
Onset	Sudden	More gradual
Duration	Minutes	Seconds
Jerks	Frequent	Rare
Headache	Frequent (after)	Occasional (before)
Confusion afterwards	Frequent	Rare
Loss of sphincter control	Frequent	Rare
Eye deviation	Horizontal	Vertical (or none)
Tongue biting	Frequent	Rare
Prodrome	Aura	Dizziness
EEG	Often abnormal	Usually normal

The physical examination is often completely normal in patients with syncope, although signs of left ventricular dysfunction or arrhythmia may be helpful both diagnostically and prognostically. An assessment of orthostatic blood pressure is essential, as is recording of a standard 12-lead ECG. It is also worth enquiring about a family history of syncope which may be present in about one-third of patients. Further evaluation may be necessary, but for many patients the diagnosis and prognosis can be clear at this stage.

□ CAUSES OF SYNCOPE

For many physicians, the names of Stokes and Adams are associated with cardiac syncope, but the eponymous syndrome relates only to those episodes associated with bradycardia. Table 2 indicates some of the commoner causes of syncope likely to present to the general physician (either acutely or electively), with indications regarding prognostic implications. It is important to exclude non-syncopal episodes such as seizure, TIA, psychogenic syncope and somatisation disorders.

Table 2 Common causes of syncope and their prognostic implications.

Cause of syncope	Possible causes/diagnoses	Prognostic implications
Neurally-mediated reflex syncopal syndromes	Vasovagal Carotid sinus hypersensitivity Situational Neuralgia	Benign, although injury may occur due to fall
Orthostatic syndromes	Iatrogenic Autonomic failure	Benign, although injury may occur due to fall
Cardiac arrhythmias	Bradycardia Tachycardia	Associated with significant risk
Structural cardiac disease or cardiopulmonary disease	Acute myocardial infarction/ ischaemia Aortic dissection Pulmonary embolism	High risk, but diagnosis usually clear from acute presentation

□ IMPACT OF SYNCOPE

Syncope has a major impact on quality of life (QoL), even when there is little prognostic effect. Recurrences will occur in about 35% of patients within three years; this has a significant negative impact on QoL in patients who are often young and otherwise fit. Because of the situation in which these episodes occur, they can result in physical injuries to the patient (eg broken bones, burns) or to the patient plus others (eg motor vehicle accidents). Recurrences of syncope often prompt hospital admission and may result in expensive (and often inappropriate) investigations. It is important, therefore, to stratify the potential risk of syncope in order to advise the patient (and family/friends) about lifestyle changes and the need for medical attention in response to syncope.

As a general rule, the following factors indicate a good prognosis with syncope, and should indicate an elective rather than emergency response to management of an acute episode:

- □ young, healthy individual with normal ECG
- □ neurally-mediated syncope
- □ orthostatic hypotension

- unexplained syncope (see section 'Causes of loss of consciousness' and Table 2).

In contrast, any episode associated with evidence of structural heart disease indicates a poor prognosis and warrants emergency or urgent review.[2]

PROGNOSTIC STRATIFICATION

Use of a simple list of risk factors allows rapid identification of those patients at risk of future events (particularly cardiac events) and, in particular, allows identification of low risk individuals in whom further investigation may not be necessary – or may, indeed, result in potentially misleading results and diagnoses. The following four factors should be assessed:

- age over 45 years
- history of congestive heart disease
- history of ventricular arrhythmia
- abnormal ECG.

Patients with none of these factors carry a 4–7% risk of death or arrhythmia during the next year, whereas the risk to patients with three or more factors is 58–80%.[1]

INVESTIGATION

The initial evaluation may provide a clear diagnosis and preclude the need for any further investigation, particularly in patients with relatively minor or infrequent symptoms and lack of injury resulting from syncope. It is always worth considering echocardiography to exclude structural heart disease. The threshold for this investigation should be low; it is mandatory in any patient with abnormal cardiac signs. If neurally-mediated syncope is suspected, tilt-testing should be considered (see below), keeping in mind that this investigation carries a relatively high false-positive rate and may not reproduce the changes associated with spontaneous syncope. Selected patients will need external or implantable loop recorders or cardiac electrophysiological studies. Holter (24-hour) monitoring is rarely of value in syncopal patients, and patient-activated devices are usually inappropriate as a syncopal patient will not be able to activate the device at the time of the event. Recording a spontaneous event, however, will always provide more information than an event associated with provoked testing (eg tilt, pharmacological or electrophysiological testing).

The following investigations are almost never of value in the investigation of syncope:

- EEG
- computed tomography and nuclear magnetic resonance scans
- carotid Doppler sonography
- ventricular signal averaged ECG

- coronary angiography
- pulmonary scintigraphy.

Tilt-testing and carotid sinus massage

Tilt-testing has become the 'gold standard' investigation for most patients with possible neurocardiogenic syncope. A number of protocols have been developed in an attempt to standardise the approach, interpretation and management decisions.[1,5,6] Most investigators are agreed upon the use of footplate (rather than saddle) support, head-up tilt angle of 60–70° and tilt duration of 20–40 minutes. The addition of pharmacological provocation undoubtedly increases sensitivity but at the cost of specificity.[7]

The importance of beat-to-beat ECG and blood pressure monitoring is clear, as is the use of a supine pretilt phase of at least 10 minutes and the provision of a suitably warm, quiet environment in which to perform the study.

The end-point of the study is reproduction of typical symptoms or completion of the protocol.

Many centres will take the opportunity to undertake carotid sinus massage (ideally in supine and upright positions), Valsalva manoeuvre and occasionally heart rate variability in order to complete the assessment of cardiovascular autonomic status.[5] Carotid sinus massage should always be preceded by auscultation and performed using firm pressure for 5–10 seconds, initially on the right, then repeated on the left after a minimum interval of one minute. A positive result is asystole for three seconds or longer or a fall in systolic blood pressure of at least 50 mmHg.

CAUSES OF LOSS OF CONSCIOUSNESS

A significant number of patients with syncope will remain undiagnosed even with extensive and structured investigation in a dedicated syncope unit. In a study presenting data on 342 patients pooled from three syncope units in Italy, Alboni *et al*[8] showed that 18% remained without diagnosis, the underlying cause was neurally-mediated and orthostatic in 58%, cardiac in 23% (of which the vast majority were arrhythmic) and 1% were of neuropsychiatric origin. In a larger study using pooled data from nearly 1,500 patients investigated during the 1980s the number undiagnosed was much greater (35%), underlining the need for specialist syncope units. However, it is important to recognise that undiagnosed syncope (even when symptoms continue) carries a good prognosis as the course is benign and patients rarely suffer harm; this reassurance should be communicated to the patient.

TREATMENT OF SYNCOPE

Class I recommendations[1]

Explanation of the diagnosis and risk, with reassurance about the prognosis form the most important part of management for most patients because ignorance and fear relating to the episodes are often major factors in persuading the patient to seek medical advice. Recognition of premonitory symptoms and description of manoeuvres to abort or minimise the episode and the consequences of a fall can also reduce the potential for injury and hospital admission. This advice should also be communicated to family and friends.

Identification and avoidance of trigger events and causal situations (when feasible) can also be of value in situational syncope. It is always appropriate to investigate and treat any underlying causal pathology in these situations.

Modification or discontinuation of hypotensive drug treatment for concomitant conditions is of especial value in elderly patients in whom orthostatic syncope is often iatrogenic.

Cardiac pacing may be of some value in patients with cardioinhibitory or mixed carotid sinus syndrome, but results of clinical trials remain somewhat confusing with evidence for a strong placebo effect.[9]

Class II recommendations[1]

Volume expansion by increasing fluid intake, avoiding caffeine-containing drinks, salt supplements, an exercise programme or head-up tilt sleeping (>10°) may all be of value in posture-related syncope.

Cardiac pacing is recommended in patients with cardioinhibitory vasovagal syncope with a frequency of more than five attacks per year, severe physical injury or accident and age over 40 years.

Tilt training is of some benefit in patients with vasovagal syncope,[10] although few centres currently have the resources to utilise this approach.

Class III recommendations[1]

There is no convincing evidence to support the efficacy of beta-adrenergic blocking drugs in patients with neurocardiogenic syncope; indeed, such drugs may aggravate bradycardia in some cardioinhibitory cases.

☐ CONCLUSIONS

Cardiovascular syncope is relatively common, affecting up to 25% of individuals at some time during their life. Initial evaluation will determine the cause in many patients. Low risk patients often require little more than explanation of the process, advice regarding management of the symptoms, and reassurance with regard to the good prognosis. Identification and referral of high risk patients (mostly those with underlying cardiac disease) improve prognosis and QoL.

REFERENCES

1 Brignole M, Alboni P, Benditt D, Bergfeldt L *et al.* Guidelines on management (diagnosis and treatment) of syncope. *Eur Heart J* 2001;22:1256–306.

2 Soteriades ES, Evans JC, Larson MG, Chen MH *et al.* Incidence and prognosis of syncope. *N Engl J Med* 2002;347:878–85.

3 Chen L, Chen MH, Larson MG, Evans J *et al.* Risk factors for syncope in a community-based sample (the Framingham Heart Study). *Am J Cardiol* 2000;**85**:1189–93.

4 Robertson D, Davis TL. Neurological and related causes of syncope: the importance of recognition and treatment. In: Grubb BP, Olshansky B (eds). *Syncope: Mechanisms and Management.* Armonk, New York: Futura Publishing Company Inc, 1998:Ch 8, 223–51.

5 Kenny RA, Ingram A, Bayliss J, Sutton R. Head-up tilt: a useful test for investigating unexplained syncope. *Lancet* 1986;**i**:1352–5.

6 Kenny RA, O'Shea D, Parry SW. The Newcastle protocols for head-up tilt table testing in the diagnosis of vasovagal syncope, carotid sinus hypersensitivity, and related disorders. *Heart* 2000;**83**:564–9.

7 Fitzpatrick AP, Lee RJ, Epstein LM, Lesh MD *et al.* Effect of patient characteristics on the yield of prolonged baseline head-up tilt testing and the additional yield of drug provocation. *Heart* 1996;**76**:406–11.

8 Alboni P, Brignole M, Menozzi C, Raviele A *et al.* Diagnostic value of history in patients with syncope with or without heart disease. *J Am Coll Cardiol* 2001;**37**:1921–8.

9 Sutton R, Brignole M, Menozzi C, Raviele A *et al.* Dual-chamber pacing in the treatment of neurally mediated tilt-positive cardioinhibitory syncope: pacemaker versus no therapy: a multicenter randomized study. The Vasovagal Syncope International Study (VASIS) Investigators. *Circulation* 2000;**102**:294–9.

10 Reybrouck T, Heidbuchel H, Van De Werf F, Ector H. Long-term follow-up results of tilt training therapy in patients with recurrent neurocardiogenic syncope. *Pacing Clin Electrophysiol* 2002;**25**:1441–6.

☐ CARDIOLOGY SELF ASSESSMENT QUESTIONS

Contemporary treatment for atrial fibrillation

1 Atrial fibrillation (AF):
(a) Is the commonest sustained arrhythmia in humans
(b) Is associated with increased mortality
(c) In most patients occurs without an identifiable aetiology
(d) Is more common in women than in men
(e) Becomes more prevalent with increasing age

2 Warfarin therapy:
(a) Is as effective as aspirin in the prevention of stroke in patients with AF
(b) Should be used in conjunction with aspirin in most patients with AF
(c) Should be routinely used in patients with AF, including young patients with no other concomitant risk factors of stroke
(d) Reduces mortality in patients with AF
(e) Should not be used in patients over the age of 70

3 Restoration of sinus rhythm:
(a) Can be achieved by electrical cardioversion, drugs, ablation or surgery
(b) With drugs is safe earlier than 72 hours after the onset of AF with or without anticoagulation
(c) Can be achieved by atrioventricular nodal ablation and pacemaker implantation in patients with AF
(d) Using intravenous flecainide is not recommended in patients with ischaemic cardiomyopathy
(e) Should be attempted in all patients with AF

Risk stratification post-myocardial infarction

1 Major adverse cardiac events after myocardial infarction (MI) can be predicted by:
(a) Exercise stress testing
(b) Coronary angiography
(c) Ventricular ectopy
(d) Sinus bradycardia
(e) Ejection fraction

2 The risk of sudden death after MI can be reduced by:
(a) Angiotensin-converting enzyme inhibitors
(b) Statins
(c) Anti-arrhythmic drugs
(d) Nitrates
(e) Beta-blockers

3 The implantable cardioverter defibrillator has been shown to reduce death in post-MI patients with:
(a) Positive signal averaged ECG
(b) Decreased heart rate variability
(c) Increased heart rate variability
(d) Non-sustained ventricular tachycardia
(e) Low ejection fraction

4 Flecainide:
(a) Increases mortality after MI
(b) Should be used to treat asymptomatic ectopy after MI
(c) Should be used to treat symptomatic ectopy after MI
(d) Should be avoided in patients with impaired ventricular function post-MI
(e) Reduces the risk of heart failure after MI

Cardiovascular funny turns

1 Vasovagal syncope in young people (<40 years):
(a) Carries a high risk of sudden death
(b) Prevents the sufferer from driving
(c) Is often best treated with reassurance
(d) Responds well to beta-blocker therapy
(e) Is likely to require pacemaker implantation

2 Useful symptoms/signs to differentiate seizure from syncope:
(a) Presence of incontinence
(b) Warning dizziness or faintness
(c) Occurrence of tongue biting
(d) Inability to stand immediately on recovery of consciousness
(e) Tonic-clonic jerking

3 Tilt-table testing for syncope:
(a) Requires an 80° head-up position
(b) Should be performed with footplate support
(c) Requires a 60-minute passive phase
(d) May require pharmacological provocation
(e) Requires beat-to-beat blood pressure and ECG monitoring

4 Carotid sinus massage:
(a) Is contraindicated in patients over 75 years
(b) Should be performed only in supine patients
(c) Carries a 0.5% risk of stroke
(d) Should be performed using firm pressure for 5–10 seconds
(e) Is positive if asystole occurs for three seconds or longer

5 The following investigations are often useful in the investigation of syncope:
(a) Echocardiogram
(b) EEG
(c) Implantable loop recorder
(d) Holter monitoring
(e) Coronary angiography

Endocrinology

What to do with thyroid nodules and goitres

Mark Vanderpump

☐ DEFINITION OF GOITRE

A goitre is an enlargement of the thyroid gland and may result from either hormonal or immunological stimulation of gland growth or the presence of inflammatory, proliferative, infiltrative or metabolic disorders.[1] A thyroid gland whose lateral lobes have a volume greater than the terminal phalanges of the thumbs of the person examined is considered goitrous. The Pan American Health Organization has defined goitre as follows:[2]

- ☐ *Grade 0*: no palpable or visible goitre.
- ☐ *Grade 1*: a mass in the neck consistent with an enlarged thyroid that is palpable but not visible when the neck is in the neutral position; it also moves upward in the neck as the subject swallows.
- ☐ *Grade 2*: a swelling in the neck visible when the neck is in the normal position and consistent with an enlarged thyroid when the neck is palpated.

Most epidemiological studies define a thyroid that is visible as well as palpable as a goitre (World Health Organization Grade 1 or above), but the clinical grading of thyroid size is subjective and imprecise. Observer variation is the greatest factor in deciding whether a thyroid that is palpable but not visible is normal or enlarged. Interobserver variation may also lead to differences in the classification of thyroid disease: for example, diffuse goitre versus multinodular goitre versus single nodule.[1] There is also considerable overlap when clinical grading of thyroid volume is compared with thyroid volume estimated by ultrasonography. Ultrasonography has been used in epidemiological studies to assess thyroid size and leads to much higher estimates of goitre prevalence than in studies in which goitre size is assessed by physical examination.[3]

☐ THE IMPACT OF IODINE DEFICIENCY

Almost one-third of the world's population live in areas of iodine deficiency and risk the consequences. Populations at particular risk tend to be remote and live in mountainous areas in South-East Asia, Latin America and Central Africa. Although most affected people live in developing countries, many in large industrialised countries of Europe are also affected. If the thyroid is threatened by hypothyroidism, it enlarges in its struggle to produce more thyroid hormone. Goitre is usually endemic where the daily iodine intake is below 50 μg; congenital hypothyroidism develops when the intake falls below 25 μg a day.[2] The prevalence of goitre in areas of severe iodine deficiency can be up to 80%. In adults, serum thyroid-stimulating hormone (TSH) concentrations are raised only in very severe iodine deficiency.

Iodisation

Iodisation programmes are of proven value in reducing goitre size and in preventing goitre development and cretinism in children. Goitrogens in the diet, such as thiocyanate in incompletely cooked cassava or thioglucosides in brassica vegetables, can explain some of the differences in prevalence of endemic goitre in areas with similar degrees of iodine deficiency. Autonomy can develop in nodular goitres, leading occasionally to thyrotoxicosis. Iodisation programmes can also induce thyrotoxicosis, especially in those aged over 40 years with nodular goitres.

□ GENETIC DEFECTS

Defects in thyroid hormone synthesis and action arising from impaired genes can result in the thyroid adapting by increasing its size to provide more cell activity and increased production of the required amount of thyroid hormone. The synthesis of thyroxine (T4) involves thyroglobulin (TG), thyroid peroxidase (TPO) and other proteins. Pendred's syndrome is characterised by defective iodide organification, goitre and congenital deafness from cochlear and endolymph defects. The genetic defect has been identified in pendrin, a protein associated with iodide transport at the apical membrane. Other genetic defects can be localised to specific mutations of the sodium-iodide symporter, TG and TPO, all of which can have goitre as a consequence, as can the thyroid hormone resistance syndrome, which is usually due to mutations in the thyroid hormone receptor β gene.

□ EPIDEMIOLOGY

Diffuse goitre

The most common thyroid disease in an iodine-replete community is simple (diffuse) goitre.[4] There are considerable regional variations in the incidence of goitre, even in non-endemic goitre areas. In cross-sectional surveys, confirmed by longitudinal studies, the prevalence of diffuse goitre declines with age. The highest prevalence is in premenopausal women (31% of all premenopausal women <45 years) and the ratio of women to men is at least 4:1 (Fig 1).[5]

A cross-sectional study performed between 1972 and 1974 in Whickham, a mixed urban and rural area in North-East England, documented the prevalence of thyroid disorders in the community. The 2,779 subjects examined in the survey (82% of the available sample) closely represented the adult population in terms of age, gender and social class. A 20-year follow-up of the Whickham cohort determined outcomes in terms of thyroid disease in 87% of the total original survey population and therefore provided longitudinal data for thyroid disease in a

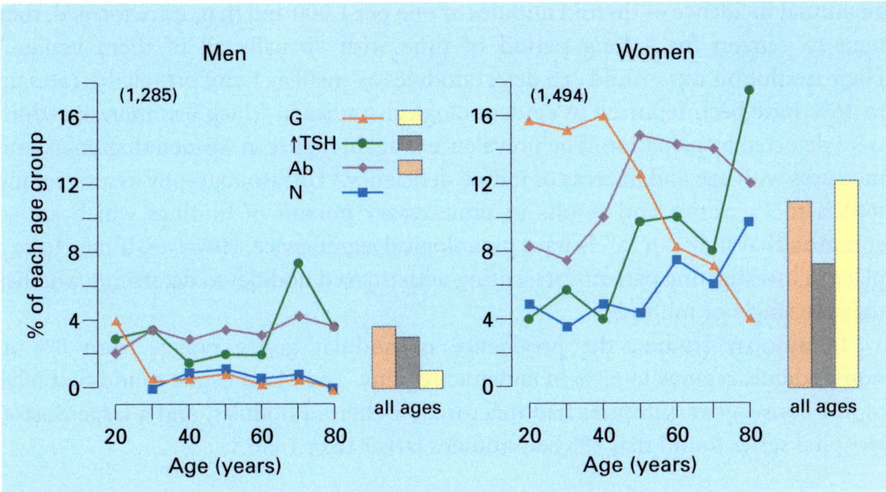

Fig 1 Age and sex distribution of thyroid microsomal antibodies (Ab), raised serum thyroid stimulating hormone (TSH) above 6 mU/l (↑TSH), visible diffuse and multinodular goitre (G) and nodules (N) in the Whickham survey (adapted from Ref 5).

representative sample of the community. In this follow-up, 10% of women and 2% of men had a goitre compared with 23% and 5%, respectively, at the first survey.[6] The presence of a diffuse goitre was not predictive of any clinical or biochemical evidence of thyroid dysfunction. In women, an association was found between the development of a goitre and thyroid antibody status at follow-up, but not initially.

Management of diffuse goitre

Conditions that may present with a diffusely enlarged thyroid gland include simple goitre, Graves' disease, Hashimoto's thyroiditis, subacute or viral (de Quervain's) thyroiditis, postpartum thyroiditis or, rarely, malignancy. Both hyper- and hypothyroidism may be difficult to diagnose from clinical findings, especially in elderly people. Biochemical evaluation of thyroid function is necessary and serum TSH measurement should be a first-line test in nearly all circumstances. If there is a high clinical suspicion of thyroid dysfunction, supplementary investigation of thyroid function should be performed with serum free T4 and TPO antibody measurement. Ultrasound examination of the thyroid gland should not be routinely performed but is occasionally helpful as an aid to clinical evaluation. Often, reassurance is all that is required.

Nodular goitre

The decline in frequency of diffuse goitre with age is in contrast to the age-related increase in frequency of thyroid nodules. In the Framingham study of subjects over 60 years, the prevalence of single and multiple thyroid nodules was 3% and 1%, respectively, as assessed by palpation.[7] Longitudinal data from Framingham suggest an annual incidence of thyroid nodules of one per 1,000 and that, once formed, they tend to remain for a long period of time with virtually all of them benign.[8] High-resolution ultrasound can detect nodules as small as 1 cm; prevalence rates up to 36% have been reported in epidemiological studies in which less than one-third were detected by palpation. The prevalence is again higher in women than men, and increases with age and in areas of iodine deficiency.[4] Ultrasonography as a screening tool is too sensitive and results in unnecessary pursuit of findings which are so common that they can rarely have pathological significance. However, it may have a place in investigating patients presenting with thyroid nodules to determine whether they are single or multiple.

In autopsy studies, the prevalence of nodular goitre ranges from 8% in non-endemic regions to 65% in endemic regions. The Mayo Clinic found that 50% of 821 consecutive autopsies had macroscopic thyroid nodules, and a large Boston Hospital series found that 8% had nodules larger than 1 cm.[9]

Thyroid cancers

The clinical presentation of thyroid cancer is usually as a solitary thyroid nodule or increasing goitre size. Thyroid nodules are common, but thyroid cancer is rare – although accounting for over 90% of the cancers of the endocrine glands[10] it comprises less than 1% of all cancers registered in the UK. The annual incidence of all thyroid cancer is 1–10 per 100,000 population in most countries and is 2–4 times more frequent in women than in men. The four major histological types are papillary, follicular, medullary and anaplastic, each of which displays a different epidemiology.

Papillary and follicular tumours

Papillary and follicular tumours, which comprise 60–90% of all thyroid cancers, are among the most curable of cancers. They are rare in children and adolescents, and their incidence increases with age in adults (Fig 2).

- *Papillary thyroid carcinoma* (PTC) is the most common thyroid malignancy, accounting for 50–90% of differentiated follicular cell-derived thyroid cancers worldwide.

- *Papillary thyroid microcarcinomas* (diameter ≤1 cm) are found in 4–36% of adults at post-mortem in population-based studies.[9] Their reported increased incidence in recent years may be attributable to improved pathological techniques. Most diagnoses of PTC occur in patients aged 30–50 years (median age 44 years), most of them in women (60–80%).

- *Follicular thyroid cancer* is relatively infrequent compared with papillary cancer and accounts for about 15% of all thyroid cancer. However, in iodine-deficient endemic goitre areas there is an increased frequency of follicular over papillary carcinoma (5:1). It tends to be a malignancy of older people, with a mean age of 50 years in most studies.

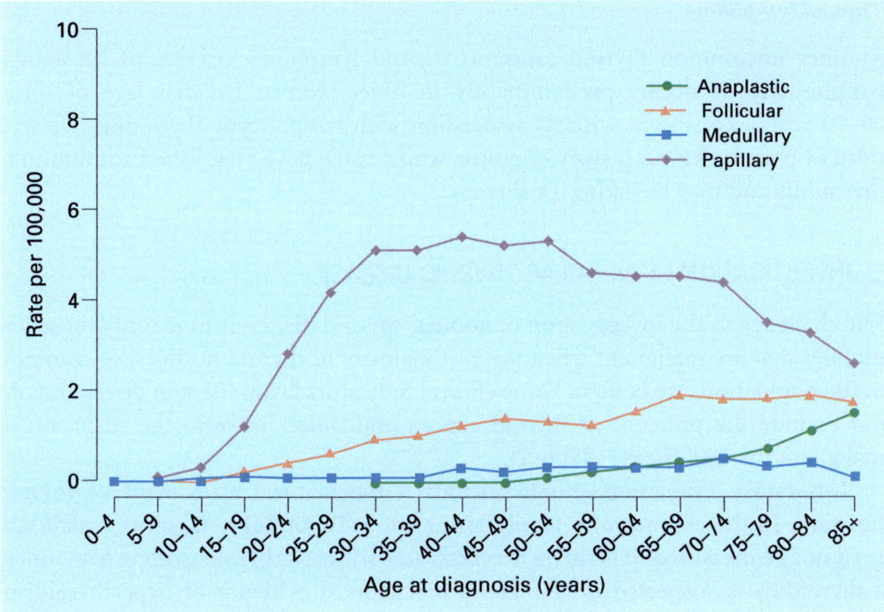

Fig 2 Thyroid cancer: age-specific incidence rates by histological type for men and women from the Surveillance Epidemiology End Results programme population registries, 1973–1987 (adapted from Ref 10).

In addition to female gender, advanced age and low iodine intake, external radiation exposure, particularly in childhood, is a major risk factor for papillary cancer. Some studies suggest that follicular cancer may also be affected in this way. There is no documented association between radioiodine therapy for thyrotoxicosis and subsequent development of thyroid cancer in adults.[4]

Medullary thyroid cancer

Medullary thyroid cancer (MTC), a rare calcitonin-secreting tumour of the thyroid C cells, is found in both sporadic and hereditary forms. The highest incidence of sporadic disease occurs in the fifth decade. Hereditary MTC can be inherited as an autosomal dominant trait with a high degree of penetrance associated with multiple endocrine neoplasia type 2 (MEN II) syndrome or as familial MTC without any other endocrinopathies. It can be diagnosed before clinical presentation by genetic and biochemical screening.[4]

Anaplastic thyroid cancer

A rare thyroid cancer, more frequent in populations with endemic goitre, is anaplastic thyroid cancer. Anaplastic change also occurs rarely in a long-standing benign thyroid adenoma or differentiated carcinoma. The women to men ratio is less pronounced, and the peak incidence is in the 70s.

Thyroid lymphoma

Another uncommon thyroid cancer is thyroid lymphoma (ca 2% of extranodal lymphomas). It occurs predominantly in older women (median age of onset 60–70 years), consistent with its association with lymphocytic thyroiditis. Up to a third of patients have a history of goitre, whilst some have established autoimmune thyroiditis and may be taking T4 therapy.

□ INVESTIGATION OF NODULAR THYROID DISEASE

The challenge in the investigation of nodular thyroid disease is to identify those few nodules that are malignant when the vast majority of thyroid nodules, so common in the population, are benign. Some clinical indicators favour benign disease but do not exclude the presence of thyroid cancer, and others increase the suspicion of malignant thyroid disease (Table 1).

Laboratory evaluation should include a biochemical assessment of thyroid function. In the absence of a family history of MTC or MEN II, serum calcitonin need not be measured. It is rarely necessary to perform a thyroid isotope scan unless a thyroiditis is suspected or if there is biochemical evidence of hyperthyroidism (ie suppressed serum TSH). Thyroid ultrasound is not routinely recommended in the initial evaluation of thyroid nodules. However, it may be useful to determine if there is a dominant nodule within a multinodular goitre, as the latter has been reported to have the same malignancy risk as a solitary thyroid nodule.

Fine-needle aspiration biopsy

The key investigation of nodular thyroid disease is fine-needle aspiration (FNA) biopsy which is most effective for distinguishing benign from malignant disease. In large series of FNA biopsies, approximately 70% were reported as benign, 4% malignant and 26% suspicious. Half the suspicious nodules were non-diagnostic and 10–30% of these were ultimately malignant. In centres reporting large series, the FNA biopsy sensitivity is 68–98% (mean 83%) and the specificity 72–100% (mean 92%),

Table 1 Clinical indicators in the investigation of nodular goitres.

Factors that favour benign disease	Factors that increase suspicion
Family history: autoimmune thyroid disease benign thyroid nodule	Age <20 or >70 years Male gender
Hypo/hyperthyroidism	Associated dysphagia/hoarseness
Associated pain or tenderness	History of external neck radiotherapy
Soft, smooth, mobile nodule	Family history of thyroid cancer
Multinodular goitre without a dominant nodule	Cervical lymphadenopathy Firm, hard, irregular, fixed nodule

respectively. The surgical yield of thyroid cancer following the introduction of FNA biopsy has increased from about 15% to 45% in many centres.[11]

☐ MANAGEMENT OF THYROID NODULES

Patients with benign cytology can be safely followed without surgical intervention. Confirmation of benign cytology at repeat FNA biopsy three months later can allow the patient to be fully reassured and safely discharged. Further investigations in patients with a euthyroid multinodular goitre who have obstructive symptoms include flow-volume loop and computed tomography scan to look for tracheal compression. Both thyroidectomy and radioiodine therapy are effective in reducing symptoms, but there is no role for T4 suppressive therapy. In view of the long-term risk of thyrotoxicosis, periodic follow-up of thyroid function every 3–5 years would be a reasonable strategy.

Thyroidectomy

Total thyroidectomy is usually indicated when nodules larger than 1 cm are found to be malignant on cytology. In patients with suspicious or repeatedly non-diagnostic cytology, a thyroid lobectomy is recommended to obtain a histological diagnosis. Most suspicious nodules are follicular lesions which cytology cannot distinguish as either an adenoma or a carcinoma. Experience in performing FNA biopsy and cytology are essential; patients with thyroid nodules should preferably be investigated and managed within the setting of a thyroid cancer multidisciplinary clinic.[11]

☐ THYROID INCIDENTALOMAS

The fact that ultrasound is such a sensitive method for detection of thyroid nodules may cause problems in daily clinical practice.[12] An incidental finding of a thyroid nodule can lead to concern for patients and general practitioners, and is an increasingly frequent reason for referral to endocrinology clinics. The impalpable thyroid nodule is usually defined as less than 1.0–1.5 cm. There are few data on the clinical significance and prognosis of differentiated thyroid malignancy in impalpable nodules, and no consensus on the size criterion below which an FNA biopsy is required. Ultrasonographic criteria such as solidity, hypoechogenicity and punctate calcification within the nodule may determine selection for FNA, but may not be diagnostically reliable and the cytology also be more difficult to interpret. Observation rather than intervention may be all that is required in these clinical circumstances.

REFERENCES

1 Siminoski K. The rational clinical examination. Does this patient have a goiter? *JAMA* 1995;273:813–7.

2 Delange F. Iodine deficiency. In: Braverman LE, Utiger RD (eds). *Werner and Ingbar's the Thyroid: a Fundamental and Clinical Text*, 8th edn. Philadelphia: JB Lippincott-Raven, 2000: 467–73.

3 Peterson S, Sanga A, Eklöf H, Bunga B *et al.* Classification of thyroid size by palpation and ultrasonography in field surveys. *Lancet* 2000;**355**:106–10.

4 Vanderpump MP, Tunbridge WM. Epidemiology of thyroid disease and swelling. In: Wass JA, Shalet SM (eds). *Oxford Textbook of Endocrinology.* Oxford: Oxford University Press, 2002:339–49.

5 Tunbridge WM, Evered DC, Hall R, Appleton D *et al.* The spectrum of thyroid disease in a community: the Whickham Survey. *Clin Endocrinol (Oxf)* 1977;**7**:481–93.

6 Vanderpump MP, Tunbridge WM, French JM, Appleton D *et al.* The incidence of thyroid disorders in the community: a twenty-year follow-up of the Whickham Survey. *Clin Endocrinol (Oxf)* 1995;**43**:55–68.

7 Sawin CT, Bigos ST, Land S, Bacharach P. The aging thyroid. Relationship between elevated serum thyrotropin level and thyroid antibodies in elderly patients. *Am J Med* 1985;**79**:591–5.

8 Vander JB, Gaston EA, Dawber TR. The significance of nontoxic thyroid nodules. Final report of a 15-year study of the incidence of thyroid malignancy. *Ann Intern Med* 1968;**69**:537–40.

9 Mazzaferri EL. Management of a solitary thyroid nodule. Review. *N Engl J Med* 1993;**328**:553–9.

10 Correa P, Chen VW. Endocrine gland cancer. *Cancer* 1995;**75**(Suppl):338–52.

11 British Thyroid Association. *Guidelines for the management of thyroid cancer in adults.* London: Royal College of Physicians, 2002.

12 Topliss D. Thyroid incidentaloma: the ignorant in pursuit of the impalpable. *Clin Endocrinol (Oxf)* 2004;**60**:18–20.

New management strategies for osteoporosis

Richard Eastell

□ INTRODUCTION

Osteoporosis is a major public health problem, but there are now a number of treatments that are safe and effective in reducing the risk of subsequent fracture.[1] UK evidence-based guidelines have been developed by the Royal College of Physicians, updated in conjunction with the Bone and Tooth Society in 2000, for measurement of bone density using dual-energy X-ray absorptiometry (DXA) and subsequent treatment (Fig 1).[2]

Osteoporosis is defined as a bone mineral density (BMD) T-score below –2.5 (a T-score is the number of standard deviations from the mean for healthy young women). In the evaluation of osteoporosis, it is important to consider the risk of fracture in the near future and to examine for secondary osteoporosis.

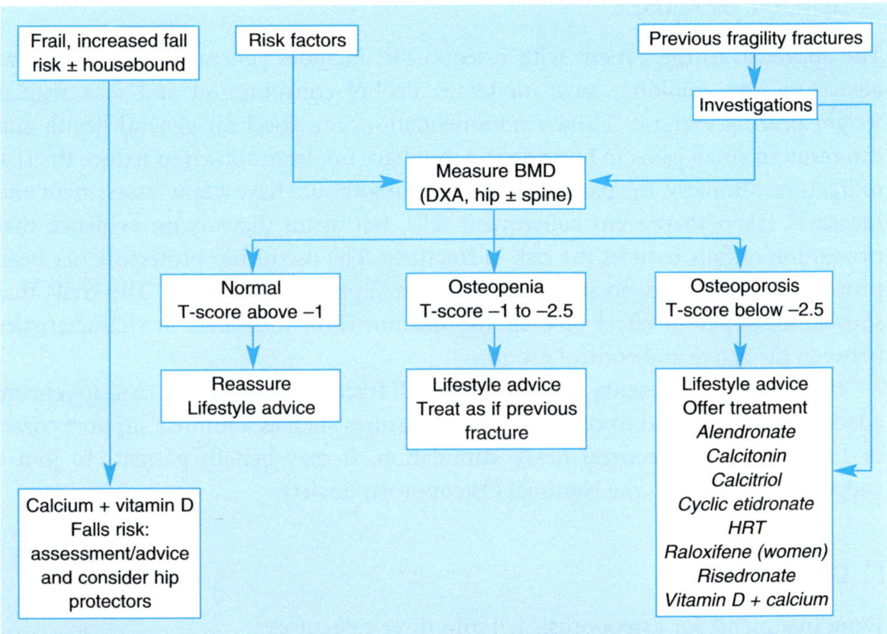

Fig 1 Treatment algorithm for the management of postmenopausal osteoporosis prepared by the Royal College of Physicians and the Bone and Tooth Society of the UK (BMD = bone mineral density; DXA = dual-energy X-ray absorptiometry; HRT = hormone replacement therapy).[2]

Fracture risk is increased by many factors, but the common risk factors for fracture include:

- □ low BMD
- □ the presence of a fracture after the age of 40 years
- □ family history of fracture (particularly maternal history of hip fracture before the age of 80)
- □ slender habitus (weight less than 58 kg), and
- □ current smoking habit.

Fracture risk is also greater in those at increased risk of falling and those taking glucocorticoids.

The importance of examination for secondary osteoporosis is because treatment of the underlying condition may result in a reduction in fracture risk. For example, treatment of primary hyperparathyroidism decreases bone turnover, increases BMD and reduces risk of fracture. However, some conditions may impair the response to osteoporosis treatment, for example vitamin D has been reported to impair the response to bisphosphonates.

□ GENERAL MEASURES

The approach to the patient with osteoporosis includes general measures such as advice to stop smoking, have moderate alcohol consumption and take regular weight-bearing exercise. These recommendations are good for general health and can result in small gains in bone density but have not been shown to reduce the risk of fracture. Similarly, the patient at risk of falling should have a falls' assessment and measures taken to prevent subsequent falls, but again there is no evidence that prevention of falls reduces the risk of fractures. The use of hip protectors has been proposed, but there is no strong evidence in support of their use. The trials that showed an apparent effect of their use did not show a balance in characteristics between the active and control groups.

If the patient presents after a vertebral fracture, it is important to ensure adequate analgesia and to consider other measures such as a lumbar support corset or transcutaneous electrical nerve stimulation. It may benefit patients to join a support group such as the National Osteoporosis Society.

□ DRUG THERAPY

Drug treatments for osteoporosis fall into three categories:[3]

1. *Antiresorptive drugs* that inhibit bone resorption, for example bisphosphonates, hormone replacement therapy (HRT) and raloxifene.
2. *Anabolic drugs* stimulating bone formation, for example parathyroid hormone (PTH) and its 1-34 amino acid peptide, teriparatide.

3 *Mixed antiresorptive and anabolic drugs* that both inhibit bone resorption and stimulate bone formation, for example strontium ranelate.

The main mechanism by which these treatments reduce the risk of fracture was thought to be through an increase in BMD. However, it has become apparent that the increase in BMD with antiresorptive drugs such as risedronate, alendronate and raloxifene accounts for only 10% of the fracture benefit. It is more likely that the most important effect of these treatments is to decrease the rate of bone turnover to healthy premenopausal women levels. Indeed, the change in bone turnover markers accounts for up to 70% of the fracture risk reduction with risedronate.[4] The way in which anabolic agents reduce fracture risk is less well studied, but it might include qualitative improvement to bone such as increases in cortical bone thickness and better connectivity of trabecular bone.

☐ SPECIFIC TREATMENTS

Calcium and vitamin D

In most of the clinical trials to date calcium and vitamin D were administered with the other treatments. Older women commonly have both low dietary calcium and vitamin D insufficiency. The latter may impair response to antiresorptive therapy. It is difficult to assess dietary calcium or vitamin D status accurately in clinical practice, so it may be sensible to give calcium and vitamin D supplements to all patients receiving therapy for osteoporosis. Indeed, in certain populations such as the housebound elderly this may reduce the risk of hip fracture without the need for further therapy.

Bisphosphonates

The commonest treatment for osteoporosis in the UK is bisphosphonates, particularly alendronate and risedronate. These drugs are poorly absorbed and so must be taken in the fasting state at least half an hour before breakfast. Following reports of oesophagitis with alendronate, the recommendation is that it must be taken with a full glass of water and the patient be advised to remain upright until after breakfast.

Bisphosphonates are well tolerated, with occasional skin rash, and are effective in reducing the risk of vertebral fractures by 40–50%, with the effect present within the first year of therapy. They reduce the risk of non-vertebral fracture, including hip fracture, by 30–50%, and also fractures in women with vertebral fractures and in women with BMD T-scores below –2.5. There is no evidence for efficacy in patients with T-scores above this threshold or in patients with fractures other than vertebral fracture.

The complicated instructions for taking bisphosphonates may reduce compliance. Both alendronate and risedronate are now available as once a week preparations, a form of administration that has proven popular with patients. Intravenous forms of bisphosphonates are being evaluated as intravenous injections at three-monthly (ibandronate) or annual (zoledronate) intervals.[5]

It is not known for how long treatment should be given. There is persistent suppression of bone turnover markers after 3–5 years of alendronate therapy, so it might be worth stopping alendronate after five years and watching for bone loss or an increase in bone turnover before reinstating therapy. It is also not yet known whether there is persistent suppression of bone turnover markers after long-term risedronate therapy.

Hormone replacement therapy

HRT has been used for many years for the prevention of fractures. The evidence for fracture risk reduction was based on cohort and case-control studies. The Women's Health Initiative study[6] then showed a clear reduction in all fractures, including hip fracture, to the same extent as bisphosphonates. However, this large randomised controlled trial reported increased cardiovascular and stroke risk in addition to the known side effects of breast cancer and venous thromboembolic disease. HRT is not commonly recommended for the prevention of fracture risk due to this adverse event profile.

Raloxifene

Raloxifene binds to the oestrogen receptor, like the oestrogen in HRT, but acts as an oestrogen agonist in some tissues and as an oestrogen antagonist in others. Long-term treatment with this drug reduces the risk of breast cancer, particularly oestrogen receptor-positive cancers, and the risk of vertebral fracture but not the risk of non-vertebral fracture. Raloxifene has minor side effects such as hot flushes and leg cramps, and rare but important side effects such as venous thromboembolic disease. It does not increase the risk of cardiovascular disease or stroke; indeed, it might reduce the risk in women at high risk of these conditions.

Calcitonin

Calcitonin, a peptide hormone made by the thyroid gland, acts directly on osteoclasts to reduce bone resorption. However, the effect of bone resorption with chronic therapy is quite small and the peptide has to be given by subcutaneous injection or nasal spray. It may cause nausea and a metallic taste when given by subcutaneous injection, and may also have an analgesic effect. It has been used in the setting of acute vertebral fracture, as well as for long-term treatment for fracture risk reduction.

Teriparatide

PTH, a peptide hormone (84 amino acids) made by the parathyroid glands, or the 1-34 amino acid peptide (teriparatide) when given as daily subcutaneous injections is anabolic to bone. In clinical trials it reduced the risk of further vertebral fractures in women with vertebral fractures prior to treatment and also reduced non-vertebral fractures.[7] The latter effect may be more potent than for the antiresorptive drugs but there has been no direct comparison. The side effects are mainly those of hypercalcaemia such as nausea and headache. Neither the optimum duration of therapy (the teriparatide trials lasted 1–2 years) nor the best treatment to use after stopping therapy is known. Prior use of bisphosphonates such as alendronate may attenuate the increase in BMD with teriparatide.[8]

Strontium

Strontium ranelate appears to have weak antiresorptive and anabolic effects. It is not clear how it exerts these actions. The increase in BMD with this compound may be misleading: strontium replaces calcium in the hydroxyapatite crystal and attenuates X-rays to a greater extent than calcium, thus giving a false reading of a great increase in bone mass. The treatment reduces the risk of vertebral fractures;[9] the results of trials for non-vertebral fracture are awaited.

□ DISCUSSION

There are now a number of effective treatments for reducing fracture risk, but it is unclear how best to use these treatments and several questions remain:

1 It is usual to give one treatment alone (plus calcium and vitamin D). Would it be better to combine treatments?

2 Some treatments appear to exert their effects long after stopping treatment (eg alendronate). Would it be better to give intermittent treatment?

3 Should therapy be monitored?

Most patients in clinical trials are likely to have a favourable reduction in fracture risk, but in clinical practice all patients may not benefit from the treatments if they do not comply fully with instructions or have coexistent disease.

Treatment can be monitored in two ways:

1 *BMD of the spine*, usually measured after 1–2 years. An increase of more than 3–6% probably indicates a favourable response.

2 *Bone turnover markers*: bone resorption markers such as N- or C-telopeptide fragments of type I collagen, NTX and CTX are usually measured. A decrease with antiresorptive therapy of more than 30–50% probably indicates a favourable response.

□ CONCLUSIONS

The major challenge in the field of osteoporosis is to identify those patients at high risk of fracture and treat them appropriately. Groups of patients likely to need treatments include those attending a fracture clinic or receiving long-term glucocorticoids. However, the use of treatments in these groups is currently limited: almost no patients receive treatment following a fracture of the hip or forearm and only one-third following a fracture of the spine.[10] There is much to be done.

REFERENCES

1 Eastell R. Treatment of postmenopausal osteoporosis. Review. *N Engl J Med* 1998;**338**:736–46.

2 Royal College of Physicians, Bone and Tooth Society. *Osteoporosis. Clinical guidelines for prevention and treatment. Update on pharmacological interventions and an algorithm for management.* London: RCP, 2000.

3 Delmas PD. Treatment of postmenopausal osteoporosis. Review. *Lancet* 2002;**359**:2018–26.

4 Eastell R, Barton I, Hannon RA, Chines A *et al.* Relationship of early changes in bone resorption to the reduction in fracture risk with risedronate. *J Bone Miner Res* 2003;**18**:1051–6.

5 Reid IR, Brown JP, Burckhardt P, Horowitz Z *et al.* Intravenous zoledronic acid in postmenopausal women with low bone mineral density. *N Engl J Med* 2002;**346**:653–61.

6 Rossouw JE, Anderson GL, Prentice RL, LaCroix AZ *et al.* Risks and benefits of estrogen plus progestin in healthy postmenopausal women: principal results from the Women's Health Initiative randomized controlled trial. *JAMA* 2002;**288**:321–33.

7 Neer RM, Arnaud CD, Zanchetta JR, Prince R *et al.* Effect of parathyroid hormone (1-34) on fractures and bone mineral density in postmenopausal women with osteoporosis. *N Engl J Med* 2001;**344**:1434–41.

8 Black DM, Greenspan SL, Ensrud KE, Palermo L *et al.* The effects of parathyroid hormone and alendronate alone or in combination in postmenopausal osteoporosis. *N Engl J Med* 2003;**349**:1207–15.

9 Meunier PJ, Roux C, Seeman E, Ortolani S *et al.* The effects of strontium ranelate on the risk of vertebral fracture in women with postmenopausal osteoporosis. *N Engl J Med* 2004;**350**:459–68.

10 Torgerson DJ, Dolan P. Prescribing by general practitioners after an osteoporotic fracture. *Ann Rheum Dis* 1998;**57**:378–9.

How to manage hypercalcaemia

Peter Selby

☐ INTRODUCTION

Hypercalcaemia is one of the most common metabolic emergencies encountered in general medical practice. It has been estimated to occur in approximately 5% of acute hospital admissions.[1] Its management is therefore an important part of the armamentarium of any general admitting physician. This chapter seeks to review the mechanisms underlying hypercalcaemia and to devise a management strategy that will be applicable in most situations.

Calcium is important for a variety of different bodily functions, including neuromuscular transmission, stimulus-secretion coupling and structural integrity, but it is not usually failure of any of these systems that makes hypercalcaemia potentially dangerous. In severe hypercalcaemia the body attempts to eliminate excess calcium via the kidneys and, in so doing, there is a concomitant loss of sodium in the urine. This in turn leads to a depletion of the circulating volume together with a reduction in glomerular filtration rate. The combination of these two processes causes a further increase in plasma calcium and a stress on renal excretion, with progressive deterioration in renal function and circulating volume. The overall effect of these changes is to lead to circulatory collapse and death in a manner analogous to that seen in conditions such as diabetic ketoacidosis. This condition is known as 'disequilibrium hypercalcaemia' and is potentially life-threatening. These cases are generally associated with plasma calcium levels above 3.0 mmol/l, together with renal impairment and clinical evidence of hypovolaemia. Their management represents a medical emergency.

Most cases of hypercalcaemia are not associated with such potential for circulatory collapse. Their assessment and treatment can be undertaken at a more leisurely pace.

☐ CAUSES OF HYPERCALCAEMIA

Many causes of hypercalcaemia are listed in standard textbooks (Table 1) but the vast majority of cases will be due to either hyperparathyroidism or malignancy. A small proportion of cases may be the result of vitamin D intoxication or abnormal activation of vitamin D by granulomatous tissue, thyrotoxicosis or the abnormality of calcium sensing known as familial hypocalciuric hypercalcaemia (FHH).[2] The other causes of hypercalcaemia are vanishingly rare.

The most important clinical question to ask when confronted with a patient suffering from hypercalcaemia is whether this is dangerous disequilibrium

Table 1 Causes of hypercalcaemia.

Common	Less common	Uncommon
Hyperparathyroidism:	Vitamin D intoxication	Thiazide diuretics
• Primary	Familial hypocalciuric hypercalcaemia	Lithium
• Tertiary	Sarcoidosis and other	Immobilisation
Malignancy	granulomatous diseases	Hyperthyroidism
• Humoral hypercalcaemia	Thyrotoxicosis	Milk-alkali syndrome
• Multiple myeloma		Post-transplant
• Bony metastases		Renal failure
		Addison's disease
		Phaeochromocytoma
		Vitamin A intoxication

hypercalcaemia. The most useful clinical feature indicating this are signs of hypovolaemia; if present, it is likely that the patient has disequilibrium hypercalcaemia and requires urgent treatment to prevent deterioration.

In addition to information regarding the severity of the hypercalcaemia, clinical assessment may also reveal important information about the presence of symptoms of hypercalcaemia or of its complications. There may also be clues to its cause such as ingestion of drugs that can raise the plasma calcium. Clinical examination may also help in the identification of the underlying cause of the hypercalcaemia; in particular, it may reveal signs suggestive of malignancy. Although clinical assessment of a patient with hypercalcaemia is important, this usually needs to be accompanied by a variety of investigations.

□ HOW DOES HYPERCALCAEMIA DEVELOP?

To understand the causes and treatment of hypercalcaemia it is necessary to review the way in which hypercalcaemia develops. In normal circumstances, plasma calcium levels are maintained by a balance between, on the one hand, calcium flowing into the plasma from the diet and as a result of bone resorption and, on the other, calcium leaving the plasma either to form new bone or through the urine. Most of these fluxes are of a similar magnitude (ca 6 mmol per day (Fig 1). The amount filtered in the urine is considerably greater (ca 226 mmol per day), most of which (ca 220 mmol per day) is reabsorbed in the renal tubules, giving an overall daily loss in the urine of approximately 6 mmol. The huge difference between the amounts filtered at the glomerulus and lost in the urine means that the kidney is the main organ for calcium homeostasis, and slight changes in renal handling of calcium can have major effects on the plasma calcium level.

Parathyroid hormone

By comparing the plasma and urine concentrations of calcium and creatinine it is possible to calculate whether hypercalcaemia in any individual is due to increased tubular reabsorption of calcium or increased throughput of calcium as a result of

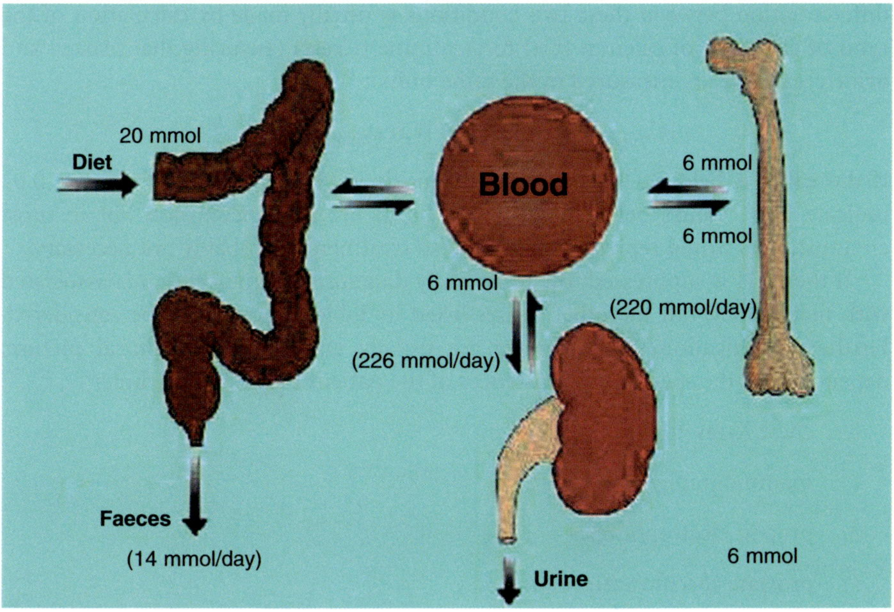

Fig 1 Diagram showing daily calcium fluxes.

either dietary calcium absorption or excessive bone resorption.[3] The major influence on the reabsorption of calcium at the renal tubule is the presence of parathyroid hormone (PTH). Increasing concentrations of PTH lead to increasing reabsorption of calcium from the urine. In most circumstances, the most important investigation in the assessment of the cause of hypercalcaemia is measurement of PTH concentration. This needs to be undertaken in a fasting state (dietary calcium will suppress PTH) and before treatment is instituted (agents such as bisphosphonates will elevate PTH). Hypercalcaemia would be expected to suppress PTH secretion by the usual feedback loop, so a PTH level above the middle of the normal range in the presence of hypercalcaemia is generally accepted to be abnormal.[4]

Familial hypocalciuric hypercalcaemia

PTH-dependent hypercalcaemia is usually the result of hyperparathyroidism (primary or tertiary) but FHH also needs to be considered. In FHH, the calcium sensing receptors are subject to an inactivating mutation, causing the body to 'believe' that the prevailing calcium level is lower than it really is. It is an important differential diagnosis to recognise because it is almost always benign and does not require treatment.[2]

Differential diagnosis

FHH is differentiated from primary hyperparathyroidism (PHP) by the amount of tubular reabsorption of calcium; this is considerably higher in FHH. The differentiation between these two conditions is usually made by calculation of the ratio of clearance of calcium (Ca) to creatinine (Creat) (ensuring that plasma and urine creatinine are measured in the same units):

$$[Ca_{urine}]/[Creat_{urine}] \times [Creat_{blood}]/[Ca_{blood}]$$

If the value is below 0.01, the likely diagnosis is FHH, whilst values above 0.02 indicate PHP. Values between these two limits are not uncommon but in most circumstances would represent mild PHP so treatment is probably not necessary.

If the PTH is suppressed, the most likely diagnosis is hypercalcaemia associated with malignancy, but the other causes listed in Table 1 should also be considered. Further investigations at this stage are usually guided by the clinical picture; depending on the specific circumstances of the patient they might include:

- chest X-ray
- mammography
- protein electrophoresis
- prostate specific antigen, or
- angiotensin-converting enzyme.

TREATMENT OF HYPERCALCAEMIA

Specific treatment will depend on the underlying cause of hypercalcaemia, but several general principles can be applied.

Emergency treatment

For a patient suffering from severe life-threatening hypercalcaemia, the most important management is the institution of rehydration using large volumes of intravenous saline. Typically, 6–8 litres will be needed over the first 24 hours. It is often taught that the addition of a loop diuretic such as furosemide will increase calcium clearance in the urine. This is probably true, but benefit is achieved at the expense of further compromising the circulating volume. Loop diuretics are therefore best reserved for those patients unable to tolerate the quantities of fluid necessary to stabilise the situation.

No treatment

In patients with less severe hypercalcaemia, the most important clinical question is often whether the hypercalcaemia needs treating. This treatment option has been best worked out for mild PHP. Two separate consensus development conferences by the US National Institutes of Health have produced guidance on when it is acceptable to leave PHP untreated.[5] More recently, a working party set up by the Bone and Tooth Society in the UK has produced guidelines for the same situation developed along evidence-based lines.[4] This guidance is summarised in Table 2.

Table 2 Guidelines for intervention in hypercalcaemia.*

	Guidelines	
Indication	**UK**	**US**
Plasma calcium	3.0 mmol/l	ca 2.85 mmol/l
Urine calcium	10 mmol/l/day (possibly)	10 mmol/l/day
Creatinine clearance	Not discussed	Reduced by 30%
Bone density	T-score <–2.5	T-score <–2.5
Age	<50 years	<50 years

*These recommendations apply in the absence of any end-organ damage such as renal stones, bone disease or pancreatitis which are themselves indications for treatment.

No specific guidance has been put forward for the management of other forms of hypercalcaemia, but it would seem reasonable to apply similar principles to the management of raised calcium of other origins.

Removing the cause of hypercalcaemia

If it is decided that the hypercalcaemia should be treated, a number of strategies are available. First, it may be possible to remove the underlying cause. This is most commonly undertaken in PHP when parathyroidectomy is usually curative. It is also possible to remove the cause if the hypercalcaemia is due to medication or a readily treatable underlying condition such as Addison's disease or hyperthyroidism. In patients with multiple myeloma or other malignant conditions, treatment of the underlying disease may also effect removal of the cause of hypercalcaemia even if the benefit is only temporary.

Neutralising the mechanism of hypercalcaemia

If the *underlying* cause of hypercalcaemia cannot be removed, an attempt is usually made to neutralise the *mechanism* causing the hypercalcaemia. Thus, in patients with increased absorption of calcium from the gut (as may be seen in sarcoidosis), administration of steroids together with a low calcium diet will reduce calcium absorption and lower the plasma calcium level.

Bisphosphonates

By far the most common way of neutralising the mechanism of hypercalcaemia is with bisphosphonates. Bisphosphonates are a group of chemically related compounds which become incorporated into the hydroxyapatite crystals of bone and block bone resorption. When this bone is resorbed by osteoclasts, the bisphosphonate poisons them and leads to inhibition of resorption.

Several bisphosphonates are available for treatment of hypercalcaemia (Table 3), all given initially by intravenous infusion. It is important not to give bisphosphonates until adequate rehydration has been achieved since there is a risk of renal damage in volume depleted patients.

Table 3 Bisphosphonates available in the UK for the management of hypercalcaemia.

Bisphosphonate	Dosing schedule
Disodium pamidronate	15–60 mg as single infusion no faster than 1 mg/min
Sodium clodronate	Single slow infusion 1.5 g Can be given orally 800 mg bd for maintenance
Zoledronic acid	4 mg in 100 ml saline given over 15 min
Ibandronic acid	2–4 mg in single infusion

Bisphosphonates are most effective in patients in whom there is increased bone resorption, perhaps as a result of malignant disease, but they are often used with other causes of hypercalcaemia. Successful treatment with bisphosphonates has been reported in sarcoidosis and vitamin D intoxication.

In patients with PHP, bisphosphonates lead to transient calcium level reduction which may be helpful in those with severe disease waiting for surgery. Unfortunately, this fall in plasma calcium is not sustained and the previous level is rapidly resumed. However, these agents continue to suppress bone resorption and may be useful in managing the osteoporosis sometimes seen as a consequence of PHP.

Glucocorticoids

If hypercalcaemia does not respond to bisphosphonates, glucocorticoid treatment may be beneficial. This is most useful in inhibiting hypercalcaemia associated with increased calcium absorption but it also suppresses hypercalcaemia in many cases of malignant disease. In general, fairly high doses of steroids are necessary (eg prednisolone 40 mg daily).

Direct reduction of plasma calcium

If the measures described above fail to reduce calcium levels, it may be possible to achieve a short-term benefit by direct reduction of plasma calcium. This can be achieved by chelating agents such as EDTA and phosphate or by dialysis against a low calcium dialysate. With the possible exception of dialysis, none of these offers a long-term solution and both EDTA and phosphate are potentially toxic. At best, these can be seen only as first-aid measures that might be useful whilst the underlying cause of hypercalcaemia is sought and definitive treatment instituted.

□ CONCLUSIONS

Hypercalcaemia is a common metabolic disorder. An understanding of its causes and mechanisms allows a systematic approach to investigation and treatment.

REFERENCES

1 Fisken RA, Heath DA, Bold AM. Hypercalcaemia – a hospital survey. *Q J Med* 1980;**49**:405–18.

2 Marx SJ, Attie MF, Levine MA, Spiegel AM *et al.* The hypocalciuric or benign variant of familial hypercalcemia: clinical and biochemical features in fifteen kindreds. *Medicine (Baltimore)* 1981;**60**:397–412.

3 Nordin BE. Diagnostic procedures. In: Nordin BE (ed). *Calcium, Phosphate and Magnesium Metabolism.* Edinburgh: Churchill Livingstone, 1976:469–524.

4 Davies M, Fraser WD, Hosking DJ. The management of primary hyperparathyroidism. Review. *Clin Endocrinol (Oxf)* 2002;**57**:145–55.

5 Bilezikian JP, Potts JT Jr, Fuleihan Gel-H, Kleerekoper M *et al.* Summary statement from a workshop on asymptomatic primary hyperparathyroidism: a perspective for the 21st century. Review. *J Clin Endocrinol Metab* 2002;**87**:5353–61.

☐ ENDOCRINOLOGY SELF ASSESSMENT QUESTIONS

What to do with thyroid nodules and goitres

1 The following statements apply to goitre:
 (a) A goitre can be present if it is not visible
 (b) A goitre is usually associated with biochemical dysfunction
 (c) It is present in 25% of women aged over 65 years
 (d) It requires investigation in all cases
 (e) Ultrasound investigation is rarely required

2 In the management of thyroid nodules:
 (a) Serum thyroglobulin should be measured at presentation if malignancy is suspected clinically
 (b) Fine-needle aspiration (FNA) biopsy should be performed in most cases
 (c) Approximately 5% will be malignant on cytology
 (d) The presence of follicular cells requires total thyroidectomy in most cases
 (e) Tenderness increases the suspicion of malignancy

3 Thyroid incidentalomas:
 (a) Require FNA biopsy in all nodules larger than 1.5 cm
 (b) Are effectively treated by thyroxine therapy
 (c) May be present in one-third of middle-aged women
 (d) The absence of punctate calcification excludes malignancy
 (e) Require thyroid lobectomy to obtain histology if FNA biopsy inadequate

New management strategies for osteoporosis

1 Bisphosphonate therapy:
 (a) May be given as a daily tablet before breakfast
 (b) May be given as a weekly tablet with breakfast
 (c) Prevents fractures of the spine and hip
 (d) Reduces the risk of breast cancer

2 Hormone replacement therapy (HRT):
 (a) Decreases the risk of hip fractures
 (b) Increases the risk of colon cancer
 (c) Decreases the risk of cardiovascular disease
 (d) Decreases the risk of stroke

3 Raloxifene:
 (a) Works by binding to the oestrogen receptor
 (b) Decreases the risk of spine and hip fracture
 (c) Decreases the risk of oestrogen-receptor negative breast cancer
 (d) Can increase the risk of hot flushes, leg cramps and venous thrombo-embolism

How to manage hypercalcaemia

1 Hypercalcaemia may be due to:
(a) Multiple myeloma
(b) Secondary hyperparathyroidism
(c) EDTA infusion
(d) Lithium therapy
(e) Carcinoid syndrome

2 Renal excretion of calcium is increased by:
(a) Sodium depletion
(b) Loop diuretics
(c) Parathyroid hormone (PTH)
(d) Phosphate infusion
(e) Bisphosphonate infusion

(3) A 58-year-old woman is found on routine screening to have a plasma calcium of 2.8 mmol/l, creatinine 87 μmol/l and a PTH 42 pg/ml (normal range 10–60 pg/mol):
(a) The diagnosis is unlikely to be primary hyperparathyroidism
(b) Detectable PTH excludes a diagnosis of malignancy
(c) She requires urgent rehydration
(d) She should have renal ultrasound examination
(e) Family history is unlikely to be helpful

4 A 46-year-old woman with known disseminated breast cancer presents with worsening symptoms of tiredness and polyuria for two weeks. Her plasma calcium is 3.87 mmol/l:
(a) She requires urgent treatment with bisphosphonates
(b) Corticosteroids are likely to help the hypercalcaemia
(c) She should have dietary calcium restriction
(d) Renal ultrasound examination is important in deciding therapy
(e) In the absence of bone disease or renal stones no treatment for the hypercalcaemia is indicated

Neurology

Should transient ischaemic attack and minor stroke be managed as a medical emergency?

Peter Rothwell

☐ INTRODUCTION

There are about 125,000 strokes each year in the UK; 25% of people who live to 85 years old will have a stroke. Stroke is second only to coronary heart disease as a cause of death worldwide, but only 10–20% are fatal. In the UK alone, there are 250,000 disabled stroke survivors. Stroke is also a common cause of dementia, depression and epilepsy. It accounts for 6% of total NHS expenditure in the UK. Without more effective prevention, both the cost and burden of stroke will increase because of the ageing population.

About 30% of patients with a disabling ischaemic stroke have a preceding transient ischaemic attack (TIA) or minor ischaemic stroke. These 'warning' events provide an opportunity to reduce the risk of stroke and guidelines highlight the need for rapid-access TIA clinics.[1,2] Although much work has been done on the causes and dangers of delayed assessment of patients with acute major stroke, until recently there were few studies in patients with TIA or minor stroke. It has therefore been uncertain how urgently patients must be seen in order for such clinics to be effective. North American guidelines suggest that assessment and investigation should be completed within one week of the TIA,[1] while UK guidelines recommend assessment within 2–4 weeks,[2] but there is great variation in routine practice.

☐ WHAT IS THE EARLY RISK OF STROKE?

The danger of delaying investigation and treatment after a TIA depends on the early risk of stroke. Risks of about 1–2% and 2–4% at seven and 30 days, respectively, are usually quoted; similarly low risks can be derived from cohort studies and clinical trials in patients with TIA.[3] These risks are likely to be underestimates because in these studies patients were not recruited immediately after the TIA (median delay from last event to study entry 12–47 days).[3] Any patients who had a major stroke during this period were excluded.

A study of patients presenting to an emergency department, almost all of whom were enrolled within 24 hours of the TIA, reported a stroke risk of 5.3% at two days.[4] However, this population was somewhat selected.

The Oxford Community Stroke Project

Data from the Oxford Community Stroke Project (OCSP), an unselected population-based study in the 1980s, were recently used to estimate the very early stroke risk after a TIA and to investigate the potential effects of delay before specialist assessment.[5] The stroke risk from the date the patient was assessed in clinic was 1.9% (95% confidence interval (CI) 0.1–3.8) and 4.4% (95% CI 1.6–7.2) at seven and 30 days, respectively. The median delay to assessment was six days. The equivalent risks from the date of onset of first-ever TIA were 8.6% (95% CI 4.8–12.4) and 12.0% (95% CI 7.6–16.4), respectively. The conclusion was that the true early risk of stroke from date of first-ever TIA is likely to be higher than commonly quoted.

Oxford Vascular Study

In 2003, a population-based prospective cohort study, the Oxford Vascular Study, estimated the very early stroke risk after a TIA or minor stroke.[6] The recurrent stroke risks at seven days, one month and three months were 8.0% (95% CI 2.3–13.7), 11.5% (95% CI 4.8–18.2) and 17.3% (95% CI 9.3–25.3), respectively, after a TIA, and 11.5% (95% CI 4.8–11.2), 15.0% (95% CI 7.5–22.5) and 18.5% (95% CI 10.3–26.7), respectively, after a minor stroke (Fig 1).

□ DOES THE VASCULAR TERRITORY MATTER?

It seems clear that the risk of stroke after a TIA or minor ischaemic stroke is much higher than previously supposed, but not all TIAs and minor strokes have the same long-term prognosis and there may also be differences in the early risk. For example, amaurosis fugax and retinal infarction are consistently associated with a lower risk of subsequent stroke than carotid territory cerebral TIAs.[7] Such differences in

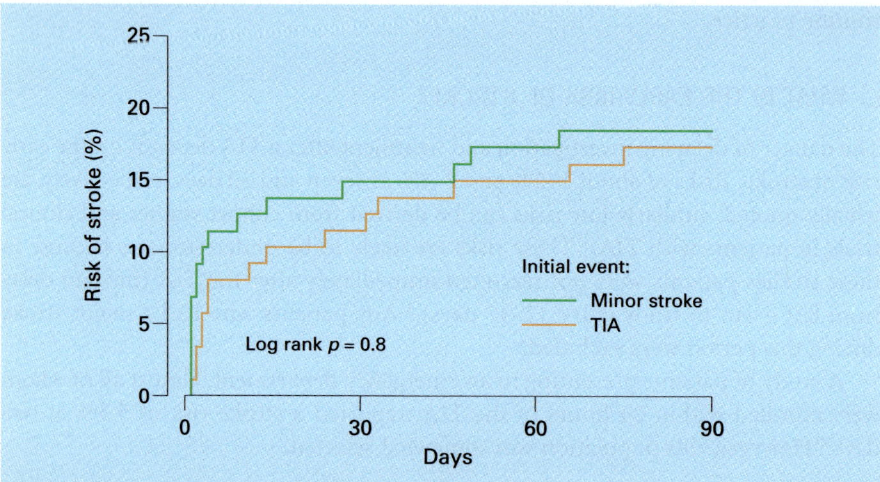

Fig 1 Cumulative risk of stroke following a transient ischaemic attack (TIA) or minor stroke in the Oxford Vascular Study.[6]

prognosis may influence treatment decisions and it is important that they are determined reliably. There were no early strokes in patients presenting with ocular TIAs in the OCSP analysis of the early risk of stroke after a TIA, thus confirming the relatively benign prognosis.[3]

Vertebrobasilar territory events

Vertebrobasilar (VB) territory events, which account for about 30% of all TIAs and minor strokes, are also thought to have a good prognosis. However, in contrast to carotid events, for which research has been stimulated by the development of carotid endarterectomy (CEA), there has been relatively little systematic research into the prognosis and risk factors for recurrent vascular events, specifically in patients with VB territory TIAs and minor strokes. Despite this, there is a widely held view that VB territory events have a more benign prognosis than carotid territory events. This stems from the results of a small number of early cohort studies in the 1960s and 1970s, many of which do not satisfy modern methodological standards. Partly as a consequence of these early studies, patients with VB events are often investigated less rigorously than patients with carotid events and may not always receive as aggressive preventive treatment against future vascular events.

Prognosis of vertebrobasilar events

The prognosis of VB events was determined in a recent systematic review of 37 published cohort studies reporting the risk of stroke after a TIA or minor stroke by territory of presenting event.[8] Individual patient data from five unpublished studies were also included. Studies that included the acute phase (up to 7 days) after the presenting event found a higher relative risk of subsequent stroke in patients with VB events than with carotid events (odds ratio (OR) 1.47, 95% CI 1.1–2.0, $p = 0.014$). Conversely, studies mainly recruiting after the acute phase found a lower relative risk (OR 0.74, 95% CI 0.7–0.8, $p = 0.00001$). In population-based studies, patients with VB events also had a higher risk of stroke (OR 1.48, 95% CI 1.1–2.0, $p = 0.025$).

Thus, there is no evidence that patients with VB events have a lower risk of subsequent stroke or death than patients presenting with carotid TIA or minor stroke. Indeed, their risk of stroke is probably higher in the acute phase, although more research is required to confirm this.

☐ WHICH AETIOLOGICAL SUBTYPES ARE AT HIGHEST RISK OF STROKE?

The early risk of stroke after a TIA or minor stroke may also differ between aetiological subtypes. Knowledge of any such differences would be important in order to organise stroke prevention effectively. However, there are few population-based data on the early risk of recurrent stroke by aetiological subtypes. Furthermore, for those studies that do exist, the numbers of early recurrent strokes are too small for reliable comparison of subtypes or to determine the risk of recurrence within seven days.

In a recent meta-analysis of data on the early risk of recurrent stroke by aetiological subtype, data from four population-based stroke incidence studies were pooled. There were 1,709 strokes, with 30, 72 and 113 recurrences at seven days, 30 days and three months, respectively.[9] Recurrent stroke risk varied significantly between subtypes ($p < 0.001$). Patients with stroke due to large artery atherosclerosis (LAA) (mainly symptomatic carotid bifurcation stenosis) had the highest odds of recurrence at seven days (OR 3.3, 95% CI 1.5–7.0), 30 days (OR 2.9, 95% CI 1.7–4.9) and three months (OR 2.9, 95% CI 1.9–4.5), respectively. Odds of recurrence at 30 days for other subtypes were:

- cardioembolic (CE): (OR 1.0, 95% CI 0.6–1.7)
- undetermined: (OR 1.0, 95% CI 0.6–1.6)
- small vessel (lacunar) stroke (SVS): (OR 0.2, 95% CI 0.1–0.6).

The early risk of recurrence was eight times higher in patients with LAA aetiology than in those with SVS and three times higher than CE stroke (Table 1, Fig 2). Although only 14% of strokes were associated with LAA, this subtype accounted for 37% of recurrences within seven days. These data highlight the importance of urgent carotid imaging.

Table 1 Actuarial risks of recurrent stroke according to aetiological subtype of transient ischaemic attack or minor stroke.

	7 days		**1 month**		**3 months**	
	Risk (%)	95% CI	Risk (%)	95% CI	Risk (%)	95% CI
SVS	0		2.0	0–4.2	3.4	0.5–6.3
CE	2.5	0.1–4.9	4.6	1.3–7.9	11.9	6.4–17.4
UND	2.3	0.5–4.1	6.5	3.4–9.6	9.3	5.6–13.0
LAA	4.0	0.2–7.8	12.6	5.9–19.3	19.2	11.2–27.2

CE = cardioembolic; CI = confidence interval; LAA = large artery atherosclerotic; SVS = small vessel (lacunar) stroke; UND = undetermined.

IS THERE ANY EVIDENCE THAT EARLY TREATMENT IS MORE EFFECTIVE?

In order to justify calling TIA and minor stroke 'medical emergencies', it needs to be shown that urgent treatment could prevent some of the early recurrent strokes, or at least that there is a reasonable potential that future research will identify effective preventive treatments. It is likely that antiplatelet therapy will reduce the early risk and trials of combination therapy are ongoing. There is no evidence that the benefits of heparin would outweigh the risks, although there have been no large trials in patients with TIA and minor stroke. Further trials are required of blood pressure lowering in the acute phase, and there is a potential for trials of neuroprotective agents to take advantage of the opportunity to 'pretreat' patients prior to any recurrent stroke.

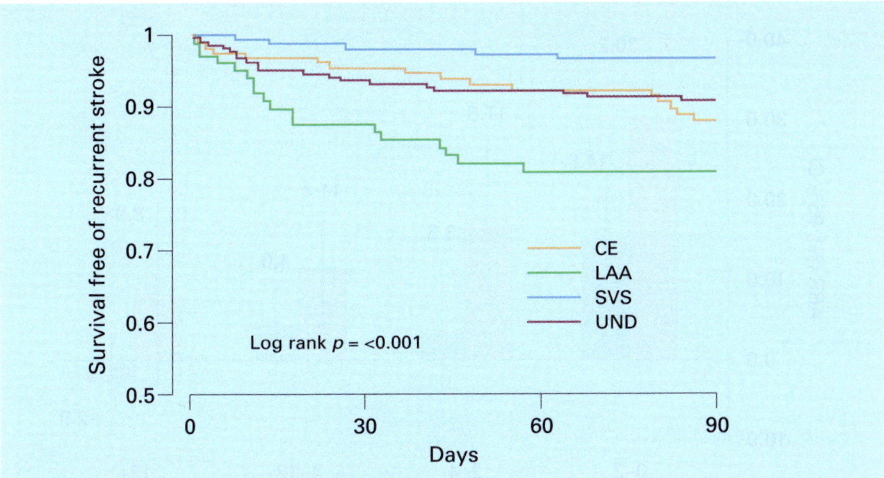

Fig 2 Cumulative survival free of recurrent stroke by aetiological subtype of the presenting stroke in a pooled analysis of data from the Oxford Vascular Study and the Oxfordshire Community Stroke Project (CE = cardioembolic; LAA = large artery atherosclerotic; SVS = small vessel stroke; UND = undetermined).[9] The corresponding actuarial risks of recurrent stroke with 95% confidence intervals in each subtype are shown in Table 1.

Surgery

Of particular importance is the observation that the subgroup of patients with carotid stenosis account for the highest proportion of early recurrent strokes.[9] CEA reduces the risk of stroke in patients who have had recent symptomatic stenosis. A recent meta-analysis of individual patient data from 5,893 patients with 33,000 patient-years of follow-up in randomised controlled trials showed that surgery was harmful in patients with less than 30% stenosis, of no benefit in patients with 30–49% stenosis, of some benefit for 50–69% symptomatic stenosis and highly beneficial for patients with 70% or more stenosis without near-occlusion.[10]

Timing of surgery

The urgency with which CEA should be performed has been much debated. In early studies the operative risk was increased if surgery was performed as an emergency, particularly in patients with major cerebral infarction. The risk of stroke on medical treatment falls rapidly over the subsequent months, possibly because of 'healing' of the unstable atheromatous plaque or an increase in collateral blood flow to the symptomatic hemisphere. Clinical guidelines simply state that patients should be operated within six months of their presenting event.

A further analysis of data from the relevant randomised trials showed that benefit from surgery depended highly on the time from the last symptomatic event to randomisation (Fig 3).[11] Benefit from surgery was greatest in patients randomised within two weeks of their last ischaemic event, falling rapidly with increasing delay. For patients with 50% or more stenosis, the number of patients needed to undergo

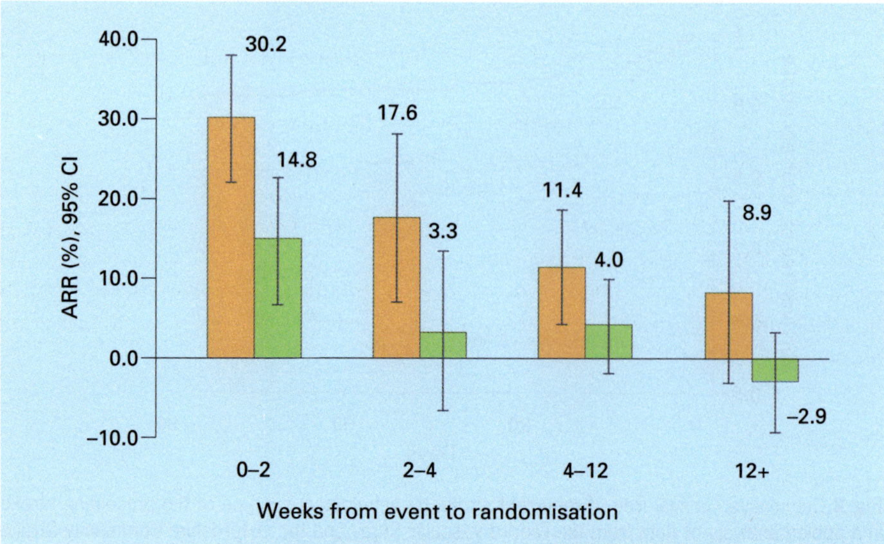

Fig 3 The absolute risk reduction (ARR) with surgery in the five-year risk of stroke and operative death in patients with 50–69% stenosis (yellow) and 70% or more stenosis without near-occlusion (blue), stratified by time from last symptomatic event to randomisation in endarterectomy trials for recently symptomatic carotid stenosis (CI = confidence interval, represented by the vertical lines within each bar).[11] The numbers above the bars indicate the actual ARR.

surgery to prevent one ipsilateral stroke in five years was five for patients randomised within two weeks after their last ischaemic event versus 125 for patients randomised more than 12 weeks later. This trend was partly because the operative risk of CEA in the trials (1% risk of death, 5–6% risk of stroke) was not increased in patients operated early.

These data suggest that CEA should be performed within days of a TIA or minor ischaemic stroke. Patients randomised in trials are different from those not randomised, so it is important to determine whether early surgery is safe in routine clinical practice. A recent systematic review of the published surgical case series that reported data found that emergency CEA for patients with evolving symptoms had a much higher risk (19.2%, 95% CI 10.7–27.8) than surgery in patients with stable symptoms (OR 3.9, 95% CI 2.7–5.7, p <0.001, 13 studies), but there was no difference between early (<3–6 weeks) and late (>6 weeks) surgery for stroke in stable patients (OR 1.13, 95% CI 0.79–1.62, p = 0.62, 11 studies).[12]

Thus, for neurologically stable patients with TIA and minor stroke, benefit from CEA is greatest if performed within two weeks of the event. The same is likely to be the case for carotid angioplasty. However, the vast majority of patients who undergo endarterectomy for symptomatic stenosis in Europe and North America are currently operated more than two weeks after their presenting event, many more than 12 weeks after the event when benefit is considerably reduced in patients with at least 70% stenosis and absent in those with 50–69% stenosis (Fig 3).

□ CONCLUSIONS

The studies outlined above show that the early risk of stroke after a TIA or minor stroke is high and that there is a short time window for prevention of stroke. Only if medical services are set up to assess and investigate patients urgently can prevention be most effective. Ideally, patients should be seen on the day they present to medical attention. Whether anything would be gained by changing the name of TIA to 'acute brain syndrome', 'impending stroke syndrome' or 'emergency prestroke syndrome' – all of which have been suggested – is uncertain. What is needed is more research, particularly randomised trials of preventive treatment, to demonstrate the benefits of urgent intervention. Public education is also needed to persuade people to present immediately to medical attention.

REFERENCES

1. The Intercollegiate Working Party for Stroke. *National Clinical Guidelines for Stroke.* London: Royal College of Physicians of London, 2002.
2. Wolf PA, Clagett GP, Easton JD, Goldstein LB *et al.* Preventing ischemic stroke in patients with prior stroke and transient ischemic attack: a statement for healthcare professionals from the Stroke Council of the American Heart Association. *Stroke* 1999;**30**:1991–4.
3. Rothwell PM. Incidence, risk factors and prognosis of stroke and TIA: the need for high-quality, large-scale epidemiological studies and meta-analyses. Review. *Cerebrovasc Dis* 2003;**16**(Suppl 3):2–10.
4. Johnston SC, Gress DR, Browner WS, Sidney S. Short-term prognosis after emergency department diagnosis of TIA. *JAMA* 2000;**284**:2901–6.
5. Lovett JK, Dennis MS, Sandercock PA, Bamford J *et al.* Very early risk of stroke after a first transient ischemic attack. *Stroke* 2003;**34**:e138–40.
6. Coull AJ, Lovett JK, Rothwell PM; Oxford Vascular Study. Population based study of early risk of stroke after transient ischaemic attack or minor stroke: implications for public education and organisation of services. *BMJ* 2004;**328**:326–8.
7. Hankey GJ, Slattery JM, Warlow CP. The prognosis of hospital-referred transient ischaemic attacks. *J Neurol Neurosurg Psychiatry* 1991;**54**:793–802.
8. Flossman E, Rothwell PM. Prognosis of vertebrobasilar transient ischaemic attack and minor stroke. *Brain* 2003;**126**:1940–54.
9. Lovett JK, Coull AJ, Rothwell PM. Early risk of recurrence by subtype of ischemic stroke in population-based incidence studies. *Neurology* 2004;**62**:569–73.
10. Rothwell PM, Eliasziw M, Gutnikov SA, Fox AJ *et al*; Carotid Endarterectomy Trialists' Collaboration. Analysis of pooled data from the randomised controlled trials of endarterectomy for symptomatic carotid stenosis. *Lancet* 2003;**361**:107–16.
11. Rothwell PM, Eliasziw M, Gutnikov SA, Warlow CP *et al*; Carotid Endarterectomy Trialists' Collaboration. Endarterectomy for symptomatic carotid stenosis in relation to clinical subgroups and timing of surgery. *Lancet* 2004;**363**:915–24.
12. Bond R, Rerkasem K, Rothwell PM. Systematic review of the risks of carotid endarterectomy in relation to the clinical indication for and timing of surgery. Review. *Stroke* 2003;**34**:2290–301.

Epilepsy: update on new therapies

John Duncan

□ INTRODUCTION

This overview of epilepsy will consider the following topics:

- □ The extent of the problem of epilepsy in the UK.
- □ The currently available medications and treatment strategies.
- □ Forthcoming medical therapies and disease-modifying medications.
- □ Surgical treatment.
- □ Some future possibilities.

□ THE PROBLEM OF EPILEPSY IN THE UK

The lifetime prevalence of epilepsy is 5% – that is, the risk of having a seizure some time during life. There are peaks in the first decade and in later life. A demographic shift is taking place: with improved antenatal and obstetric care, the incidence of childhood epilepsy is decreasing but, as people live longer and more people survive stroke, there is an increase of epilepsy in the older age groups.

Prevalence and incidence

There are about 350,000 people with epilepsy in the UK at the present time, some 100,000 of whom are troubled with recurrent seizures despite treatment. In terms of incidence, 30,000 people develop epilepsy every year in the UK (ca 80 a day). Those diagnosed with epilepsy at specialist neurology clinics are about one-quarter of those referred with 'possible epilepsy'. A clinic would expect to see four or five people presenting with 'possible epilepsy' to diagnose one with the condition – illustrating the huge potential for misdiagnosis. Of people who start anti-epileptic medication, about two-thirds will go into remission fairly easily. For them, epilepsy will be an episode in their life, not a lifelong problem.[1]

Mortality

Of the 30,000 people who develop epilepsy each year, about 5,000 will die in the first year, mainly from the cause of the epilepsy: stroke, trauma, encephalitis, head injury, tumour and so on. In the UK, about 1,000 of those who do not die of the aetiology and continue with seizures will die each year as a direct result of a seizure.

About half (ca 500 deaths a year) are the direct consequence of seizures, for example, falling in the road and being run over, drowning or vomiting and aspirating. The other 500 deaths are what are called 'sudden unexpected deaths', where presumably the individual has a seizure, witnessed or unwitnessed, and, secondary to that, has either respiratory depression or asystole and succumbs.[2]

□ CURRENT MEDICATIONS

In the mid-1850s, Edward Sieveking observed that there was hardly a substance in the world capable of passing through the gullet of man that has not at one time or other enjoyed the reputation of being an anti-epileptic. That was the starting position about 150 years ago.

Conventional anti-epileptic drugs

The first drugs for epilepsy were bromide (1857), phenobarbitone (1912), phenytoin (1938), primidone and ethosuximide. These were followed by the more recent development of the newer anti-epileptic drugs.

Recent developments

What has happened more recently? Two drugs that might have been helpful, but turned out not to be, were progabide, marketed in France, and vigabatrin. Vigabatrin was really the first of the new rational anti-epileptic drugs; it was potentially a promising medication with good efficacy and often good tolerability. Unfortunately, however, in the late 1990s it became apparent that as many as 40% of people who take vigabatrin long term develop retinal toxicity, manifest as a peripheral visual field constriction that is largely permanent. As a result, although vigabatrin is still licensed, it is used nowadays only for infantile spasms or as a drug of last resort for adults.

In the early 1990s, oxcarbazepine, a derivative of carbamazepine, was developed and zonisamide and lamotrigine came on stream. In early 1998, felbamate, gabapentin and piracetam became available. When felbamate was marketed it became evident that about one person in 5,000 would have fatal liver failure and aplastic anaemia so, although still obtainable, it is again only a drug of last resort. Tiagabine, topiramate and levetiracetam were developed later. These are the ten drugs that have become of use over the last decade.

□ TREATMENT STRATEGIES

Seizure freedom

What are we trying to do in treating epilepsy? Complete seizure freedom is what matters to individuals who have seizures because then they can drive and life can return to more or less normality. Although a 50% seizure reduction is commonly used as an end-point in therapeutic trials, this really is of no benefit to the patient. If the patient has one seizure a month rather than two, little benefit is conferred.

Absence of adverse effects

Medication for epilepsy will be long-term therapy, usually for years, so a lack of adverse effects is important. The long-term effects of these medications are of concern. Although cognitive effects may not be severe, they can be debilitating for someone trying to work and think for their living. Increasingly, both in the press and in terms of public awareness, the issue of teratogenicity is key. The experience with valproate, with which teratogenicity has been appreciated only 20 years after the drug became available, is an important message.

Lifestyle

It is important that the treatment is not obtrusive, so there should be once or twice a day dosing, drug interactions should be avoided and maintenance of a normal lifestyle possible.

Reduction of mortality and morbidity

Treatment should also reduce the morbidity and mortality. Reduction of mortality from epilepsy stems from complete seizure freedom: most of the mortality in people with established epilepsy is a direct consequence of a seizure (see above).

Guidelines

The Scottish Intercollegiate Guidelines Network 70, revised in 2003 (updated June 2004),[3] give guidelines on how epilepsy should be treated with the currently available medication. The National Institute for Clinical Excellence (NICE) has recently produced the Health Technology Assessment of the newer versus the older anti-epileptic drugs.[4] For NICE, 'newer' means anything available in about the last 12 years, so 'new' is up to 12 years old. The NICE epilepsy guidelines are currently going through the drafting stage and should be published in September 2004.

The criticism that may be made of all these guidelines is that they underestimate the heterogeneity of the epilepsies. Epilepsy is as heterogeneous as cancer or anaemia in aetiology and manifestation. The guidelines underestimate the heterogeneity of seizure types, epilepsy syndromes, aetiologies, comorbidity, lifestyle and impact of adverse effects. Nevertheless, they end up with a sensible list of first- and second-line therapies that can at least guide physicians in primary and secondary care.

Results of therapy

How helpful are the therapies? Of people with epilepsy presenting with their first seizures and prescribed their first first-line drug, 47% will go into remission with the first drug prescribed; 32% of those for whom seizures continue despite that first drug will go into remission with a second drug. As is intuitively obvious, if the first anti-epileptic drug is pushed up to a full dose, the second drug is effective in perhaps only about 11%; if, on the other hand, the first drug is not tolerated, perhaps because of an allergic reaction, dizziness or some other problem, the second drug has a much better chance of being helpful (55%). If full doses of two drugs have been tried, the chances of a third medication stopping seizures is 9%. After that, there is a law of diminishing returns: for people who have had three drugs at full doses, the chances of going into remission subsequently with a further agent is less than 5%. The prognosis of the epilepsy is determined early in the course of treatment.[5]

□ CURRENT TREATMENT

First-line drugs

At the present time, carbamazepine, lamotrigine and oxcarbazepine would be the commonly used first-line medications for somebody presenting with partial or secondary generalised seizures. Valproate is added to this list for those with generalised tonic-clonic seizures. The absence of valproate from the list for partial seizures reflects the increasing concerns about the teratogenic potential of sodium valproate, such that nowadays valproate would probably not be prescribed to women of childbearing potential if there was a reasonable alternative. For myoclonic seizures, valproate and clonazepam are the most effective and, for absences, valproate, lamotrigine and ethosuximide.

Second-line drugs

The order of preference for the second- and third-line drugs changes from month to month. Levetiracetam and topiramate, two of the recently available drugs, appear to show more efficacy – on the whole – than the other agents. For somebody with troublesome epilepsy despite trying three of the first-line drugs, those two will be fairly high up the list of the next drugs to try. In contrast, it is probably fair to say that there would be fewer expectations of benefit with gabapentin, tiagabine and acetazolamide. Phenytoin, phenobarbitone and vigabatrin are now relegated to being drugs of last resort, not because they lack efficacy but because of their increased side effects.

The impact on chronic epilepsy of the newer drugs is slightly disappointing. At best, 10-20% of people with seizures that have continued despite the regular therapies become seizure-free with levetiracetam and topiramate – two of the most potent of the newer medicines.

Head-to-head comparisons in patients with newly diagnosed epilepsies show no difference in terms of efficacy between the newer drugs and the conventional drugs; for example, lamotrigine versus carbamazepine shows no real difference in efficacy. However, the newer drugs are better tolerated on the whole and have fewer side effects; thus, a retention-on-therapy analysis shows that people are more likely to stay on the newer drugs than the older ones.

None of the current medicines has any effect on the prognosis of epilepsy: the medication is simply seizure-suppressant and does nothing to the underlying condition, the underlying tendency to have seizures.

☐ FUTURE THERAPIES

There is a need for new medicines to improve both the prognosis of those with chronic epilepsy – the 100,000 people in the country who continue to have recurrent seizures – and first-line therapy in terms of efficacy, safety, pharmacokinetics and cost-effectiveness.

Pregabalin

Of the newer medicines that are coming, pregabalin (Lyrica) will be marketed by Pfizer in the summer of 2004. It is derived from gabapentin and binds to the δ2 subunit of the calcium channel. It looks fairly potent in partial seizures: clinical trials in people with refractory epilepsy show a 49% seizure reduction and (the more interesting figure) a seizure-free rate of 8%. Given that this medication would have been tried in people who have failed many of the 12 or 13 drugs previously available – a difficult group in whom to try a new medicine – 8% seizure-free is quite impressive. Pregabalin lacks drug interactions and is generally well tolerated. The main adverse effect, which will probably limit its long-term use, is weight gain. As many as one person in five may have a 10 kg weight gain over some months, which is significant. The prime marketing goal is likely to be neuropathic pain, where it looks highly effective, and generalised anxiety disorder.

Zonisamide

Zonisamide is undergoing something of a renaissance. It was trialled in the 1980s, but the trials were held up in Europe and the US because of a 1% incidence of renal calculi attributed to the fact that it is a carbonic anhydrase inhibitor. It has however now been resuscitated and shows about 30% reduction in partial seizures, with 2% seizure-free. It is not a dramatic new therapy but will slightly increase the armamentarium. Its clearance is increased by enzyme inducers so it is difficult to use, and there is a concern that about 10% of patients report anorexia and cognitive slowing on zonisamide.

☐ DISEASE-MODIFYING MEDICATIONS

All medications to date have simply been seizure suppressant; nothing has been available that is proven to modify the course of the disease in terms either of preventing the process of developing epilepsy or of neuroprotection – preventing the secondary brain damage that may occur as the result of seizures.

Any insult to the brain may result in the process of epileptogenesis which gives rise to epilepsy. An insult may also give rise to neuronal damage, which itself can contribute to the development of epilepsy. However, this is not entirely straightforward: for example, if neuronal damage is prevented, this may not necessarily prevent the neuronal rewiring that continues to occur. The patient's genetic make-up is clearly a major factor in this.[6]

Primary prevention

In terms of modifying the occurrence of epilepsy, primary prevention is fundamental. As stated earlier, improved obstetric and neonatal care has led to almost a halving of childhood epilepsy in the UK over the last 10-15 years. Wearing motorcycle helmets is important in preventing epilepsy from head trauma. Globally, cysticercosis is probably one of the most common causes of refractory focal epilepsy. Simple attention to sanitation and hygiene would have a major impact there.

Secondary prevention

Nothing is proven about secondary prevention. Studies are looking at the role of interleukins, protein kinases, neurotrophic factors and ion channel modifications, but there is nothing clinically usable at the present time.

Surgical treatment

One way in which epilepsy can be modified is by surgery. It is worth considering the risks and benefits of surgical treatment compared with medical therapy in somebody with refractory epilepsy.

For refractory partial seizures – that is, seizures clearly arising from one part of the brain – which have carried on for two or three years despite two or three medications having been tried, the chance of being seizure-free with drugs is less than 5%. In addition, there is the risk of morbidity from seizures, the psychosocial handicap of recurrent seizures and the one in 100 annual mortality rate suffered by this population. In contrast, with appropriate surgical therapy, the chance of being seizure-free is about 70%.[7]

The risks of surgery are about one in 100 of long-lasting neurological impairment, at worst a hemiparesis or aphasia, and one in 20 of a quadrantanopia with a temporal lobe resection that may prevent driving.

The way to balance up these risks when advising patients is to explain that for somebody with refractory epilepsy the risks of surgery are equivalent to living with the epilepsy for a year – and, of course, the chances of a good result are much better with surgery.

The most common surgical target is hippocampal sclerosis; this may be demonstrated on coronal magnetic resonance imaging (MRI) (Fig 1).This is a key reason for insisting that patients with refractory epilepsy have good quality MRI to identify whether it is surgically curable. Following surgery, the right patients have a 70% chance of being rendered entirely seizure-free and effectively cured of their epilepsy (Fig 2).

A group of patients who have refractory partial seizures have normal MRI. This is a difficult group to evaluate. A lot of work has been done to try to develop new MR tools for identifying focal pathology in the brain that underlies seizures not evident on conventional imaging. For example, in somebody with right frontal lobe epilepsy with normal conventional imaging, the tools of diffusion tensor imaging, magnetisation transfer imaging and T2 mapping can all show abnormality in the

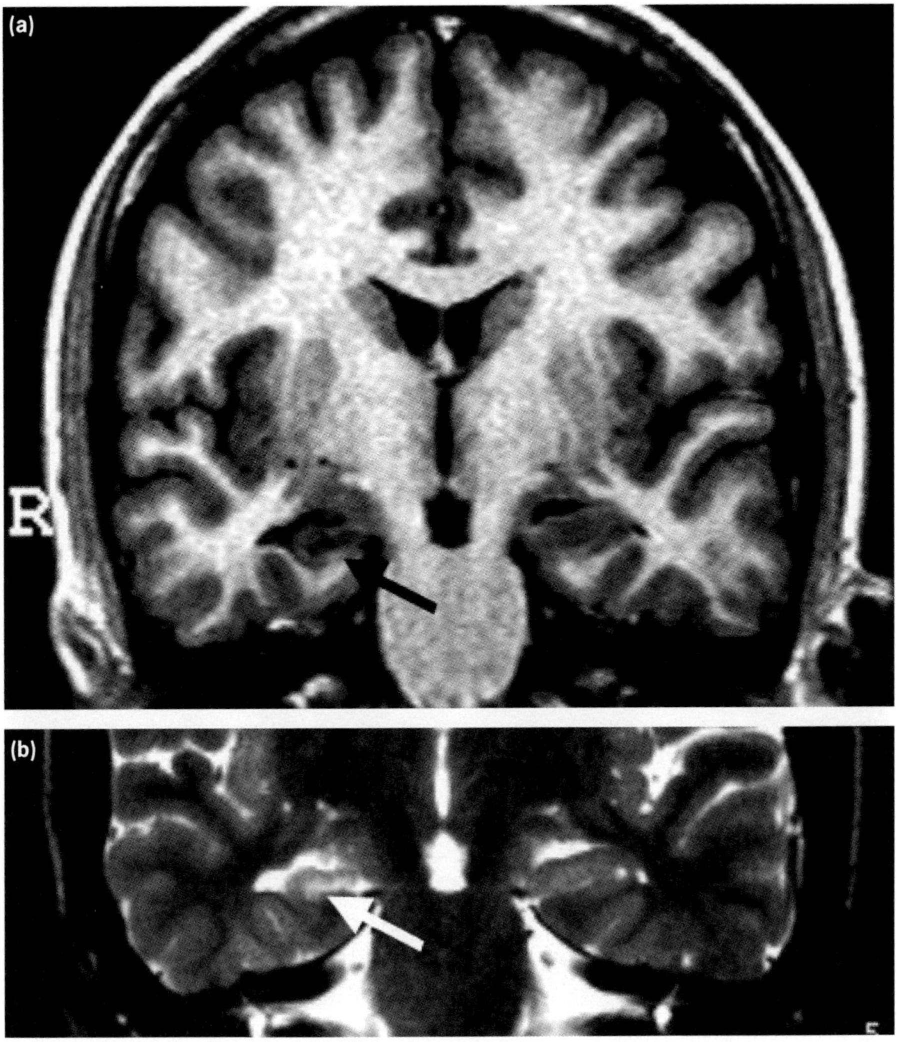

Fig 1 Coronal magnetic resonance imaging (MRI) scan showing **(a)** right hippocampal sclerosis with **(b)** reduced volume and increased signal evident on T2-weighted image.

right frontal pole. This can then be used as a target for depth electrodes to prove that is indeed the area from where the seizures are arising, potentially leading to a resection.

Vagal nerve stimulation

Vagal nerve stimulation (VNS) has been mentioned in both the lay press and the medical press over the last few years. Essentially, this is a device like a cardiac pacemaker in which the wire is wrapped around the left vagus nerve rather than going into the heart.

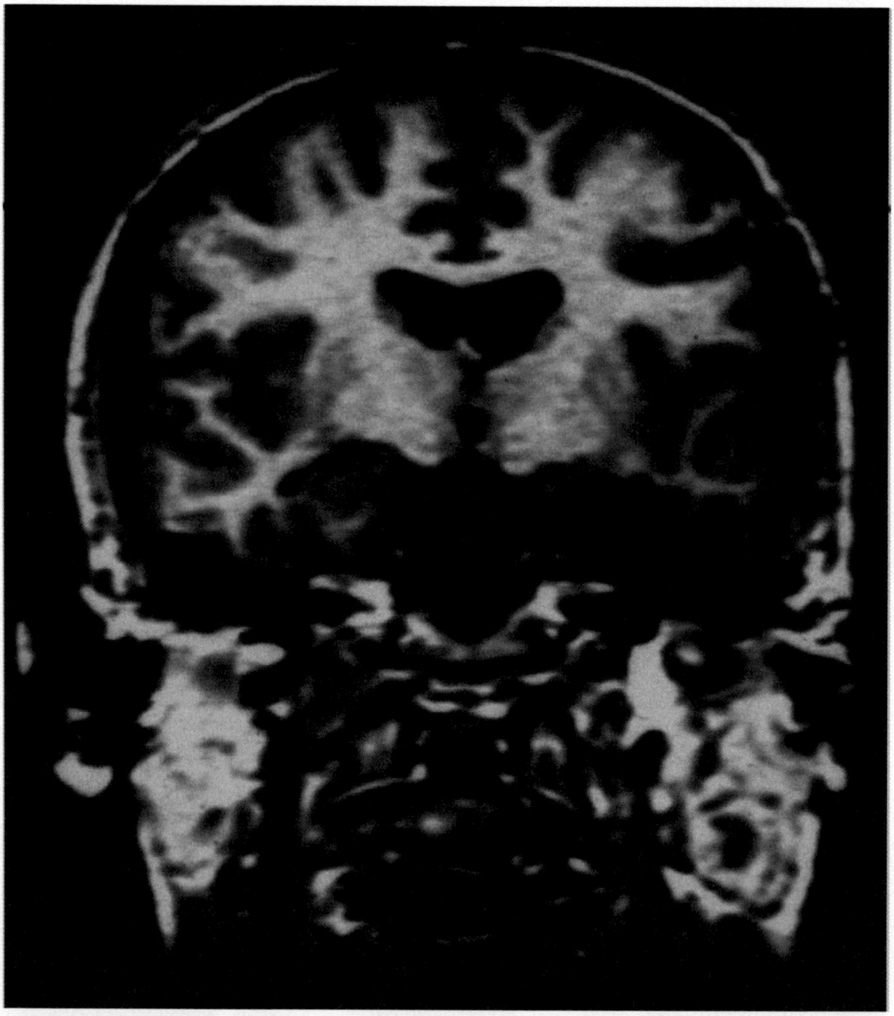

Fig 2 Coronal magnetic resonance imaging scan following left anterior temporal lobe resection.

In refractory patients, VNS has a similar efficacy to a new anti-epileptic drug. It is palliative; people do not become seizure-free with VNS and the median seizure reduction is about 30%. These comments might seem rather negative, but one positive observation is that with a vagal nerve stimulator people may be able to reduce the amount of medication they take without their seizures worsening and so become more alert and less sedated.[8]

Deep brain stimulation

Deep brain stimulation is being trialled, with stereotactic stimulation in the subthalamic nucleus. High-frequency stimulation at this site is inhibitory. It is still really in the anecdotal phase, with few reports, but 30-50% seizure reduction has been found. It is uncertain whether or not this will turn out to be useful for refractory epilepsy in the same way that deep brain stimulation may be useful for some refractory movement disorders, but trials are in progress and this should become clear in about the next five years.[8]

□ FUTURE TREATMENT POSSIBILITIES

One of the key aspects of epilepsy that perhaps marks it out from any other condition is that people are well most of the time, then abruptly have a seizure. They do not know when it will happen. What bothers patients most often is the unpredictability of their seizures. If it were possible to predict when seizures would occur, life would be much easier and might also lead to the possibility of giving treatment to prevent development of the seizures.

Interesting work is ongoing with non-linear analysis of EEG patterns, both intracranial recordings and scalp recordings, which some optimists think may allow identification of patterns in some people that could predict seizures 10–15 minutes ahead of time. Clearly, it would be helpful for patients to know this was going to happen so that they could get to a place of safety, get off their bicycle or whatever. If this could be combined with the local application of a drug or local neural stimulation, it would have the potential for a reactive anticipatory system that would prevent seizures occurring. It would also avoid exposing those patients to chronic medication that may have adverse side effects and which they are taking all the time, whereas in fact they need medication perhaps only once every few months.

□ CONCLUSIONS

In conclusion, epilepsy is a common problem. This review has considered the currently available medications, current treatment strategies, forthcoming therapies, disease-modifying medications and surgical treatment. It should be stressed that one of the main difficulties with surgical treatment is the delay in appropriate referral. In our centre at the moment the median time for which people have had epilepsy when they come for surgery is 18 years. About 10 years ago it was 21 years, so the delay has been slightly reduced. The problem is that there are many thousands of people with refractory epilepsy who have low expectations, as perhaps the treating physicians also have, and they are not referred for potential curative treatment.

REFERENCES

1 Sander JW. The epidemiology of epilepsy revisited. Review. *Curr Opin Neurol* 2003;**16**:165–70.

2 Gaitatzis A, Sander JW. The mortality of epilepsy revisited. Review. *Epileptic Disord* 2004; **6**:3–13.

3 Scottish Intercollegiate Guideline Network. *Epilepsy guidelines.* SIGN guidelines no. 70, 2003; updated June 2004.

4 National Institute for Clinical Excellence. *Epilepsy guidelines,* 2004. www.nice.org.uk

5 Kwan P, Brodie MJ. Early identification of refractory epilepsy. *N Engl J Med* 2000;**342**:314–9.

6 Duncan JS. The promise of new antiepileptic drugs. Review. *Br J Clin Pharmacol* 2002; **53**:123–31.

7 Wiebe S, Blume WT, Girvin JP, Eliasziw M; Effectiveness and Efficiency of Surgery for Temporal Lobe Epilepsy Study Group. A randomized, controlled trial of surgery for temporal-lobe epilepsy. *N Engl J Med* 2001;**345**:311–8.

8 Theodore WH, Fisher RS. Brain stimulation for epilepsy. Review. *Lancet Neurol* 2004;**3**:111–8.

Diagnosis and management of motor neurone disease

Karen Morrison

□ INTRODUCTION

Motor neurone disease (MND) is the most common disorder of motor nerves of adults, with a prevalence of 4–6 per 100,000. Approximately three people die each day from MND in the UK, and each general practitioner (GP) will, on average, care for one person with MND during a lifetime of practice.

MND is a disorder steeped in negative publicity, feared by the public and a condition that physicians are reluctant to diagnose. On giving the diagnosis, the doctor is frequently confronted by the response 'Isn't that the disease suffered by Diane Pretty?',[1] and 'Isn't that the disease that raises the issue of assisted suicide?'. Unfortunately, there is still no cure for MND or any treatment that greatly affects prognosis, but much progress has been made in the last 10 years towards understanding the mechanism of motor nerve degeneration in the disease, particularly in its familial forms.

□ TYPES OF MOTOR NEURONE DISEASE

Several subtypes of MND are recognised (Table 1):[2]

1. The commonest variety, accounting for 70% of cases, is the classical or 'Charcot' *amyotrophic lateral sclerosis*, with upper and lower motor neurone features manifesting in the limb muscles. It presents with asymmetrical weakness, wasting, fasciculation and cramping.

2. About 20% of all MND patients present with *bulbar involvement*, with symptoms of dysarthria and/or dysphagia.

Table 1 Clinical subtypes of motor neurone disease.

Clinical subtype	Main features
'Classical' amyotrophic lateral sclerosis	Combined LMN and UMN limb involvement
Progressive bulbar palsy	Dysarthria with or without dysphagia
Primary lateral sclerosis	UMN features in limb and bulbar muscles
Progressive muscular atrophy	LMN involvement of the limbs

LMN = lower motor neurone; UMN = upper motor neurone.

3 *Primary lateral sclerosis* describes a disorder of solely upper motor neurone involvement, with prominent limb stiffness and spasticity.

4 *Progressive muscular atrophy* (PMA) is the term reserved for the lower motor neurone variant. PMA nearly always begins in the limbs and spreads later to the bulbar muscles, and most cases also develop upper motor neurone features as the disease progresses.

☐ WHAT CAUSES MOTOR NEURONE DISEASE?

The causes of MND are unknown. Current hypotheses suggest that its development involves both genetic and environmental factors, with proposed pathogenic mechanisms that include oxidative stress, mitochondrial dysfunction, abnormal intracellular calcium handling, abnormalities in cytoskeletal proteins, glutamate excitotoxicity, and eventually cell death via apoptosis.[6]

☐ GENETIC FACTORS

Familial motor neurone disease and superoxide dismutase-1 mutations

Most MND occurs sporadically. Approximately one patient in ten will have a family history of the disease, most likely consistent with autosomal dominant inheritance. A huge breakthrough in MND research occurred in 1993 with the identification of mutations in the gene encoding the enzyme copper-zinc superoxide dismutase-1 (SOD-1) in some familial cases. Such mutations are found in 20% of autosomal dominant cases and occasionally in sporadic cases, and are responsible for 2–3% of MND cases overall.[7] Evidence from SOD-1 gene 'knock-out' studies in animals suggests that mutant SOD-1 in familial MND exerts its effect through a gained toxic function rather than through a decrease in the normal function of the enzyme to detoxify free radicals.

Over 100 different SOD-1 mutations have been identified in different MND kindreds. There is usually a poor correlation between a specific SOD-1 mutation and a particular phenotype, with much intrafamilial variation in age at onset and speed of disease progression. The variable penetrance of SOD-1 mutations within kindreds and the lack of effective disease-modifying therapies mean that presymptomatic SOD-1 gene screening is not generally recommended in familial MND kindreds with identified SOD-1 mutations.

Other forms of familial motor neurone disease

Various other rare forms of familial MND are recognised. Mutations in the gene encoding alsin, a guanosine triphosphatase regulator, are found in a rare, juvenile onset form in individuals of Middle Eastern descent, with prominent upper motor neurone features.[8] Many other loci have been linked to familial MND in individual pedigrees, but no other disease-causing mutations have been identified to date.

□ ENVIRONMENTAL FACTORS

Various environmental factors have been proposed to have a causative role in MND. These include:

- exposure to metals, including lead, manganese and aluminium
- exposure to solvents and agricultural chemicals
- excessive physical exercise
- dietary glutamate intake
- trauma, and
- residence in rural areas.

So far there is no good evidence to support any of these as exogenous risk factors. There are some data in support of smoking as a risk factor.

□ PRESENTATION AND PROGRESSION

Most people with MND present between the ages of 50 and 70 years, although onset as young as the late teens and in those older than 80 years is well recognised. The usual pattern is for the spread of the symptoms and signs to adjacent muscle segments. In patients who present with the bulbar form, the disease usually eventually spreads to the limbs; likewise, in those presenting with limb disease, eventual involvement of speech and swallowing muscles is the rule. Most patients with MND die from complications due to respiratory muscle involvement.

□ PROGNOSIS

Prognosis in MND remains poor, although it has improved in the last 10 years. A study of Scottish patients with MND in 1993 found average survival from diagnosis to be only 14 months, with 50% survival from symptom onset less than three years. More recent retrospective studies suggest that average survival is now 3–4 years following the introduction of features such as disease management by specialised multidisciplinary teams, intervention with enteral feeding and respiratory support, and the introduction of the disease-modifying drug riluzole. Certain subtypes of MND are associated with a better prognosis (Table 2). One study suggested that as

Table 2 Features of motor neurone disease associated with a better prognosis.

- Primary lateral sclerosis (average survival 20 years plus)
- Pure lower motor neurone forms
- Limb rather than bulbar onset
- Some familial forms (eg those with G37R, H46R, D90A SOD-1 mutations)
- Younger age at onset (familial and sporadic cases)

many as 10% of those with a diagnosis of MND will be alive 10 years after diagnosis; it is useful to mention this figure to patients and their families when giving the diagnosis as a glimmer of hope in an otherwise gloomy discussion.

☐ HOW TO DIAGNOSE MOTOR NEURONE DISEASE

Diagnosis of MND is based on clinical examination and investigation suggesting a disorder of upper and/or lower motor neurones, with progression over time and the absence of identifying any other cause for the symptoms. A useful pointer is the finding of brisk reflexes in a weak, wasted and fasciculating limb. Prominent fasciculations can occur in other disorders, such as the 'benign fasciculation syndrome' (in which they are unaccompanied by weakness), but the presence of widespread fasciculations with weakness is highly suggestive of MND. Table 3 lists some of the features **not** seen in MND to bear in mind when considering this diagnosis.

Most patients do not develop significant cognitive impairment or dementia, other than those suffering from the syndrome of 'MND-dementia', a rare disorder that is often familial with dementia as a prominent and early feature and thought to be closely related to frontotemporal dementia.

Table 3 Clinical features not seen in motor neurone disease (MND).

- Sensory symptoms and signs
- Autonomic dysfunction
- Eye movement abnormalities
- Bladder or bowel symptoms
- Marked cognitive impairment*

* Dementia is a prominent and early symptom in MND-dementia (see text).

☐ DIFFERENTIAL DIAGNOSIS

Cervical spondylotic myelopathy

Some disorders that may mimic MND are listed in Table 4. For example, cervical spondylotic myelopathy, although usually presenting with sensory and motor symptoms and signs, can present with purely motor features and cause diagnostic uncertainty. Unless an individual has prominent symptoms and signs above the neck (tongue or facial fasciculation and/or evidence of denervation of facial muscles on electromyography (EMG)), magnetic resonance imagining (MRI) of the cervical spine is recommended to exclude compressive spinal cord pathology.

Adult onset spinal muscular atrophy

It can be difficult to distinguish adult onset spinal muscular atrophy (SMA) from the PMA variant of MND. In SMA, the history is likely to have been one of gradual progression over a number of years, and a family history of the disorder (autosomal

Table 4 Differential diagnosis of motor neurone disease.

- Cervical spondylotic myelopathy
- Other cervical myelopathies
- Lumbosacral radiculopathy
- Syringomyelia
- Radiation myelopathy
- Kennedy's disease
- Adult-onset spinal muscular atrophy
- Endocrine diseases (thyrotoxicosis, hyperparathyroidism)
- Multifocal motor neuropathy
- Benign fasciculation syndrome
- Lead, mercury poisoning
- Lymphoma

dominant, recessive or X-linked) is much more likely than in MND. The genetic defect in childhood onset autosomal recessive SMA has been identified as deletions or mutations in the survival motor neurone gene, *SMN*, on chromosome 5. Cases of homozygous *SMN* deletion are occasionally found in adult onset SMA, and thus *SMN* screening may be warranted in adults presenting with purely lower motor neurone features.

X-linked spinobulbar muscular atrophy

X-linked spinobulbar muscular atrophy (Kennedy's disease) should be considered in males presenting with lower motor neurone facial and upper limb weakness. The genetic mutation here is an expansion of a CAG trinucleotide repeat within the first exon of the androgen receptor gene on the X chromosome. The importance of diagnosing SMA in the context of considering a differential diagnosis of MND is not that any specific treatment is implied but rather that a guide to prognosis can be given (much slower progression than MND), and genetic counselling may be appropriate.

Multifocal motor neuropathy

An important disorder not to be confused with MND is multifocal motor neuropathy (MMN). This disorder usually presents in middle age with asymmetrical weakness of the upper limbs out of proportion to the degree of wasting and is more common in men. The key point in the diagnosis of MMN is the electrophysiological finding of motor nerve conduction block, with a significant drop in amplitude of the compound muscle action potential recorded in a muscle when the innervating nerve is stimulated distally compared with proximally in the absence of nerve compression. It is thought that MMN arises due to autoimmune attack of peripheral motor nerves. Some 70% of cases have plasma antibodies to the ganglioside GM1, but this finding is not specific for MMN. The disorder is treatable with intravenous immunoglobulin therapy, sometimes with a dramatic response in patients who have been severely disabled. It is of interest that the disorder does not respond to either oral or intravenous steroids, which indeed may worsen the condition.

Other disorders

Occasionally, thyrotoxicosis or hyperparathyroidism can present with weakness, wasting and fasciculation, so these should be excluded.

□ ANIMAL MODELS OF MOTOR NEURONE DISEASE

There are a few spontaneously occurring animal models of MND (eg the progressive motor neuronopathy mouse and the 'wobbler' mouse) that mimic some, but not all, of the features of MND. An important benefit of finding SOD-1 mutations in some MND cases has been the development of an animal model of the disease. Mice and, more recently, rats expressing human mutant SOD-1 develop an adult-onset syndrome of progressive muscle weakness and wasting leading to early death, with neuropathological features similar to human MND. Many theories of pathogenesis of the disease have come from studies of these animals and, importantly, the animals have provided a tool for treatment screening. Unfortunately, many of the therapies beneficial in the mouse model have not proven effective in controlled clinical trials in human MND. Possible reasons for this difference include:

- not using equivalent doses in mouse and man
- species-dependent differences in central nervous system drug penetration, and
- the timing of drug delivery, which may be started too late in the human disease.[9]

□ INVESTIGATION

Investigation is aimed towards excluding alternative diagnoses and trying to confirm the diagnosis of MND. There is still no surrogate marker for the disease. All patients in whom the diagnosis is being considered ought to undergo both peripheral nerve electrophysiology to confirm the presence of a motor rather than a sensory neuropathy and EMG to confirm changes of neuronal degeneration and reinnervation. Studies should also be undertaken specifically to exclude 'conduction block' (see above).

Should serum creatine kinase be measured? The level may be high in MND (signifying very active muscle loss), normal or low (when extreme muscle atrophy has already occurred). A single serum creatine kinase estimation is thus not useful. An extremely high level would be more in keeping with a primary muscle disorder and should prompt investigation towards an alternative diagnosis.

As yet, there is no brain imaging tool that allows specific accurate diagnosis of MND. Increased signal in the corticospinal tracts is sometime seen on T2-weighted and proton density MRI, but these changes are not sufficiently sensitive to be used diagnostically.

□ MANAGEMENT

An important element in the management of MND is the initial telling of the diagnosis. The Motor Neurone Disease Association (MNDA), the main lay support organisation for people with MND and their carers in the UK, has highlighted that this aspect is often badly handled by medical professionals. The MNDA has suggested guidelines for how this should be undertaken, including the diagnosis being given by a physician experienced in MND care, in privacy with the spouse or another appropriate person present, and with written information about MND provided.

In the UK, increasing numbers of MND patients are cared for within the setting of a multidisciplinary team. This team may include a neurologist, a specialist nurse, an occupational therapist, a physiotherapist, a speech and language therapist, a dietitian, a respiratory physician and a social worker. Our clinic also has representatives from the Citizens Advice Bureau and the MNDA. A recent paper suggested that management within a team skilled in MND care has a significant effect in terms of improving not only patients' quality of life but also their survival.[3]

□ SYMPTOMATIC TREATMENTS

Some of the possible symptomatic therapies are listed in Table 5.

Tube feeding

Recent years have seen an increase in the provision of tube feeding and assisted ventilation in MND patients in the UK. There is reasonable evidence that enteral feeding, via either a percutaneous endoscopically inserted gastrostomy tube or a radiologically inserted gastrostomy, improves quality of life and survival.[2] Indications for considering such tube feeding include poor dietary intake, dehydration, falling weight, significant dysphagia and risk of aspiration.

Assisted ventilation

Assisted ventilation is usually supplied in the form of a non-invasive positive pressure system via a nasal or face mask. Symptoms suggestive of respiratory muscle compromise include shortness of breath at rest, on speaking or minimal exertion, and orthopnoea. Nocturnal hypoventilation may manifest as frequent night-time wakening, night-time sweating or the early morning presence of a throbbing headache due to carbon dioxide retention. Positive pressure ventilation is generally most successful if the patient has respiratory rather than marked bulbar weakness, as the risk of aspiration with ventilation is increased with the latter. Only a few centres in the

Table 5 Possible symptomatic therapies in motor neurone disease.

Symptom	Therapy
Cramps	quinine sulphate carbamazepine phenytoin
Spasticity	baclofen tizanidine dantrolene
Sialorrhoea	atropine eye drops (sublingually) atropine tabs hyoscine (transdermal patches or tabs) glycopyrrolate liquid home suction machine botulinum toxin injection (into salivary gland)
Thick secretions	pineapple juice carbocisteine syrup
Emotional lability	amitriptyline SSRI
Anxiety	lorazepam (sublingual or oral) diazepam suppositories
Depression	psychological support SSRI
Respiratory distress	non-invasive ventilation morphine (oral) benzodiazepines morphine/diamorphine (subcutaneous infusion) 'breathing space kit'*

*Available on request from the Motor Neurone Disease Association. Kit consists of box with suggestions for drug management of acute respiratory symptoms, obtained through prescription via the general practitioner.
SSRI = selective serotonin reuptake inhibitor.

UK offer specialist assisted ventilation services to people with MND, so in this country such ventilation is still offered to only a small proportion of those who might benefit.[4]

Tracheostomy

Invasive ventilation via tracheostomy is rarely performed for MND patients in the UK, although in some other countries, notably Japan, nearly 25% of all MND patients are so ventilated. A recent study suggests that tracheostomy ventilation increases stress in the carers and families of patients, with minimal overall improvement in the quality of life of the latter.[5] Tracheostomy ventilation should not be undertaken lightly.

Advance directives

More patients in the UK are now writing 'advance directives', indicating their preferences for treatment in the terminal stages of the disease. The number of occasions is decreasing when a patient with MND is rushed to casualty due to a chest infection and, without adequate forethought, is intubated and ventilated as an emergency.

☐ DISEASE-MODIFYING THERAPIES

Riluzole

Based on data from human cerebrospinal fluid and post-mortem studies and from the SOD-1 animal model, a number of possible therapeutic agents have been tested in MND.[10] To date, riluzole (Rilutek) is the only one shown to prolong life in MND, with an average improvement in survival of about three months if the drug is taken for 18 months.[11] The effect of riluzole in MND is thought to result from its antiglutamatergic effects, both pre- and post-synaptically. National Institute for Clinical Excellence guidelines for riluzole in the UK[12] include prescription of the drug from a specialist in MND care and shared care between the prescriber and the local GP. The drug slows progression of the disease, but patients do not notice any subjective improvements in symptoms. Despite this lack of obvious symptomatic benefit, most MND patients in the UK opt to take riluzole in the hope that other effective treatments will become available within their lifetime.

Stem cell therapy

With the advent of high-throughput drug screening strategies in animal and cell culture models, it is anticipated that many more agents will come to clinical trial within the next few years. Stem cell therapy is also being raised as a possibility in MND,[13] the concept being that motor neurone precursor cells could be delivered to the appropriate sites in the nervous system and coaxed to differentiate into functioning motor neurones with appropriate synaptic connections. Other approaches are to target stem cells already present in the adult nervous system to differentiate into new motor neurones to replace those lost in the disease or to use stem cells as sources of neuroprotective or neurotrophic factors. At present, much basic research is required before stem cell treatment trials should be performed in MND.

☐ CONCLUSIONS

Efforts in a multidisciplinary MND clinic are currently concentrated on giving an accurate diagnosis as soon as possible, and initiating a package of care and support to people with the disease and their families. Symptomatic treatments abound, but there are still no truly effective disease-modifying therapies. Animal and cell culture models have recently been developed, and for the first time high-throughput screening of compounds to treat MND is underway. Stem cell therapy may offer an effective approach in the future, but this is still some time away from being translated into clinical practice.

Much has been said in the press about the importance of recognising the 'right to die' in conditions such as MND. Those in the field of caring for people with MND are working unstintingly towards promoting the 'right to live' with dignity and quality when this dreaded disease has struck.

Useful motor neurone disease websites

1. www.mndassocation.org: the website of the Motor Neurone Disease Association, the main national lay organisation in the UK offering support and advice to people with MND and their carers.
2. www.mdausa.org: the website of the Muscular Dystrophy Association USA, with clinical and research information on various neuromuscular diseases including MND.
3. www.alsa.org: the website of the largest US national health organisation dedicated solely to MND. This is particularly useful for information on current clinical trials and reviews of research developments.

REFERENCES

1 BBC News, Health. Diane Pretty dies. news.bbc.co.uk/1/hi/health/1983457.htm 2002

2 Leigh PN, Abrahams S, Al-Chalabi A, Ampong MA *et al.* The management of motor neurone disease. Review. *J Neurol Neurosurg Psychiatry* 2003;**74**(Suppl 4):iv32–iv47.

3 Traynor BJ, Alexander M, Corr B, Frost E, Hardiman O. Effect of a multidisciplinary amyotrophic lateral sclerosis (ALS) clinic on ALS survival: a population based study, 1996–2000. *J Neurol Neurosurg Psychiatry* 2003;**74**:1258–61.

4 Bourke SC, Williams TL, Bullock RE, Gibson GJ, Shaw PJ. Non-invasive ventilation in motor neuron disease: current UK practice. *Amyotroph Lateral Scler Other Motor Neuron Disord* 2002;**3**:145–9.

5 Kaub-Wittemer D, Steinbuchel N, Wasner M, Laier-Groeneveld G, Borasio GD. Quality of life and psychosocial issues in ventilated patients with amyotrophic lateral sclerosis and their caregivers. *J Pain Symptom Manage* 2003;**26**:890–6.

6 Rowland LP, Shneider NA. Amyotrophic lateral sclerosis. Review. *N Engl J Med* 2001;**344**: 1688–700.

7 Andersen PM, Sims KB, Xin WW, Kiely R *et al.* Sixteen novel mutations in the Cu/Zn superoxide dismutase gene in amyotrophic lateral sclerosis: a decade of discoveries, defects and disputes. *Amyotroph Lateral Scler Other Motor Neuron Disord* 2003;**4**:62–73.

8 Shaw PJ. Genetic inroads in familial ALS. *Nat Genet* 2001;**29**:103–4.

9 Rothstein JD. Of mice and men: reconciling preclinical ALS mouse studies and human clinical trials. Review. *Ann Neurol* 2003;**53**:423–6.

10 Morrison KE. Therapies in amyotrophic lateral sclerosis – beyond riluzole. Review. *Curr Opin Pharmacol* 2002;**2**:302–9.

11 Miller RG, Mitchell JD, Lyon M, Moore DH. Riluzole for amyotrophic lateral sclerosis (ALS)/motor neuron disease (MND). Review. *Cochrane Database Syst Rev* 2000;**2**:CD001447.

12 National Institute for Clinical Excellence. Riluzole for motor neurone disease; full guidance. *Technology Appraisal* no.20, 2001.

13 Svendsen CN, Langston JW. Stem cells for Parkinson disease and ALS: replacement or protection? *Nat Med* 2004;**10**:224–5.

☐ NEUROLOGY SELF ASSESSMENT QUESTIONS

Should transient ischaemic attack and minor stroke be managed as a medical emergency?

1 The early risk of stroke after a transient ischaemic attack (TIA):
- (a) Is greatest in the second week
- (b) Is about 12–15% during the first 30 days
- (c) Is higher in patients with ocular TIAs than in those with cerebral TIAs
- (d) Is higher in patients with vertebrobasilar territory events than carotid territory events
- (e) Is best estimated from data collected in randomised controlled trials

2 The early risk of recurrence after a first-ever stroke:
- (a) Is greatest in patients with cardioembolic events
- (b) Is lowest in patients with lacunar events
- (c) Is confined to patients with large artery atherosclerosis
- (d) Is most effectively reduced by treatment with heparin
- (e) Is much lower than after a TIA

3 Carotid endarterectomy:
- (a) Reduces the risk of stroke in patients with 50–69% recently symptomatic carotid stenosis
- (b) Has an operative risk of stroke and death of 5–7%
- (c) Is associated with a higher operative risk if performed as an emergency in patients with acute ischaemic stroke
- (d) Should not be performed for at least two weeks after a TIA or minor ischaemic stroke
- (e) Is effective only in patients with recently symptomatic 70–99% stenosis if performed within four weeks of the event

Epilepsy: update on new therapies

1 Epilepsy in the UK:
- (a) Develops in 3,000 people every year
- (b) Affects approximately 350,000 people at the present time
- (c) Causes 1,000 deaths per year
- (d) Is the diagnosis in most patients referred to 'first seizure clinics'

2 Anti-epileptic drug (AED) treatment:
- (a) The first AED used will control seizures in 40–50% of patients
- (b) If the first AED fails, the second AED tried will control seizures in 30–35%
- (c) If the first two AEDs fail, the third AED tried will control seizures in 20%
- (d) In a population with refractory epilepsy, a new AED will give control of seizures in 20%

3 Surgical treatment of epilepsy:
(a) Gives seizure control in 90% of those selected for surgery
(b) Vagal nerve stimulation results in a mean 30% seizure reduction
(c) Resection carries a 1% risk of severe morbidity
(d) For those with refractory partial seizures, the risk of surgery is similar to the risks due to epilepsy over 10 years

Diagnosis and management of motor neurone disease

1 Features seen in more than one-third of motor neurone disease (MND) patients include:
(a) Autonomic symptoms
(b) Diplopia
(c) Brisk reflexes in a wasted limb
(d) Survival of 10 years or more
(e) Family history of the disease

2 Regarding multifocal motor neuropathy:
(a) Females are frequently affected
(b) The upper limbs are usually involved
(c) Antiganglioside GM1 antibodies are specific for the disease
(d) The disease may respond to intravenous (iv) immunoglobulin therapy
(e) The disease usually responds to iv steroid therapy

3 The following interventions prolong life in MND:
(a) Enteral feeding
(b) Non-invasive ventilation
(c) Riluzole therapy
(d) Regular exercise
(e) Management in a multidisciplinary MND clinic

Renal

Uraemia and cardiovascular risk

David Wheeler

☐ INTRODUCTION

Premature death from cardiovascular disease is well recognised in dialysis patients, but it also occurs in the much broader group of individuals with milder forms of chronic kidney disease (CKD). Although exposed to 'traditional' risk factors such as hypertension and dyslipidaemia, these CKD patients have generally been excluded from large-scale clinical trials of risk factor modification, so the benefits of accepted interventions such as lowering of serum cholesterol are unproven. In addition, uraemia is associated with a variety of functional and metabolic abnormalities, some of which may increase the risk of cardiovascular disease and be worthwhile targets for therapy. There is now a growing appreciation that 5–10% of the general population has mild CKD, and that undiagnosed kidney dysfunction may represent an important cause of cardiovascular morbidity and mortality in patients unlikely to be under the care of a nephrologist. Early detection of CKD may provide opportunities for intervention both to slow progression of kidney failure and to reduce the associated risk of cardiovascular morbidity and mortality. The key messages in this chapter are summarised in Table 1.

Table 1 Key messages about the interrelationship between cardiovascular disease (CVD) and chronic kidney disease (CKD).

- CKD is more common than widely appreciated
- A rise in serum creatinine is a late event in CKD progression
- CKD is associated with an increased risk of CVD even in the early stages
- CKD is a marker of poor prognosis in patents with established CVD
- Therapies that reduce cardiovascular risk may also slow progression of kidney disease
- Early detection of CKD may enhance opportunities for reducing cardiovascular risk

CKD = chronic kidney disease; CVD = cardiovascular disease.

☐ CLASSIFICATION OF CHRONIC KIDNEY DISEASE

The management of patients with CKD has already been greatly helped by the development of a classification system by the US Kidney Disease Outcomes Quality Initiative (K/DOQI) which is gaining international acceptance (Table 2). The K/DOQI working group has promoted use of the term 'chronic kidney disease' (as used in this chapter) in place of 'chronic renal failure'. Recognising that serum

Table 2 New classification of chronic kidney disease.

Stage	Description	GFR (ml/min)	Prevalence* (%)
1	Kidney damage	>90	3.3
2	Mildly reduced GFR	60–89	3.0
3	Moderately reduced GFR	30–59	4.3
4	Severely reduced GFR	15–29	0.2
5	Kidney failure	<15 or receiving dialysis	0.2

* Estimated prevalence in US as percentage of total population (from Ref 1).
GFR = glomerular filtration rate.

creatinine is a poor marker of kidney function, particularly in early CKD, the K/DOQI classification is based on glomerular filtration rate (GFR). GFR can be readily calculated using serum creatinine in an equation that takes into account factors such as weight, age and sex (Table 3). This new classification also includes patients with kidney damage but normal creatinine clearance, some of whom will eventually progress to require dialysis. The K/DOQI guidelines stress that specific groups of patients at high risk of developing both CKD and cardiovascular diseases (such as those with diabetes) require appropriate screening.

Whilst the K/DOQI project will help to focus attention on the problem of undiagnosed kidney disease, the prevalence has not yet been properly established. Large observational studies in the US indicate that, overall, 11% of the population have CKD according to the new K/DOQI definitions (Table 2).[1] The best available data in the UK (from the National Diet and Nutrition Survey) are broadly consistent, with an elevated serum creatinine (compatible with K/DOQI stage III-V disease) detected in 10% of a population over 65 years old. Other studies, which will also assess the impact of early referral to a nephrologist, are ongoing.

□ CARDIOVASCULAR DISEASE RISK IN ADVANCED CHRONIC KIDNEY DISEASE

The outlook for patients with CKD in developed countries has been dramatically improved over about the last 30 years, mainly due to the expansion of dialysis programmes and advances in kidney transplantation. Such patients are now unlikely

Table 3 Calculation of glomerular filtration rate by estimation of creatinine clearance from a patient's age, weight and serum creatinine.

Men	Creatinine clearance =	$\dfrac{1.23 \times (140 - \text{age}) \times \text{weight (kg)}}{\text{Serum creatinine } (\mu\text{mol/l})}$
Women	Creatinine clearance =	$\dfrac{1.04 \times (140 - \text{age}) \times \text{weight (kg)}}{\text{Serum creatinine } (\mu\text{mol/l})}$

to die as a result of uraemia when they reach 'end stage', but their life expectancy is still dramatically reduced compared with age- and sex-matched healthy controls and may be shorter than that of individuals with certain common malignancies. The major causes of premature death among CKD patients are cardiovascular diseases, with younger patients being at highest relative risk.[2] As an example, the risk of cardiovascular mortality in a 45-year-old CKD patient receiving dialysis is approximately 100 times greater than for a healthy individual of similar age and gender. Unfortunately, kidney transplantation does not solve this problem, although individuals who receive transplants are generally at lower risk of major cardiovascular events than those remaining on dialysis.[2]

Outcomes for CKD patients receiving renal replacement therapy (ie dialysis or kidney transplantation) might therefore be further improved by the development of preventive therapies aimed at reducing cardiovascular risk. Such strategies could be based in part on our understanding of the pathophysiology of cardiovascular diseases in the general population. However, there is a growing appreciation that the functional and metabolic changes that complicate uraemia (Table 4) may damage the heart and arteries.[3] This is reflected by differences in the pathological changes that characterise cardiovascular diseases in CKD patients and in the general population. For example, the arteries of CKD patients may be heavily calcified (Fig 1), even in areas where overt

Table 4 Complications of uraemia that may increase cardiovascular disease risk.

- Hypertension
- Dyslipidaemia
- Intravascular volume overload
- Increased cardiac output due to presence of arteriovenous fistula
- Anaemia
- Hyperhomocysteinaemia
- Increased oxidative stress
- Chronic activation of the inflammatory response
- Elevated calcium x phosphate product
- Hyperuricaemia

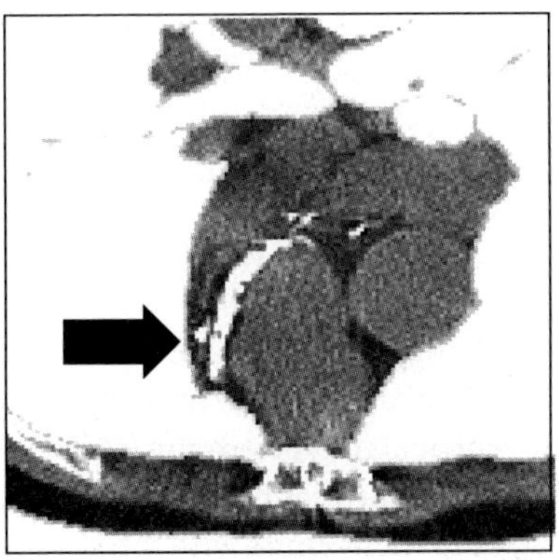

Fig 1 A computed tomography scan showing extensive calcification of the left coronary artery (arrowed) in a patient with chronic renal failure undergoing long-term haemodialysis.

atherosclerotic lesions are absent. Furthermore, epidemiological studies among CKD patients have failed to show the expected associations between risk factors such as hypertension or hypercholesterolaemia and mortality.[4] Taken together, these observations suggest that the management of cardiovascular risk in CKD may require a more specific approach than that adopted in non-uraemic individuals. Therapies of proven benefit in other groups may be less effective than expected in CKD, whilst specific targeting of uraemic risk factors could be worthwhile.

☐ RISK FACTOR MODIFICATION TRIALS IN CHRONIC KIDNEY DISEASE PATIENTS

Unfortunately, the presence of proteinuria or an elevated serum creatinine has been an exclusion criterion for many recent clinical trials examining therapies that modify cardiovascular risk, so it is not clear whether the results of these studies are applicable to patients with kidney damage. Nevertheless, nephrologists are understandably keen to demonstrate that risk factor modification is worthwhile in CKD patients. The largest ongoing trial involving patients with kidney disease, the UK-based Study of Heart and Renal Protection (SHARP), aims to randomise approximately 9,000 patients with CKD defined as serum creatinine for women above 130 μmol/l, for men above 150 μmol/l or requiring dialysis to either a combination of simvastatin 20 mg and ezetimibe 10 mg or placebo. The rate of decline of kidney function will be assessed in those not on dialysis and cardiovascular events in the whole group.

Other ongoing large trials are assessing alternative interventions such as correction of hyperhomocysteinaemia with high-dose folic acid therapy. Smaller trials that have been completed demonstrated a reduction in cardiovascular end-points among CKD patients randomly assigned to receive an antioxidant regimen rather than placebo.[5] Increased levels of oxidative stress are well recognised in uraemia, but these findings are clearly contrary to those of much larger studies in non-CKD patients. Such observations may highlight the potential benefits to be gained from specifically targeting risk factors modified by the presence of CKD, but need to be confirmed in much larger, more robust studies. In this respect, other interventions that may reduce risk in CKD include prevention of fluid overload, correction of anaemia and reduction in calcium x phosphate product.

☐ CARDIOVASCULAR DISEASE RISK AND EARLY CHRONIC KIDNEY DISEASE

Optimal therapy to reduce cardiovascular risk will need to be started early in the course of CKD. Many patients not requiring dialysis already have established cardiac and arterial pathology which may be detectable by non-invasive techniques. For example, at the point of starting dialysis, approximately three-quarters of patients in a Canadian cohort had left ventricular hypertrophy (LVH) on echocardiography.[6] In the Chronic Renal Impairment in Birmingham (CRIB) study, one-third of patients attending a UK nephrology outpatient clinic with CKD (not requiring dialysis) had vascular disease detected at baseline screening.[7] The fact that cardiovascular diseases develop early in the course of CKD suggests that mild kidney dysfunction might increase the level of risk. It is now recognised that most patients with CKD die before requiring dialysis, often as the result of a cardiovascular event.[8] It follows that early detection of kidney disease might be advantageous, providing an opportunity to institute therapies that may both slow the rate of deterioration of kidney function and reduce the risk of cardiovascular complications. Conveniently, certain therapies such as lowering blood pressure may have this dual effect.

Unfortunately however, many patients are referred to a nephrologist with end-stage kidney disease and need dialysis immediately. It is recognised that such patients have a poorer outcome than those referred with milder kidney dysfunction, possibly in part because opportunities to manage complications such as anaemia, a risk factor for the development of LVH, are missed. Efforts such as the K/DOQI project which help to demystify the diagnosis and management of early CKD, along with greater collaboration between nephrologists and other healthcare professionals might help to rectify this situation. Early diagnosis and prevention of CKD will be addressed in the second part of the Renal Services National Services Framework, which is expected to be published during 2005.

□ KIDNEY DISEASE AS A RISK FACTOR FOR CARDIOVASCULAR DISEASE IN OTHER POPULATIONS

Mild kidney dysfunction may also be an important adverse prognostic factor among patients with established cardiovascular disease. For example, several studies have shown an association between reduced GFR and poor survival following acute myocardial infarction (MI).[9] This was explained, at least in part, by the increased chances of developing heart failure, but might also reflect a reluctance by physicians to offer these patients therapies usually prescribed to those with better kidney function.

There is a similar relationship between kidney dysfunction and poor outcome in studies involving patients considered to be at high risk of developing cardiovascular disease. For example, the relative risk of a major cardiovascular event (MI, stroke or cardiovascular death) was increased 1.4-fold in individuals recruited to the Heart Outcomes and Prevention Evaluation (HOPE) study who had a raised serum creatinine (124–200 μmol/l) at baseline, even after adjustments were made for other risk factors.[10] Indeed minor kidney dysfunction conferred the same increase in risk as diabetes mellitus.

The association between impaired kidney function and cardiovascular disease in the general population has not been clearly established. Among Framingham participants, impaired kidney function (serum creatinine 120–265 μmol/l) was independently associated with an increased risk of a cardiovascular event in women but not in men.[11] In contrast, among apparently healthy individuals participating in the British Regional Heart Study, elevated serum creatinine (≥130 μmol/l) was associated with a two- to threefold increased risk of cardiovascular death, coronary heart disease events or stroke after correction for other risk factors.[12]

Increased urinary albumin excretion, another marker of kidney disease, is also a potent predictor of future cardiovascular events in high-risk populations. In patients recruited to the HOPE study, the effects of microalbuminuria and elevated serum creatinine were additive, with microalbuminuria being an equally strong renal-related risk predictor as elevated serum creatinine.[10] Similar findings have been reported in studies of diabetic populations among whom cardiovascular risk increases in relation to the level of urinary protein excretion. These observations raise the possibility that in certain groups of patients, microalbuminuria may be a manifestation of a generalised increase in the permeability of small blood vessels as the result of injury, rather than a specific indication of the presence of kidney disease.

☐ CONCLUSIONS

An increased risk of cardiovascular disease is associated with uraemia and extends to the much larger group of patients with earlier stages of CKD not requiring dialysis. Outcomes are likely to be improved by a better understanding of the pathophysiology of uraemic arteriopathy and cardiomyopathy, together with the development of effective treatment strategies. Opportunities for intervention may be greatest among those patients with mild kidney disease in whom therapeutic intervention may not only reduce cardiovascular risk, but also slow progression of kidney failure and delay the need for renal replacement therapy.

REFERENCES

1 Coresh J, Astor BC, Greene T, Eknoyan G, Levey AS. Prevalence of chronic kidney disease and decreased kidney function in the adult US population: third National Health and Nutrition Examination Survey. *Am J Kidney Dis* 2003;**41**:1–12.

2 Foley RN, Parfrey PS, Sarnak MJ. Clinical epidemiology of cardiovascular disease in chronic renal disease. Review. *Am J Kidney Dis* 1998;**32**(5Suppl3):S112–S19.

3 Baigent C, Burbury K, Wheeler DC. Premature cardiovascular disease in chronic renal failure. Review. *Lancet* 2000;**356**:147–52.

4 Kalantar-Zadeh K, Block G, Humphreys MH, Kopple JD. Reverse epidemiology of cardiovascular risk factors in maintenance dialysis patients. Review. *Kidney Int* 2003;**63**:793–808.

5 Boaz M, Smetana S, Weinstein T, Matas Z *et al.* Secondary prevention with antioxidants of cardiovascular disease in endstage renal disease (SPACE): randomised placebo-controlled trial. *Lancet* 2000;**356**:1213–8.

6 Foley RN, Parfrey PS, Harnett JD, Kent GM *et al.* The prognostic importance of left ventricular geometry in uremic cardiomyopathy. *J Am Soc Nephrol* 1995;**5**:2024–31.

7 Landray MJ, Thambyrajah J, McGlynn FJ, Jones HJ *et al.* Epidemiological evaluation of known and suspected cardiovascular risk factors in chronic renal impairment. *Am J Kidney Dis* 2001;**38**:537–46.

8 Keith DS, Nichols GA, Gullion CM, Brown JB, Smith DH. Longitudinal follow-up and outcomes among a population with chronic kidney disease in a large managed care organization. *Arch Intern Med* 2004;**164**:659–63.

9 French WJ, Wright RS. Renal insufficiency and worsened prognosis with STEMI: a call for action. *J Am Coll Cardiol* 2003;**42**:1544–6.

10 Mann JF, Gerstein HC, Pogue J, Bosch J, Yusuf S. Renal insufficiency as a predictor of cardiovascular outcomes and the impact of ramipril: the HOPE randomized trial. *Ann Intern Med* 2001;**134**:629–36.

11 Culleton BF, Larson MG, Wilson PW, Evans JC *et al.* Cardiovascular disease and mortality in a community-based cohort with mild renal insufficiency. *Kidney Int* 1999;**56**:2214–9.
12 Wannamethee SG, Shaper AG, Perry IJ. Serum creatinine concentration and risk of cardiovascular disease: a possible marker for increased risk of stroke. *Stroke* 1997;**28**:557–63.

Is proteinuria bad for the kidney?

Nigel Brunskill

□ INTRODUCTION

The provision of renal replacement therapy (RRT) in the form of dialysis imposes a major burden on patients, their families and society. Dialysis is an imperfect substitute for native renal function, dialysed patients experiencing both reduced quality and quantity of life. In Western society, dialysis populations are growing steadily. In the UK, projections indicate that the number will not plateau for a further 15–20 years; currently, around 100 individuals per million population commence dialysis each year, with annual costs per person of about £20,000.[1] This level of dialysis provision has major cost implications for the NHS.

Clearly, it would be desirable to prevent the need for dialysis in patients with renal disease, but unfortunately many individuals display a clinical course characterised by relentless loss of renal function regardless of the underlying renal diagnosis. The eventual outcome of such illnesses is end-stage renal failure (ESRF) and the need for RRT. Preventing ESRF is currently a national priority area; it is emphasised in the recently published National Service Framework for Renal Services, Part 1,[1] and will comprise a significant portion of Part 2.

Most progressive renal diseases are associated with the development of a common renal histological pattern known as the end-stage kidney, characterised by prominent interstitial inflammation and scarring, together with fibrosis and gross tubular atrophy. Declining renal function correlates extremely closely with these developing changes in the renal tubulointerstitium. These observations have led to the hypothesis that, whatever the initiating renal insult, a common pathophysiological process is precipitated which culminates in the development of the end-stage kidney.

□ PROTEINURIA

Urinalysis is a useful tool to predict the risk of renal disease progression. Proteinuria is a universal finding in patients with progressive renal diseases, and is associated with a greatly increased risk of development of renal failure.[2] It has been postulated therefore that excess protein may exert a toxic effect on the proximal tubular epithelial cells (PTC), damaging the cells and thus initiating a process of interstitial inflammation and scarring: the concept of proteinuric nephropathy.[3,4] Proteinuric PTC injury is readily appreciated by examination of renal biopsies from patients with nephrosis. Prominent vacuolation of PTC is observed in these heavily proteinuric patients, the vacuoles containing protein reabsorbed from the proximal tubular fluid. Such is the severity of structural disruption to the PTC in this situation that disturbance of cell function must also be present. Indeed, proteinuric patients exhibit elevated urinary levels of N-acetyl-β-glucosaminidase, an enzyme released from damaged PTC, indicative of PTC injury.

□ ANGIOTENSIN-CONVERTING ENZYME INHIBITORS

Not only is heavy proteinuria associated with a poor renal prognosis, but reduction of proteinuria by blockade of the renin angiotensin system is protective of renal function. A renoprotective effect of angiotensin-converting enzyme inhibitors (ACEIs) in renal disease began to be investigated in a variety of animal models of renal disease in the mid- to late 1980s. The landmark study by Lewis *et al*[5] established the utility of captopril as a renoprotective agent in diabetic nephropathy, independent of its effect on blood pressure control but in association with reduced proteinuria. Since then, many studies have reported beneficial effects of ACEIs, and indeed of angiotensin receptor antagonists (ARAs), in a multiplicity of proteinuric renal diseases.

The Ramipril Efficacy in Nephropathy (REIN) study examined the effect of ramipril or placebo on proteinuria and renal disease progression in non-diabetic renal disease in patients with equivalent blood pressure control.[6] Ramipril produced a significant antiproteinuric renoprotective effect, suggesting that reduced proteinuria and improved renal prognosis are causally related. As a consequence of this and other studies, ACEIs and/or ARAs are now regarded as mandatory in patients with persistent proteinuria.

□ PROTEINURIC RENAL INJURY

The role of albumin

Several investigators have looked for effects of components of proteinuric proximal tubular fluid on cultured PTC function *in vitro*. Albumin has been best studied as it is the most prevalent protein in this fluid. Albumin is taken up into PTC by receptor-mediated endocytosis, but it is now clear that albumin can also behave as a signalling molecule in PTC. Studies have demonstrated that albumin activates many intracellular signalling cascades in PTC, including enzymes such as p85/p110 phosphatidylinositide 3-kinase (PI 3-kinase), pp70^{s6} kinase, p42/p44 extracellular signal regulated kinase, p38 mitogen-activated protein kinase, c-jun terminal kinase and protein kinase C.[4,7]

Many of these enzymes are involved in regulation of cell growth survival. Not surprisingly, therefore, one functional consequence of PTC albumin signalling is proliferation.[7] Albumin stimulates PTC proliferation via a kinase cascade involving PI 3-kinase, pp70^{s6} kinase and extracellular signal regulated kinase.[7] *In vivo* hyperplasia of PTC in rats with protein overload proteinuria has also been demonstrated, and recently PTC hyperplasia has been confirmed in proteinuric humans.[8] Not surprisingly, however, the *in vivo* situation is more complex, with proteinuric animals also demonstrating significant PTC apoptosis in addition to proliferation. Careful examination of kidneys from rats with protein overload nephrosis suggests that the balance of PTC hyperplasia/apoptosis favours cell deletion, so continuing loss of tubular cells by apoptosis may contribute to tubular atrophy.

Other consequences of PTC albumin signalling include activation of a variety of transcription factors such as NFκB, AP-1, and JAK/STAT.[3,4] As a result, cultured PTC produce a cocktail of chemoattractants and profibrotic cytokines in a dose-dependent manner in response to albumin.[3] *In vivo* models of proteinuric renal disease demonstrate prominent interstitial accumulation of macrophages particularly associated with those proximal tubules displaying the most marked accumulation of intracellular protein. These heavily protein overloaded tubules also demonstrate the greatest chemokine expression.[3] This evidence indicates that albuminuria may, via PTC, also induce a pro-inflammatory scarring environment in the kidney, with altered growth of PTC contributing to the development of proteinuric nephropathy.

Because glomerular damage may have indirect effects on aspects of tubular physiology such as peritubular haemodynamics and peritubular oxygen tension, it has been suggested that proteinuria does not have either a directly toxic effect in PTC or a causal role in progressive renal disease.

Gross *et al*[9] used the axolotl as a model to address this issue. The axolotl kidney possesses both closed nephrons and nephrons with ciliated peritoneal funnels called nephrostomes that have access to the peritoneal fluid. Injection of protein into the peritoneal cavity of these animals, thus exposing only nephrons with nephrostomes to a protein load, confirmed a direct pro-inflammatory, profibrotic effect of proteins in the kidney acting via PTC in the absence of glomerular damage or pathology.

The role of lipids

Other molecules also enter the proximal tubule in proteinuria. Circulating albumin is a carrier for many serum-derived molecules; in particular, albumin possesses 5–7 high–affinity binding sites for fatty acids which are carried with albumin into the proximal tubule. Long-chain fatty acids are poorly soluble, and filtered albumin thus has the capacity to present these molecules to PTC in an unregulated manner at concentrations far above that normally determined by their solubility in aqueous solution. Furthermore, in nephrosis the fatty acid load per albumin molecule is markedly increased, with a molar ratio of about 6 (fatty acid:albumin) compared with a ratio of 1 in health. Lipid accumulation in PTC can be demonstrated by Oil Red O staining and results in considerable metabolic perturbation. If proximal tubular segments are exposed to fatty acid-bearing albumin *in vitro*, PTC will elaborate a lipid chemoattractant that has a potentially key role in the induction of interstitial inflammation. This response is not observed in proximal tubular segments exposed to fatty acid-free albumin. Further evidence of the potential nephrotoxicity of albumin-bound fatty acid comes from the observation that urinary albumin in the relatively benign minimal change disease is devoid of fatty acid compared with that found in other nephrotic conditions.

The pathophysiological importance of lipid in progressive glomerular and tubular disease has been suggested by several authors, recently confirmed by studies demonstrating that PTC growth, survival and fibronectin matrix protein secretion are modulated by albumin-bound fatty acid. In *in vivo* studies, protein overload proteinuria in rats induced by fatty acid-carrying albumin evoked more severe tubulointerstitial inflammation, PTC apoptosis and injury than that induced by fatty acid-free albumin. Subsequent work demonstrated that these adverse effects occur, at least in part, as a result of fatty acid activation of peroxisome proliferator activated receptor-γ (PPARγ) in PTC.[10]

□ PEROXISOME PROLIFERATOR ACTIVATED RECEPTORS

The PPARs, PPARα, -β/δ and -γ, are ligand activated transcription factors that regulate the expression of genes with specific PPAR response elements in their promoter regions, and consequently diverse cell functions including adipocyte differentiation, control of inflammation, fatty acid metabolism, cell cycle control and the development of atherosclerosis.[11] A variety of endogenous and exogenous ligands for PPARs have been identified. PPARα is the target for fibrate drugs, and PPARγ the target for the antidiabetic thiazolidinediones (TZD) and the eicosanoid 15-deoxy-$\Delta^{12,14}$-prostaglandin J_2. Most fatty acids also activate PPARs.

All three PPAR subtypes have been identified in mammalian kidneys, but their role in regulating renal (patho)physiology has only recently begun to be examined. PPARγ is the isoform best studied in this context, and some animal work has suggested a protective effect of TZD in both diabetic and non-diabetic models of renal disease. However, transcriptional activation by different PPAR agonists is ligand- and depot-specific; different PPARγ ligands may induce differential gene transcription, so the effects of PPARγ agonists are likely to vary between cell types. Accordingly, glomerular cells respond differently to different PPARγ activators and some, but not all, PPARγ agonists potentially augment detrimental inflammatory responses in glomerulonephritis.

The effects of PPARγ activation in cells of the kidney are therefore likely to be complex and context dependent. It remains unclear in what circumstances PPARγ activation in the kidney may be beneficial or deleterious. Recent experiments using various PPARγ agonists have demonstrated differential effects of these PPARγ ligands in PTC where the antidiabetic TZDs behave as partial agonists; this suggests a pharmacological basis for their use to combat progressive proteinuric renal disease,[12] such that a partial agonist TZD may be employed to inhibit the detrimental effects of other PPARγ ligands such as albumin-bound fatty acids.

□ ANTIPROTEINURIC STRATEGIES

There is now powerful clinical and experimental evidence to support a causal role for proteinuria *per se* in the development of progressive renal scarring. How does this evidence translate into practical benefits for patients?

1 Antiproteinuric strategies targeting the renin angiotensin system have already demonstrated success in slowing progression, but more needs to be done.

2 The roles of lipids in progression are also likely to be key. All the major lipid-lowering studies in cardiovascular disease excluded patients with significant renal disease, but meta-analysis of a number of small lipid-lowering studies in renal disease has suggested a significant benefit.

3 The optimum lipid-lowering agent also requires some consideration. In this regard, there is developing evidence that pleiotropic effects of 3-hydroxymethylglutaryl co-enzyme A (HMG-CoA) reductase inhibitors (ie effects unrelated to cholesterol lowering) may also confer significant protection on the failing kidney.

4 Finally, agents that modulate the activity of PPAR also hold some promise as renoprotective agents for clinical use.

□ CONCLUSIONS

It seems that proteinuria *is* bad for the kidney, and that therapies specifically aimed at modifying proteinuria hold considerable promise for the treatment of progressive renal failure.

REFERENCES

1 The National Service Framework for Renal Services, Part 1. London: Department of Health, 2004. http://www.dh.gov.uk/assetRoot/04/07/05/25/04070525.pdf

2 Cameron JS. Proteinuria and progression in human glomerular diseases. Review. *Am J Nephrol* 1990;**10**(Suppl 1): 81–7.

3 Remuzzi G. Nephropathic nature of proteinuria. Review. *Curr Opin Nephrol Hypertens* 1999;**8**:655–63.

4 Brunskill NJ. Albumin signals the coming of age of proteinuric nephropathy. *J Am Soc Nephrol* 2004;**15**:504–5.

5 Lewis EJ, Hunsicker LG, Bain RP, Rohde RD. The effect of angiotensin-converting-enzyme inhibition on diabetic nephropathy. *N Engl J Med* 1993;**329**:1456–62.

6 Randomised placebo-controlled trial of effect of ramipril on decline in glomerular filtration rate and risk of terminal renal failure in proteinuric, non-diabetic nephropathy. The GISEN Group (Gruppo Italiano di Studi Epidemiologici in Nefrologia). *Lancet* 1997;**349**:1857–63.

7 Dixon RJ, Brunskill NJ. Activation of mitogenic pathways by albumin in kidney proximal tubule epithelial cells: implications for the pathophysiology of proteinuric states. *J Am Soc Nephrol* 1999;**10**:1487–97.

8 Hebert LA, Agarwal G, Sedmak D, Mahan JD *et al.* Proximal tubular epithelial hyperplasia in patients with chronic glomerular proteinuria. *Kidney Int* 2000;**57**:1962–7.

9 Gross ML, Hanke W, Koch A, Ziebart H *et al.* Intraperitoneal protein injection in the axolotl: the amphibian kidney as a novel model to study tubulointerstitial activation. *Kidney Int* 2002;**62**:51–9.

10 Arici M, Chana R, Lewington AL, Brown J, Brunskill NJ. Stimulation of proximal tubular cell apoptosis by albumin-bound fatty acids mediated by peroxisome proliferator activated receptor-gamma. *J Am Soc Nephrol* 2003;**14**:17–27.

11 Guan Y, Breyer MD. Peroxisome proliferator-activated receptors (PPARs): novel therapeutic targets in renal disease. Review. *Kidney Int* 2001;**60**:14–30.

12 Chana RS, Lewington AJ, Brunskill NJ. Differential effects of peroxisome proliferator activated receptor-gamma (PPARgamma) ligands in proximal tubular cells: Thiazolidinediones are partial PPARgamma agonists. *Kidney Int* 2004;**65**:2081–90.

Primary small vessel vasculitis

Lorraine Harper

☐ INTRODUCTION

Inflammation and necrosis of blood vessel walls occur in about a dozen primary vasculitic disorders. An attempt to classify these diverse forms of vasculitis resulted in the Chapel Hill international consensus definitions which used vessel size as the determinant of classification. Wegener's granulomatosis (WG) and microscopic polyangiitis (MPA) are described as small vessel vasculitides commonly associated with antineutrophil cytoplasmic antibodies (ANCA). These diseases share a common pathology:

- focal necrotising lesions affecting many different vessels and organs
- capillaritis in the lungs which may cause alveolar haemorrhage
- pauci-immune crescentic glomerulonephritis within the glomerulus of the kidney which may cause acute renal failure (ARF)
- there may be a purpuric rash or vasculitic ulceration in the dermis, and
- WG may have granulomatous lesions.

The incidence of these diseases is increasing with more than 20 per million affected, and they occur more frequently in an elderly population (peak age 55–70 years).[1]

☐ PATHOGENESIS

Antineutrophil cytoplasmic antibodies

Understanding the pathogenesis of ANCA-associated vasculitis is important for the development of novel therapeutic agents, and important advances have been made in recent years.[2] The causes of ANCA-associated vasculitis are unknown, but the presence of ANCA suggests an autoimmune basis. How ANCA are produced and initiate autoimmunity are also unknown, but both genetic and environmental influences are important. Proteinase 3 expression on the cell surface is genetically determined, and there is higher expression in individuals who have WG. Patients with WG who have inherited α1-antitrypsin deficiency (the main inhibitor of proteinase 3) have more severe disease and higher mortality. Environmental factors include a now well reported link with antithyroid medication, particularly propylthiouracil. Cases tend to be associated with myeloperoxidase (MPO)-ANCA, although clinical vasculitis is rare. Silica is another environmental insult associated with development of ANCA. It is unclear how these insults induce ANCA.

ANCA are present in 90% of patients with pauci-immune vasculitis and the level appears to reflect disease activity. *In vitro*, ANCA can bind to its antigens, proteinase 3 and MPO, present in the azurophil granules of neutrophils and monocytes when they are surface expressed following cytokine priming. Binding of ANCA to neutrophil Fcγ receptors causes neutrophil activation with a respiratory burst and release of granule enzymes and cytokines, inducing endothelial cell damage. ANCA also interfere with the normal processes of resolution of inflammation. Neutrophil apoptosis is dysregulated by ANCA activation of neutrophils, preventing apoptotic cell removal; this in turn allows progression to secondary necrosis, a highly inflammatory event.

An animal model has recently provided direct evidence of the pathogenicity of ANCA. Immunisation of MPO knock-out mice with MPO produced anti-MPO antibody (ANCA), and transfer of splenocytes or isolated immunoglobulin (Ig) into two types of mice which express MPO – Rag2 deficient mice (which do not produce functioning T or B lymphocytes) and wild type B6 mice – caused a necrotising crescentic glomerulonephritis similar to the human disease.[3]

Endothelial cells

The endothelial cell is also important for localising inflammation. Endothelial cells develop an activated phenotype in ANCA-associated vasculitis, with enhanced expression of adhesion molecules that promote interaction with circulating inflammatory cells. ANCA activation can convert rolling neutrophils to stationary adherent cells well placed to mediate endothelial damage. Release of pro-inflammatory mediators, including nitric oxide, reactive oxygen species and proteolytic enzymes, might all directly contribute to damaging the endothelium. Studies measuring abnormal vasodilatation of the brachial artery and dermal microvessels provide evidence of widespread endothelial dysfunction in patients with vasculitis.

T cells

Activation of endothelial cells and neutrophils is important for the early development of vasculitic lesions; their progression is accompanied by T cell and monocyte recruitment. T cell-mediated immunity is thought to contribute to the pathogenesis of ANCA-associated vasculitis. Several studies have shown that peripheral T cells from patients with active or quiescent disease can proliferate in response to proteinase 3 or MPO. T cell activation also persists after disease remission, suggesting that T cells contribute to the remitting/relapsing nature of ANCA-associated vasculitis and show the failure of current therapies to suppress immune disease processes and induce tolerance.

☐ CLINICAL FEATURES

In WG there is a predilection for the upper and lower respiratory tracts and the kidneys to be involved, typically with granuloma and small vessel vasculitis. Upper respiratory tract symptoms include rhinorrhoea, sinusitis, otitis media and tracheal stenosis. Lung disease can progress to life-threatening pulmonary haemorrhage. Renal manifestations are common, with microscopic haematuria, proteinuria and red cell casts, and there can be a rapid deterioration in renal function. Other systems commonly involved include the eyes and peripheral nervous system with mononeuritis multiplex.

MPA is similar to WG, but there is no granuloma formation and upper airway involvement is rare. So-called idiopathic rapidly progressive glomerulonephritis, without immune deposits and no systemic features of systemic vasculitis, is now considered part of the spectrum of MPA. Constitutional symptoms are common. Differentiation between WG and MPA is often difficult, but this distinction is not important clinically because treatment and prognosis are similar.[4]

□ DIAGNOSIS

Diagnosis is made on the basis of clinical findings, by biopsy of a relevant involved organ and the presence of ANCA. Testing for ANCA using both indirect immunofluorescence and antigen-specific enzyme-linked immunosorbent assay is recommended and provides high sensitivity and specificity.[5] WG and MPA are commonly associated with ANCA directed against proteinase 3 and MPO, respectively, although other specificities may be found.

□ TREATMENT[6]

The prognosis of untreated ANCA-associated vasculitis is poor, with up to 90% of patients dying within two years, usually due to respiratory failure. The introduction of treatment with cyclophosphamide and high-dose corticosteroids in the 1970s markedly reduced mortality and converted this acutely fatal disease into a chronic relapsing disorder. The combination of prednisolone and cyclophosphamide, now viewed as standard therapy, leads to control of disease in 80–90% of patients. There appears to be little role for prednisolone alone – it is associated with a lower remission rate, and higher relapse and mortality rates than when combined with cyclophosphamide.

Current treatment is toxic, with treatment-related morbidity in over 50% of patients. Steroid-induced diabetes, bladder and lymphoproliferative malignancy and infertility contribute to both morbidity and mortality. Treatment must be tailored to the stage and severity of disease, balancing the dangers of the disease against those of treatment. For successful treatment, vasculitis must be recognised and treated early before permanent scarring occurs.

Induction therapy

Initial therapy of systemic disease with vital organ involvement such as kidney or lung requires cyclophosphamide and corticosteroids and can achieve a 93% remission rate at six months. Treatment is usually given as a daily oral dose of cyclophosphamide and a tapering dose of steroids. Encouraged by the success of pulsed cyclophosphamide in the treatment of systemic lupus erythematosus (SLE), several small studies addressed the question of efficacy of a pulsed regimen in ANCA-associated vasculitis. A meta-analysis of three randomised trials comparing daily oral with pulsed cyclophosphamide found no difference in mortality or renal survival but there was a higher relapse rate following the latter. However, these studies were flawed and may reflect an insufficient dose of cyclophosphamide. In a recent report, the French Co-operative Polyarteritis Study Group found 12 monthly pulses of cyclophosphamide superior to six pulses with regard to remission and subsequent relapse in polyarteritis with poor prognostic factors.[7] To address this question, a multicentre randomised trial is ongoing comparing pulsed cyclophosphamide and an oral regimen using a consensus protocol designed by the European Vasculitis Study Group.

In those with milder disease (non-critical organ involvement), azathioprine or methotrexate has been used in an attempt to avoid the toxicity of cyclophosphamide. In a study of patients with early systemic, but non-renal, involvement patients were randomised to receive cyclophosphamide or methotrexate with prednisolone for one year.[8] Preliminary results suggest that methotrexate is as good as cyclophosphamide at inducing remission, but there was an increased relapse rate in the methotrexate limb. Also, rapid taper of steroids and withdrawal of all immunosuppressants at one year resulted in an unacceptable relapse rate in both limbs: 70% after methotrexate and 45% after cyclophosphamide induction treatment by 18 months. Methotrexate should not be used in those with renal impairment (serum creatinine >177 μmol/l) because of increased risk of hepatic and marrow toxicity.

Additional therapy is required in those with more severe disease, either life- or organ-threatening (serum creatinine >500 μmol/l or pulmonary haemorrhage).[8] Preliminary results of a recent multicentre randomised controlled trial (RCT) have suggested that plasma exchange is more beneficial than methylprednisolone. Patients who received plasma exchange were more likely to be dialysis independent at three months than those who received methylprednisolone, especially those who were dialysis dependent at presentation. In addition to the removal of pathogenic autoantibodies, plasma exchange removes coagulation factors and cytokines and also has effects on immunoregulation and endothelial activation.

Maintenance therapy

The risks of maintenance therapy have to be balanced against the risks of disease relapse (25–50% over 3–5 years). A combination of cyclophosphamide with low-dose corticosteroids was previously used to maintain remission, but recent studies support less toxic immunosuppressants following disease remission. Azathioprine has been extensively used. In a recently reported trial comparing azathioprine with cyclophosphamide in the maintenance of remission, it was found to be as effective as continued cyclophosphamide.[9] Studies switching from cyclophosphamide to methotrexate after remission have shown similar results.

These studies do not provide information on how long immunosuppression should be continued beyond 24 months because, despite continued immunosuppression with azathioprine or cyclophosphamide, relapse remains high (15% and 50% at 18 months and five years, respectively).

☐ DISEASE MONITORING AND RELAPSE

There is a strong association between primary small vessel vasculitis and the presence of ANCA, the detection of ANCA in patients facilitating diagnosis. Recent large multicentre studies combining immunofluorescence and enzyme immunoassays have demonstrated a specificity approaching 99% for WG, MPA or their renal limited form.[5] In the correct clinical setting, the positive predictive value is high. In patients with proteinuria, renal failure and haematuria the positive predictive value of ANCA is over 80% with a negative predictive value of 95%.

The high frequency of late relapse necessitates prolonged therapy with all its complications, but the usefulness of measuring ANCA titres in predicting disease activity and guiding therapy is controversial. Relapse is more common in patients with WG than in those with MPA, and those with a predominantly renal presentation relapse less often. Persistence of ANCA is strongly associated with relapse when immunosuppression is withdrawn. However, absolute titres correlate only weakly with disease activity. Rising titres of ANCA are predictive of relapse, but the positive predictive rate varies from 25–100%. Evidence to support pre-emptive treatment based on a rising ANCA titre is limited, most studies being retrospective or non-randomised, so this cannot be currently recommended.

☐ RESCUE THERAPY FOR REFRACTORY AND RELAPSING DISEASE

Standard induction therapy fails to induce remission in approximately 10% of patients. A further difficult patient group comprises those who frequently relapse, necessitating recurrent use of cyclophosphamide. Both these groups have a high risk of side effects due to the high cumulative dose of cyclophosphamide.

Tumour necrosis factor blockade

The success of tumour necrosis factor (TNF) blockade in rheumatoid arthritis (RA) has paved the way for the use of similar exciting therapeutic strategies in patients with ANCA-associated vasculitis.[10] There are strong reasons for believing that TNF may be pivotal in sustaining ongoing inflammation in systemic ANCA-associated vasculitis. Granuloma formation, a characteristic of WG, is completely inhibited in the absence of TNF. Increased circulating TNF levels have been detected during active vasculitis and TNF-α mRNA and protein are markedly increased at vasculitic sites. TNF primes neutrophils increasing surface expression of ANCA antigens. TNF is also a potent endothelial cell activator, inducing increased adhesion molecule expression and promoting a pro-adhesive state for neutrophils and other leukocytes.

Trials with anti-TNF specific antibody in patients with RA showed significant reduction in cytokine-induced vascular adhesion molecules (E-selectin, intercellular adhesion molecule-1 and vascular cell adhesion molecule-1) and reduction in leukocyte trafficking. Indeed, in ANCA-associated vasculitis, upregulation of adhesion molecules on endothelial cells correlates with disease activity. Recent evidence has shown benefit of TNF blockade in an animal model of acute crescentic glomerulonephritis, a model of human renal vasculitis.

Anti-tumour necrosis factor treatment

Anti-TNF treatments approved for clinical use in RA include:

- *monoclonal antibodies*: infliximab, a chimeric antibody composed of a murine anti-TNF antibody grafted on to a human IgG1κ which is approximately two-thirds murine, and adalimumab, a fully humanised IgG1 anti-TNF monoclonal antibody, and
- *soluble TNF receptor fusion protein*: etanercept, a protein produced by fusion of the Fc portion of human IgG1 to two TNF-R75 molecules.

Both infliximab[11] and etanercept[12] have been used in Phase 1 trials involving patients with ANCA-associated vasculitis. The drugs are well tolerated with few adverse events, but there were relapses despite improvements in disease activity. The results of these studies have prompted larger RCTs.

Safety of anti-tumour necrosis factor blockade

Concerns have been raised regarding the safety of these treatments. There appears to be a clear increase in the risk of reactivation of tuberculosis (TB). In the US, the incidence of TB among rheumatoid patients treated with infliximab is approximately four times higher than in rheumatoid patients not receiving infliximab.[13] The effect is greater with infliximab than with etanercept.

Development of antinuclear antibodies is common, but their pathogenicity is unclear and development of classical SLE is extremely rare. Patients treated with infliximab may develop antichimeric antibodies, resulting in infusion reactions and decreased treatment efficacy. Adalimumab may be anticipated to have fewer adverse effects related to immunogenicity.

□ OTHER POSSIBLE TREATMENTS

T cells play a central role in the pathogenesis of vasculitis. Depletion of T cells with monoclonal and polyclonal antibodies has been effective in refractory disease, leading to sustained treatment-free remission in some patients, but toxicity can limit their use. With increasing evidence for the pivotal role of ANCA, B cell depletion using rituximab is being considered in patients with ANCA-associated vasculitis, although only case reports currently support its use. Alternative immunosuppressants, including leflunomide, cyclosporin, mycophenolate and deoxyspergualin have shown benefit in small open-label studies.

☐ SUPPORTIVE THERAPY

Opportunistic infections are common, and prophylactic antifungal therapy and *Pneumocystis carinii* prophylaxis are useful. Common side effects of steroids include diabetes, hypertension and osteoporosis, particularly in postmenopausal women. Regular bone densitometry and bone protection or calcium supplements should be considered. Persistent endothelial dysfunction may be a risk for atherosclerosis, and hypertension or hypercholesterolaemia should be treated aggressively. Side effects of cyclophosphamide (haemorrhagic cystitis, bladder cancer, lymphoma, bone marrow suppression, infertility) are related to cumulative dose. Patients of childbearing age should be counselled about the risk of infertility and gamete storage offered. Patients on long-term azathioprine should be examined regularly for cutaneous malignancies. Regular white blood cell count monitoring is essential while patients are receiving cytotoxic therapy. Allopurinol (a xanthine oxidase inhibitor) is contraindicated in those taking azathioprine because of the high risk of bone marrow suppression.

☐ CONCLUSIONS

The advent of cyclophosphamide and corticosteroid treatment for patients with ANCA-associated vasculitis has dramatically improved their outlook. The current challenge lies in tailoring immunosuppression to reduce treatment-associated morbidity and mortality without compromising organ damage. Novel therapeutic agents, including newer immunosuppressants and biological agents, are being subjected to large RCTs using the gold standard of cyclophosphamide and corticosteroids as controls, thereby improving the evidence base for treatment of this challenging disease and continuing to improve the outlook for patients.

REFERENCES

1 Watts RA, Lane SE, Bentham G, Scott DG. Epidemiology of systemic vasculitis: a ten-year study in the United Kingdom. *Arthritis Rheum* 2000;**43**:414–9.

2 Harper L, Savage CO. Pathogenesis of ANCA-associated systemic vasculitis. Review. *J Pathol* 2000;**190**:349–59.

3 Xiao H, Heeringa P, Hu P, Liu Z *et al.* Antineutrophil cytoplasmic autoantibodies specific for myeloperoxidase cause glomerulonephritis and vasculitis in mice. *J Clin Invest* 2002;**110**:955–63.

4 Savage CO, Harper L, Adu D. Primary systemic vasculitis. Review. *Lancet* 1997;**349**:553–8.

5 Hagen EC, Daha MR, Hermans J, Andrassay K *et al.* Diagnostic value of standardized assays for anti-neutrophil cytoplasmic antibodies in idiopathic systemic vasculitis. EC/BCR Project for ANCA Assay Standardization. *Kidney Int* 1998;**53**:743–53.

6 Kamesh L, Harper L, Savage CO. ANCA-positive vasculitis. Review. *J Am Soc Nephrol* 2002;**13**:1953–60.

7 Guillevin L, Cohen P, Mahr A, Arene JP *et al.* Treatment of polyarteritis nodosa and microscopic polyangiitis with poor prognosis factors: a prospective trial comparing glucocorticoids and six or twelve cyclophosphamide pulses in sixty-five patients. *Arthritis Rheum* 2003;**49**:93–100.

8 Jayne D. Current attitudes to the therapy of vasculitis. *Kidney Blood Press Res* 2003;**26**:231–9.

9 Jayne D, Rasmussen N, Andrassy K, Bacon P *et al.* A randomized trial of maintenance therapy for vasculitis associated with antineutrophil cytoplasmic autoantibodies. *N Engl J Med* 2003;**349**:36–44.

10 Stone JH. Current status of tumor necrosis factor inhibition strategies in the treatment of vasculitis. *Kidney Blood Press Res* 2003;**26**:240–8.

11 Lamprecht P, Voswinkel J, Lilienthal T, Nolle B *et al.* Effectiveness of TNF-alpha blockade with infliximab in refractory Wegener's granulomatosis. *Rheumatology (Oxford)* 2002;**41**:1303–7.

12 Stone JH, Uhlfelder ML, Hellmann DB, Crook S *et al.* Etanercept combined with conventional treatment in Wegener's granulomatosis: a six-month open-label trial to evaluate safety. *Arthritis Rheum* 2001;**44**:1149–54.

13 Gomez-Reino JJ, Carmona L, Valverde VR, Mola EM, Montero MD; BIOBADASER Group. Treatment of rheumatoid arthritis with tumor necrosis factor inhibitors may predispose to significant increase in tuberculosis risk: a multicenter active-surveillance report. *Arthritis Rheum* 2003;**48**:2122–7.

Anaemia in renal failure

Iain Macdougall

□ INTRODUCTION

Up to 90% of patients on dialysis and up to 67% of patients starting renal replacement therapy suffer from a chronic anaemia associated with their renal failure.[1] The management of this condition has seen monumental changes over the last 10–15 years. Prior to the 1980s, many patients suffering from this condition required regular top-up blood transfusions to avoid the persistence of severe anaemia. However, this treatment improved the anaemia only transiently and, in addition, the patients were exposed to the risks of transmitting viral agents, increased susceptibility to HLA antigens and exacerbation of iron overload.

It has been recognised for over 20 years that the major factor in the pathogenesis of renal anaemia is an inappropriately low circulating erythropoietin (EPO) level for the degree of anaemia. There was clearly a rationale for administering synthetic EPO replacement therapy; the advent of recombinant DNA technology has allowed this to become a reality. There have now been further developments in the management of renal anaemia, including the synthesis of second- and third-generation erythropoietic agents, including darbepoetin alfa and continuous erythropoiesis receptor activator (CERA).

The anaemia of renal failure has many parallels with diabetes mellitus, in that both conditions have deficient secretion of a glycoprotein hormone from an endocrine organ (insulin from the pancreas versus EPO from the kidney).

The main physiological action of EPO is on the bone marrow where it acts as an anti-apoptotic agent to prolong the life of primitive erythroid progenitor cells, thus enhancing their proliferation and differentiation through various stages into mature circulating red cells in the blood. An amazing two million new red cells are manufactured every second under normal conditions, replacing the loss of the same number of red cells from the bloodstream when the more mature red cells have come to the end of their natural life (usually around 120 days). The turnover of red cells in the blood is an extremely dynamic process tightly controlled by EPO, the secretion of which is itself controlled by levels of hypoxia in the vasculature of the renal medulla. In chronic renal failure (CRF), the capacity of the kidneys to synthesise EPO *de novo* is severely reduced.

□ RECOMBINANT HUMAN ERYTHROPOIETIN (EPOETIN)

Historical background

In 1977 Miyake *et al* isolated human EPO from several thousand litres of urine obtained from patients with aplastic anaemia.[2] Over the next few years, scientists successfully isolated and cloned the gene for human EPO, finally achieving this in 1983. Because of an urgent clinical need for the availability of recombinant EPO, a remarkable fast tracking of this new therapeutic agent was initiated. Clinical trials were begun, and the first clinical report of its use in treating anaemia in dialysis patients was published in the *Lancet* towards the end of 1986.[3] The product finally became licensed as a therapeutic agent in 1989 in the US and in 1990 in Europe.

Administration

In the context of renal anaemia, EPO therapy is highly effective: about 90% of patients respond with a significant increase in their haemoglobin concentration. The drug can be administered both intravenously (iv) and subcutaneously (sc), but the iv route is practical only for patients receiving haemodialysis who have ready vascular access. The sc route is preferred for patients on peritoneal dialysis and for those not yet requiring dialysis. There is a fairly robust body of evidence to suggest that the weekly dose requirements with sc administration of epoetin may be around 30% lower than when given iv.[4] This explains why many haemodialysis patients (particularly in the UK) also receive epoetin via the sc route.

The starting dose of epoetin is around 2,000 units two or three times weekly, with the sc injection given into the thigh, arm or abdomen. The prescribing clinician usually expects a haemoglobin response of the order of 1–2 g/dl per month.

Iron balance

Many patients with CRF are in negative iron balance. The synthesis of new red blood cells generates additional iron requirements with two implications for patients receiving epoetin therapy:

- iron status should be monitored regularly, and
- many patients require iron supplementation.

Iron supplements are frequently given iv since oral iron often cannot keep pace with the demands of the bone marrow and is also poorly absorbed from the gastrointestinal tract in uraemic patients.[5]

Blood pressure

Blood pressure should be monitored regularly since up to 20% of patients may have an exacerbation of hypertension. This usually responds to fluid removal or intensification of antihypertensive medications. Severe hypertension with encephalopathy is no longer seen.

Beneficial effects of epoetin

Correction of anaemia with epoetin has proven benefits for the patient, including increased quality of life, increased exercise capacity,[6] improved cardiac function, regression of left ventricular hypertrophy (LVH),[6] reduced bleeding tendency, improved brain and cognitive function, improved sleep patterns, reduced hospitalisations and, of course, decreased requirements for blood transfusion.

The regression of LVH following epoetin therapy (Fig 1)[6] has generated particular interest among nephrologists. There is some evidence to suggest that this is an independent risk factor for mortality in dialysis patients and that decreased LV mass is associated with a reduced risk of development of new-onset cardiac failure (Fig 2).[7]

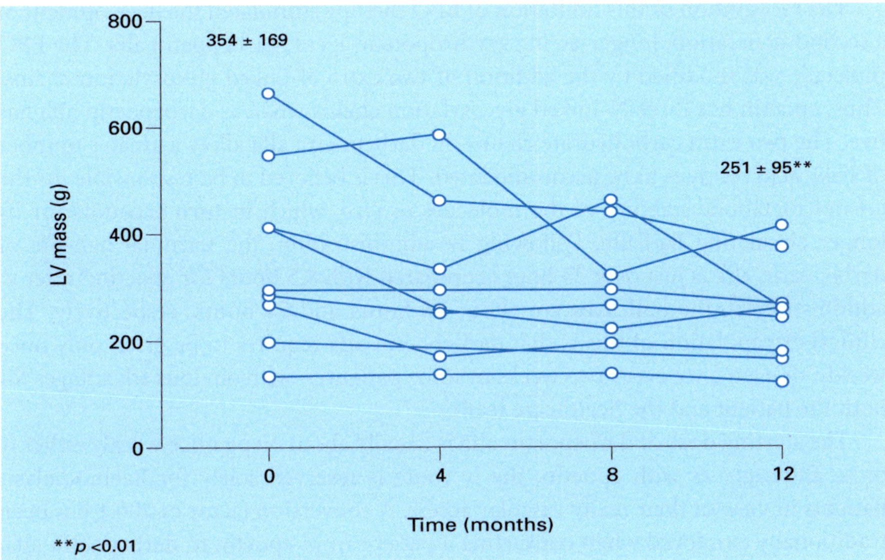

Fig 1 Effect of erythropoietin therapy on left ventricular (LV) mass.[6]

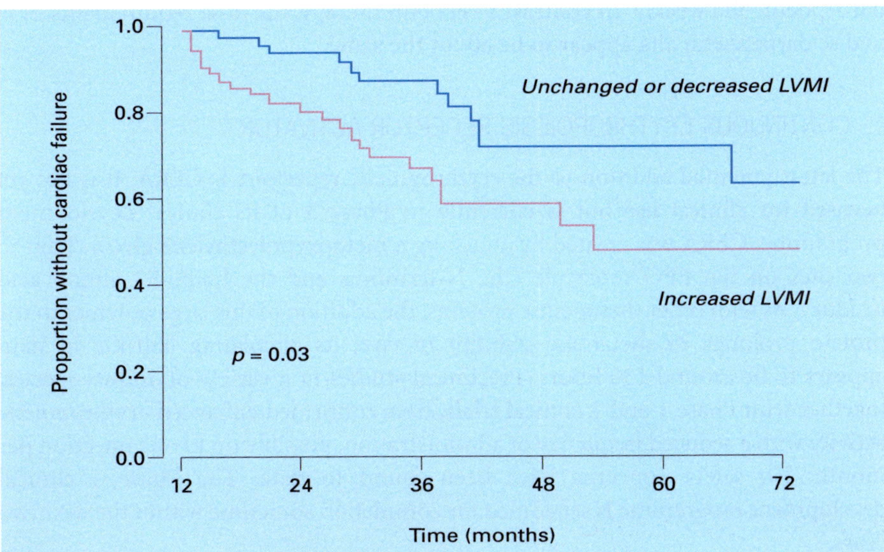

Fig 2 Regression of left ventricular (LV) hypertrophy in dialysis patients: reduced risk of new-onset cardiac failure[7] (echo= echocardiography; LVMI = LV mass index).

☐ DARBEPOETIN ALFA

Both the US and the European Best Practice Guidelines on Anaemia in Renal Failure recommend that epoetin be given three times weekly, based on its pharmacokinetic and pharmacodynamic properties. This dosing frequency allows adequate circulating EPO levels to be achieved to support erythroid cell development for most of the week, whereas twice- or even once-weekly dosing can probably achieve this only with higher dosages.

The recognition of this limitation of EPO therapy stimulated the development of a second-generation, longer-acting erythropoietic agent, darbepoetin alfa. The EPO molecule was modified by the addition of two extra N-linked glycosylation chains. Thus, epoetin has three N-linked glycosylation chains whereas darbepoetin alfa has five. The two extra carbohydrate chains on darbepoetin alfa allow a greater number of sialic acid residues to be accommodated. This is believed to be responsible for the greater metabolic stability of the molecule *in vivo*, which in turn accounts for its longer circulating half-life. Following iv administration, the terminal half-life of darbepoetin alfa is just over 25 hours compared with 8.5 hours for epoetin;[8] after sc administration, the half-lives are about 48 hours and 24 hours, respectively. The clinical extrapolation of this is that darbepoetin alfa requires to be given only once weekly, or even once every two weeks in some patients – with obvious advantages for both the patient and the healthcare team.

The starting dose of darbepoetin alfa is usually about 30 μg once weekly either iv or sc although, as with epoetin, the iv route is reserved solely for haemodialysis patients in view of their ready vascular access. A conversion factor of 200:1 has been traditionally employed when converting a patient from epoetin to darbepoetin alfa, although this has been challenged by more recent data. Thus, a patient maintained on 6,000 units of epoetin per week might convert to approximately 30 μg of darbepoetin alfa weekly. In contrast to epoetin therapy, the dose requirements of iv and sc darbepoetin alfa appear to be about the same.

☐ CONTINUOUS ERYTHROPOIESIS RECEPTOR ACTIVATOR

The latest potential addition to the erythropoietic repertoire is CERA. It is not yet licensed for clinical use but is currently in Phase 3 of its clinical development programme. CERA was created by attaching a methoxypolyethylene glycol chain to two sites on the EPO molecule (the N-terminus and the lysine-52 amino acid residue). As with other therapeutic proteins, the addition of this large polymer to the protein prolongs its metabolic stability *in vivo*; its circulating half-life in man appears to be around 130 hours. Preclinical studies in a variety of animal species, together with Phase 1 and 2 clinical trials, have confirmed enhanced erythropoietic activity with a reduced frequency of administration, possibly up to one injection per month. No safety concerns have been found to date. The Phase 3 clinical development programme is scheduled for completion sometime within the next two years.

☐ SAFETY

Epoetin-induced pure red cell aplasia

Until two years ago, there were no major safety concerns about the use of epoetin therapy or other erythropoietic agents. The adverse event profile was exemplary apart from some exacerbation of hypertension in up to 20% of patients and possibly an increased risk of vascular access clotting and skin irritation at the injection site.

It therefore came as a shock to the nephrological community when the first 13 cases of epoetin-associated pure red cell aplasia (PRCA) were described in the *New England Journal of Medicine* in February 2002.[9] This condition was associated with the development of anti-EPO antibodies which completely neutralised the biological activity of EPO and thus caused a severe transfusion-dependent anaemia.[10] The marrow aplasia was specific to the erythroid lineage so white cell and platelet maturation continued as normal. Patients with this condition usually have normal white cell and platelet counts with a profound reticulocytopenia ($<10 \times 10^9$ per litre). Bone marrow examination generally shows normal cellularity but sparse erythroblasts (<5%). Anti-EPO antibodies are detected using a radioimmune precipitation assay and the neutralising activity can be confirmed in a bioassay.[10] There has been a dramatic increase in the number of cases of antibody-positive PRCA reported since 1998.

Possible mechanisms

Various hypotheses have been generated to explain the development of PRCA including:

- removal of human serum albumin from one of the formulations (as requested by the European Union)
- a break in the cold storage chain
- the sc route of administration
- the use of polysorbate 80 as a stabilising agent, and
- extractable adjuvants from the rubber bungs in the prefilled syringes.

Almost all cases of PRCA have been observed in renal patients, although it has been described in two patients with myelodysplastic syndrome. The median time from first exposure to the development of severe anaemia is 11 months (range 2–63 months).[10]

Management

The management of epoetin-induced PRCA consists of immediate cessation of erythropoietic treatment. Immunosuppressive therapy is indicated to reduce the levels of the anti-EPO antibodies – conservative management without immunosuppressants rarely, if ever, leads to resolution of the condition.[11] Immunosuppressive therapy usually comprises corticosteroids plus cyclophosphamide or cyclosporin. Renal transplantation has also been shown to have a high success rate, although it is not clear whether this is due to the concomitant immunosuppressive therapy associated with this procedure.[11]

There is now preliminary evidence that once the anti-EPO titre has decreased to barely detectable levels, rechallenge with erythropoietic therapy while continuing immunosuppressant treatment might be effective.[12]

□ CONCLUSIONS

During the last 10–15 years there have been major developments in the manufacture of effective erythropoietic agents for the treatment of renal anaemia. Recombinant human EPO (epoetin) and darbepoetin alfa have now been available for nearly 15 years and just over two years, respectively. CERA is an exciting new agent, still in Phase 3 of its clinical development programme. The benefits of treating renal anaemia are considerable, including regression of LVH, improved quality of life and increased exercise capacity. The aim is to keep the haemoglobin concentration in all renal failure patients above 11 g/dl if possible.

Nephrologists now need to be vigilant for the possible development of epoetin-induced PRCA, which however remains an extremely rare condition.

REFERENCES

1 Pereira BJ. Introduction: new perspectives in chronic renal insufficiency. *Am J Kidney Dis* 2000;**36**(6 Suppl 3):S1–3.

2 Miyake T, Kung CK, Goldwasser E. Purification of human erythropoietin. *J Biol Chem* 1977;**252**:5558–64.

3 Winearls CG, Oliver DO, Pippard MJ, Reid C *et al.* Effect of human erythropoietin derived from recombinant DNA on the anaemia of patients maintained by chronic haemodialysis. *Lancet* 1986;**ii**:1175–8.

4 Besarab A, Reyes CM, Hornberger J. Meta-analysis of subcutaneous versus intravenous epoetin in maintenance treatment of anemia in hemodialysis patients. *Am J Kidney Dis* 2002;**40**:439–46.

5 Kooistra MP, Niemantsverdriet EC, van Es A, Mol-Beermann NM *et al.* Iron absorption in erythropoietin-treated haemodialysis patients: effects of iron availability, inflammation and aluminium. *Nephrol Dial Transplant* 1998;**13**:82–8.

6 Macdougall IC, Lewis NP, Saunders MJ, Cochlin DL *et al.* Long-term cardiorespiratory effects of amelioration of renal anaemia by erythropoietin. *Lancet* 1990;**335**:489–93.

7 Foley RN, Parfrey PS, Kent GM, Harnett JD *et al.* Serial change in echocardiographic parameters and cardiac failure in end-stage renal disease. *J Am Soc Nephrol* 2000;**11**:912–6.

8 Macdougall IC, Gray SJ, Elston O, Breen C *et al.* Pharmacokinetics of novel erythropoiesis stimulating protein compared with epoetin alfa in dialysis patients. *J Am Soc Nephrol* 1999;**10**:2392–5.

9 Casadevall N, Nataf J, Viron B, Kolta A *et al.* Pure red-cell aplasia and antierythropoietin antibodies in patients treated with recombinant erythropoietin. *N Engl J Med* 2002;**346**:469–75.

10 Rossert J, Casadevall N, Eckardt KU. Anti-erythropoietin antibodies and pure red cell aplasia. *J Am Soc Nephrol* 2004;**15**:398–406.

11 Verhelst D, Rossert J, Casadevall N, Kruger A *et al.* Treatment of erythropoietin-induced pure red cell aplasia: a retrospective study. *Lancet* 2004;**363**:1768–71.

12 Macdougall IC, Roche A, Rossert J, Casadevall N *et al.* Re-challenging a patient who developed pure red cell aplasia with epoetin: can it be done? *Nephrol Dial Transplant* 2004 (in press).

□ RENAL SELF ASSESSMENT QUESTIONS

Uraemia and cardiovascular risk

1 With respect to chronic kidney disease (CKD):
 (a) Serum creatinine may be normal in the early stages
 (b) Most patients progress to end-stage kidney failure
 (c) Cardiovascular disease risk is increased even in the early stages
 (d) Complications may be established before glomerular filtration rate falls below 30 ml/min
 (e) Patients do better if dialysis is planned in advance

2 With respect to cardiovascular risk in CKD:
 (a) Increased risk is independent of the cause of the kidney disease
 (b) Kidney transplantation has no impact on the level of risk
 (c) Early dialysis is proven to reduce the risk
 (d) Risk may be increased even when serum creatinine is below 200 μmol/l
 (e) Management of uraemic complications is proven to reduce risk

3 Potential cardiovascular risk factors that usually complicate CKD include:
 (a) Hypercholesterolaemia
 (b) Hypertension
 (c) Hyperhomocysteinaemia
 (d) Low high-density lipoprotein cholesterol
 (e) Insulin resistance

Is proteinuria bad for the kidney?

1 The following agents are renoprotective independent of blood pressure lowering effects:
 (a) Beta-adrenergic blockers
 (b) Calcium antagonists
 (c) Angiotensin-converting enzyme inhibitors
 (d) Angiotensin receptor antagonists
 (e) Alpha-adrenergic blockers

2 Proteinuria:
 (a) May be an early marker of renal disease
 (b) Is an independent risk factor for progressive renal failure
 (c) May cause renal inflammation
 (d) Results in lipid entry into the proximal tubule
 (e) Is a therapeutic target in renal disease

3 Treatment of progressive renal failure:
 (a) Is an important public health issue
 (b) May delay an individual's requirement for dialysis

(c) May be informed by understanding cell signalling effects of albumin
(d) Is already effective and achievable in most patients
(e) Treatment by statins is supported by unequivocal evidence

Primary small vessel vasculitis

1 Wegener's granulomatosis is associated with:
(a) Antinuclear antibodies
(b) Antiglomerular basement membrane antibodies
(c) Antineutrophil cytoplasmic antibodies (ANCA)
(d) Antimitochondrial antibodies

2 Systemic organ-threatening ANCA-associated vasculitis should be treated initially with:
(a) Corticosteroids alone
(b) Antibiotics
(c) Corticosteroids and cyclophosphamide
(d) Corticosteroids and azathioprine

3 Maintenance therapy for ANCA-associated vasculitis should:
(a) Be continued for at least 24 months to prevent relapse
(b) Include cyclophosphamide
(c) Include low-dose steroids
(d) Include allopurinol

4 Microscopic polyangiitis:
(a) Is associated with acute renal failure
(b) Is associated with ANCA directed against myeloperoxidase
(c) Is associated with granuloma
(d) Is commonly associated with ear, nose and throat involvement

5 Cyclophosphamide is associated with:
(a) Bone marrow suppression
(b) Hypertension
(c) Infertility
(d) Acne

Anaemia in renal failure

1 The healthy bone marrow manufactures the following number of new red blood cells every second during life:
(a) 4,000
(b) 48,000
(c) 240,000
(d) 400,000
(e) Two million

2 The following routes of administration are routinely used for erythropoietin therapy:
(a) Intravenous (iv)
(b) Intramuscular
(c) Subcutaneous (sc)
(d) Oral
(e) Intranasal

3 Comparing the dose requirements for iv and sc administration of epoietin therapy to obtain the same effect:
(a) Both are equivalent
(b) 5-10% more is required iv
(c) 5-10% more is required sc
(d) 30% more is required iv
(e) 30% more is required sc

4 Regarding darbepoietin alfa, which of the following statements are correct?
(a) It contains an extra N-linked glycosylation chain compared with epoietin
(b) It has a longer circulating half-life *in vivo* than epoietin
(c) The recommended starting dose for darbepoietin alfa in renal failure is 300 μg once weekly
(d) The conversion factor usually used when converting patients from epoietin to darbepoietin alfa is 200:1
(e) Dose requirements are very similar for both iv and sc administration

5 Regarding epoietin-induced pure red cell aplasia:
(a) The incidence of this condition has been increasing since 1995
(b) White cell and platelet counts are usually normal
(c) The reticulocyte count is usually normal or slightly increased
(d) A possible factor in the aetiology of this condition is the addition of human serum albumin to the formulation
(e) This condition is more common with iv than with sc administration of epoietin

Respiratory

Asthma or chronic obstructive pulmonary disease? Managing the acute exacerbation

Robert Stockley

☐ INTRODUCTION

Acute exacerbations of chronic obstructive pulmonary disease (COPD) are a major cause of morbidity and mortality. These episodes influence overall health status[1] and the subsequent decline in lung function,[2] they account for 10–20% of all hospital admissions and the major health costs required for COPD management are heavily biased towards these admission episodes. A priority both for the patient and healthcare resources is therefore effective management and prevention of exacerbations.

Despite the impact of these episodes, patient management has remained largely empirical until recently. COPD, by definition, is a condition of airflow limitation that is not fully reversible. However, airflow limitation is also a feature of asthma in which exaggerated changes occur during exacerbations and for which effective treatment and preventive strategies have been extensively studied. The symptoms of such asthmatic episodes (increased breathlessness, wheeze, cough and sputum production) are similar to those that occur in exacerbation of COPD. The empirical approach to management of COPD exacerbations has been mainly based on the strategies used effectively for asthmatic episodes.

The British Thoracic Society asthma guidelines[3] highlight the features of effective management of exacerbations of asthma, including:

- unrestricted oxygen supplementation
- nebulised bronchodilators *with or without* intravenous theophylline
- oral corticosteroids, and
- possible ventilatory support.

Episodes can be largely prevented by the sensible use of inhaled corticosteroids, although the role of long-acting beta2-agonists has yet to be determined. This approach for asthma is usually that used in the management of COPD, with minor differences. Patients with COPD are more likely to have type II respiratory failure, making unrestricted oxygen sometimes inappropriate. Furthermore, antibiotic therapy, not required in exacerbations of asthma,[3] is likely to be given in exacerbations of COPD.

This chapter will explore the evidence of efficacy of the therapeutic approach used, whilst acknowledging that clear differences exist between the pathophysiology of asthma and COPD.

☐ BRONCHODILATOR THERAPY

Measurement of reversibility

Asthma is a condition that usually has clear reversibility and fluctuations in airflow obstruction, whereas COPD is generally considered an irreversible condition. Reversibility refers to the ability of an inhaled bronchodilator or steroid therapy to increase lung function, specifically the FEV_1. This is a simple measure, but it is effort dependent and can vary within an individual by up to 200 ml. Thus, defining 'reversibility' presents a major problem. Patients who show a response in excess of this variability have been classified as 'asthmatic' or, at best, an 'asthmatic subgroup'. It has become accepted that COPD is largely 'irreversible' and that any physiological measure following bronchodilator therapy should not exceed the expected variability of the test.

It is also now widely accepted that COPD is present when bronchodilator therapy and a trial of corticosteroids produces an FEV_1 response less than 200 ml or 12% of the volume predicted for the patient's age, height, sex and race. However, some patients who otherwise appear clinically to have COPD show responses in excess of these limits.

The presence of sputum eosinophilia predicts the response to corticosteroids.[4] The eosinophil is the cell most associated with asthmatic airway inflammation (as opposed to the neutrophil in COPD), so it is likely that these patients represent an 'asthmatic' subgroup both physiologically and pathologically, although further characterisation studies are awaited.

Nevertheless, recent studies have shown that even the 'irreversible' group, defined as above, show responses that exceed baseline (on average) whilst remaining within the limits of 'non-reversibility' following bronchodilator (Fig 1) and steroid therapy.[5,6] Furthermore, in placebo-controlled studies of long-acting beta2-agonists, 'non-reversible' patients show a similar improvement in FEV_1 within the 12% predicted limitations on active treatment whereas placebo has no effect.[7] This improvement in average FEV_1 is noticed by the patients and recorded as improvements in their health status.[7] It would seem more appropriate to refer to COPD patients in general as 'poorly reversible' rather than 'non-reversible'.

Increased airflow obstruction

During exacerbations, patients with COPD usually complain of increased breathlessness. This may have many potential causes. Clearly, bronchospasm with increased airflow obstruction is one, but oedema of the airway wall and mucus plugging reducing functioning lung units are alternatives. A further cause could be the ambient or patient temperature, both of which can lead to hyperventilation which, in a patient with airflow obstruction, results in increased work of breathing perceived as breathlessness.

There is evidence that increased airflow obstruction is a feature of exacerbations of COPD. The peak expiratory flow rate declines with such episodes and recovers with resolution, as documented with patient diary cards.[8] Similar effects on airflow obstruction are seen in patients hospitalised for exacerbation.[9] These changes are small, but

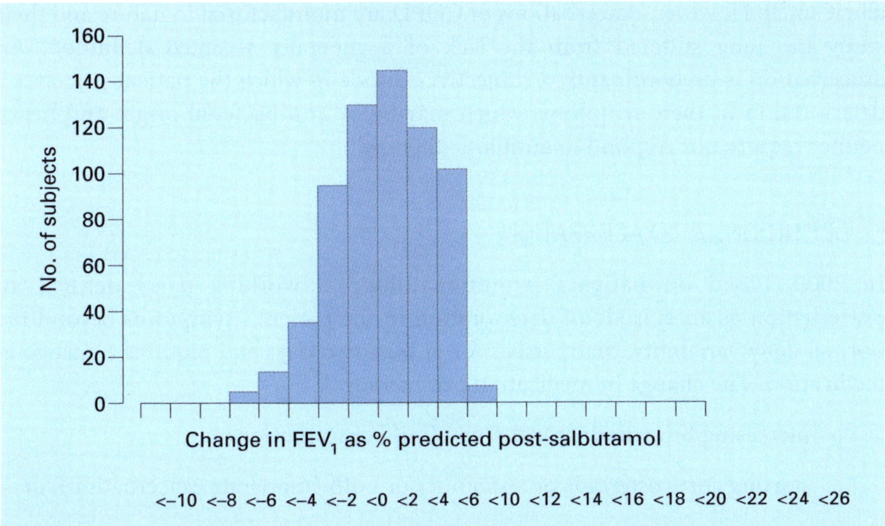

Fig 1 The response of chronic obstructive pulmonary disease patients to inhaled bronchodilator therapy shown as change in FEV_1 expressed as a percentage of the predicted value for the patient. The columns represent the number of patients showing each incremental increase (horizontal axis) (from Ref 5).

recent data have demonstrated that even small improvements in airflow obstruction tests can reflect much greater reductions in air trapping.[10] This would reduce hyper-inflation, thereby reducing the work of breathing and hence the sensation of dyspnoea.

Bronchodilator therapy therefore seems fully justified for such episodes, although there have been no controlled trials.

☐ CORTICOSTEROIDS

There are better data for the efficacy of corticosteroids: they speed up symptom resolution and lung function improvement, at least in the first few days. This again may reflect the fact that at least some of these episodes are associated with increased airway eosinophilia and therefore represent an 'asthmatic' episode.

On the basis of these studies, both inhaled bronchodilators and oral corticosteroids are recommended, and appear justifiable, in the management of acute exacerbations of COPD.[11]

☐ ANTIBIOTICS

Infection in the airways has been recognised as a factor leading to an exacerbation of both asthma and COPD, usually associated with increased cough and often sputum production as well as breathlessness. Most of the 'infective' episodes in asthma are viral in origin and do not require antibiotic therapy.[3]

The need for antibiotic therapy for exacerbations of COPD is far less clear. Meta-analysis of the best controlled trials suggests a benefit from antibiotic therapy, albeit small. However, exacerbations of COPD are multifactorial in nature and their study has long suffered from the lack of a generally accepted definition. An exacerbation is predominantly a subjective episode in which the patient perceives a deterioration in their symptoms which may be of non-bacterial origin and hence neither require nor respond to antibiotic therapy.

□ DEFINITION OF 'EXACERBATION'

In 2000, based on patients' symptomatology, a working party defined an exacerbation as an episode of deterioration in the patient's symptoms beyond the normal daily variability, that persists for at least two days and requires a change in medication. The change in medication can include:

- □ increasing bronchodilator therapy (mild exacerbation)
- □ starting corticosteroids or antibiotics or both (moderate exacerbation), or
- □ hospital admission (severe exacerbation).

Note that the severity relates to *healthcare utilisation* rather than to the *pathological process.*

With this as a background, it has become possible to study exacerbations in a more consistent way than previously – although the definition fails to give guidelines on antibiotic therapy or its role.

Sputum microbiology would seem the obvious defining feature, but this has been viewed with a degree of cynicism – mainly because bacteria can be isolated from the sputum of about 40% of patients with COPD even in the stable state and isolation rates increase only slightly (50%) during exacerbations. Nevertheless, protected brush specimens confirm increased isolation rates for these low pathogenic organisms during exacerbations suggesting that they play a role.

□ PRINCIPLES OF HOST DEFENCE IN CHRONIC OBSTRUCTIVE PULMONARY DISEASE

A clearer understanding of the role of bacteria and stable-state colonisation versus an acute episode of infection has been derived from the application of basic principles of host defences in COPD.

About 10^4 viable organisms are inhaled daily; in health, these are cleared by primary lung defences (airway macrophages, bacteriostatic and bactericidal proteins, and the mucociliary escalator). When the bacterial load becomes excessive, secondary host defences (predominantly the neutrophil) are recruited in response to inflammatory signals generated by airway macrophages and epithelial cells. The bacterial load dependency on this secondary response has been clearly demonstrated in animal models[12] and verified in studies in humans.[13] Sputum samples derived from patients show that an increased inflammatory response in the airways is generated only when the bacterial load exceeds 10^6 colony forming units per ml (Fig 2). It is not just the presence but the number of bacteria that mobilises the host

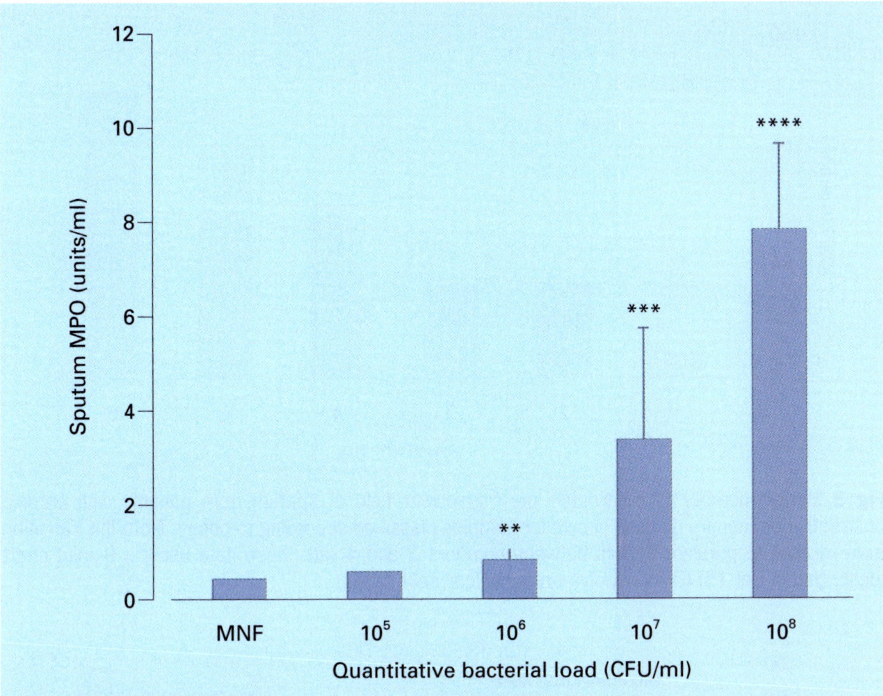

Fig 2 The average (± standard error) myeloperoxidase (MPO) concentration in sputum samples related to the absence (ie mixed normal mouth flora (MNF) or presence of a colonising organism categorised by the size of the bacterial load. MPO is a granule protein that reflects neutrophil number and activation (** = p <0.01; *** = p <0.001; **** = p <0.0001 compared with MNF) (CFU = colony forming unit) (data adapted from Ref 13).

'infection' response. Recent data have suggested that it is a change in the bacteria (detected phenotypically) that results in an exacerbation, perhaps because the new species evades local immune defences.[14]

The subsequent enhanced neutrophil response is reflected in the release of its contents, including the enzyme myeloperoxidase. This protein is green, determining the visual appreciation of purulence. This can be confirmed by comparison with a standardised colour chart;[15] when present, it visibly reflects not only the neutrophil content (Fig 3) but also the likelihood that bacteria will be isolated (Fig 4).

Clinical study of chronic obstructive pulmonary disease exacerbations

This principle has been utilised in a clinical study of exacerbations of COPD.[16] Patients presenting with purulent sputum had increased airways neutrophilia and inflammation[16] and a new or increased bacterial load.[17] These features resolved with antibiotic therapy. On the other hand, patients who presented with mucoid sputum had bacteria no more frequently than in the stable clinical state and the bacterial load (when present) was similar to the stable state.[16] These patients recovered without antibiotic therapy.

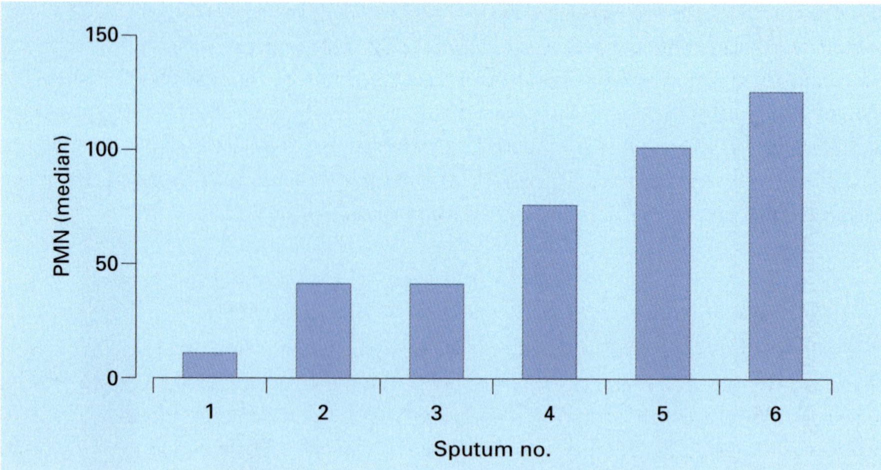

Fig 3 Median number of neutrophils per high-power field of sputum from patients with chronic obstructive pulmonary disease shown for samples classified according to colour. Note the transition from mucoid to purulent occurs between numbers 3 and 4 with these data using a 9-point chart (described in Ref 15) (PMN = polymorphonuclear neutrophils).

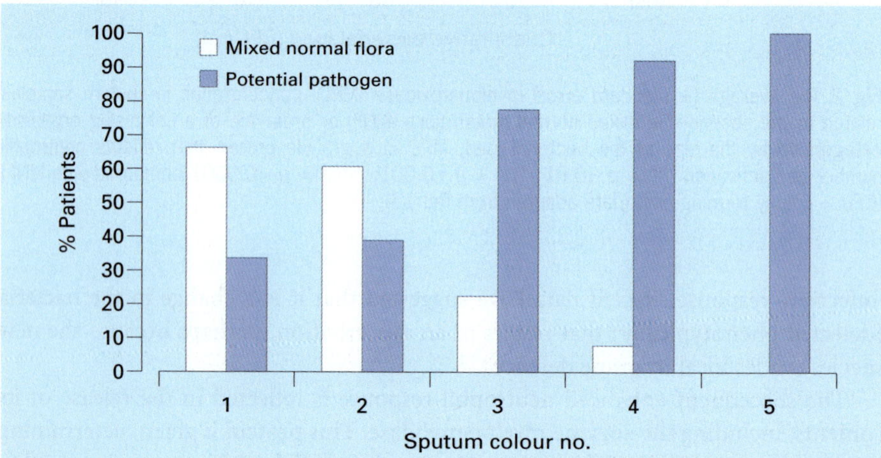

Fig 4 Isolation of bacterial species regarded as potential pathogens (solid histograms) versus negative culture or mixed normal mouth flora (open histograms) from sputum samples obtained from chronic obstructive pulmonary disease patients (indicated as percentage). The samples were classified as colour number using a simplified 5-point colour chart. Note the transition from mucoid to purulent occurs between numbers 2 and 3.

This was not a controlled clinical trial, but the results are consistent with the best such trial in which documented symptoms of exacerbations were examined both overall and in a subgroup analysis.[18] The three key symptoms were breathlessness, increased sputum volume and new or increased sputum purulence. The results for the whole group showed a benefit, but this was clear only in the subgroup with all three symptoms: that is, those who by definition also had to have purulent sputum.

The data indicate that antibiotics play a role in exacerbations of COPD, but it seems logical to restrict their use to those in whom purulent sputum is a feature, reflecting neutrophil recruitment as part of the episode. Ideally, a measure of the bacterial load should also be obtained but it is usually a reflection of the degree of visible purulence.

This overall approach is similar to that regularly employed in the assessment and treatment of urinary tract infections where the presence of both neutrophils and a bacterial load greater than 10^5 organisms per ml indicates the need for therapy.

□ PROPHYLACTIC THERAPY

The frequency of exacerbations relates both to lower health status and decline in lung function, so it seems logical to prevent such episodes where possible. Early studies suggested that prophylactic antibiotics can reduce these episodes,[19] but this approach has not been generally adopted because of concerns about bacterial resistance. More recent studies have shown that inhaled corticosteroids reduce exacerbations and they are now recommended for the most severely affected patients with frequent (>3 per year) exacerbations. Similarly, long-acting beta2-agonists[20] and anticholinergic agents[21] reduce exacerbation frequency. Many patients now take these agents because of the improvement in their health status and lung function even in the stable state.

It remains unknown which type of exacerbation these treatments prevent, but it seems likely that the main effect would be to reduce the impact of increased inflammation and bronchospasm rather than the prevention of infection.

The role and efficacy of influenza vaccination in prevention of infective exacerbations is still uncertain but is recommended for patients with COPD.[11]

□ CONCLUSIONS

Treatment and prevention of exacerbations of COPD are broadly along the lines used for asthma, but a better understanding of the pathophysiology of the episodes has led to rationalisation of antibiotic therapy, at least in COPD, and will promote the development of new therapies. Studies indicate that inhaled corticosteroids or long-acting beta2-agonists reduce the frequency and severity of exacerbations and should be prescribed for patients who have frequent or severe episodes. The efficacy of these treatments has been determined through clinical studies but it is critical to remember that significant results for a group do not indicate individual responses. The aetiology, and hence pathophysiology, of exacerbations is varied and further studies of the nature of the individual episodes may lead to more carefully targeted therapy.

REFERENCES

1 Seemungal TA, Donaldson GC, Paul EA, Bestall JC *et al.* Effect of exacerbation on quality of life in patients with chronic obstructive pulmonary disease. *Am J Respir Crit Care Med* 1998;**157**(5 Pt 1):1418–22.

2 Dowson LJ, Guest PJ, Stockley RA. Longitudinal changes in physiological, radiological, and health status measurements in alpha(1)-antitrypsin deficiency and factors associated with decline. *Am J Respir Crit Care Med* 2001;**164**(10 Pt 1):1805–9.

3 British Thoracic Society; Scottish Intercollegiate Guidelines Network (SIGN). British guideline on the management of asthma. *Thorax* 2003;**58**(Suppl 1):i1–94.

4 Pizzichini E, Pizzichini MM, Gibson P, Parameswaran K *et al.* Sputum eosinophilia predicts benefit from prednisone in smokers with chronic obstructive bronchitis. *Am J Respir Crit Care Med* 1998;**158**(5 Pt 1):1511–7.

5 Calverley PM, Burge PS, Spencer S, Anderson JA, Jones PW. Bronchodilator reversibility testing in chronic obstructive pulmonary disease. *Thorax* 2003;**58**:659–64.

6 Mahler DA, Wire P, Horstman D, Chang CN *et al.* Effectiveness of fluticasone propionate and salmeterol combination delivered via the Diskus device in the treatment of chronic obstructive pulmonary disease. *Am J Respir Crit Care Med* 2002;**166**:1084–91.

7 Jones PW, Bosh TK. Quality of life changes in COPD patients treated with salmeterol. *Am J Respir Crit Care Med* 1997;**155**:1283–9.

8 Seemungal TA, Donaldson GC, Bhowmik A, Jeffries DJ, Wedzicha JA. Time course and recovery of exacerbations in patients with chronic obstructive pulmonary disease. *Am J Respir Crit Care Med* 2000;**161**:1608–13.

9 Karpel JP, Pesin J, Greenburg D, Gentry E. A comparison of the effects of ipratropium bromide and metaproterenol sulfate in acute exacerbations of COPD. *Chest* 1990;**98**:835–9.

10 O'Donnell DE, Lam M, Webb KA. Spirometric correlates of improvement in exercise performance after anticholinergic therapy in chronic obstructive pulmonary disease. *Am J Respir Crit Care Med* 1999;**160**:542–9.

11 British Thoracic Society. BTS guidelines for the management of chronic obstructive pulmonary disease. *Thorax* 1997;**52**(Suppl 5):S1–28.

12 Onofrio JM, Toews GB, Lipscomb MF, Pierce AK. Granulocyte-alveolar-macrophage interaction in the pulmonary clearance of *Staphylococcus aureus. Am Rev Respir Dis* 1983;**127**:335–41.

13 Hill AT, Campbell EJ, Hill SL, Bayley DL, Stockley RA. Association between airway bacterial load and markers of airway inflammation in patients with stable chronic bronchitis. *Am J Med* 2000;**109**:288–95.

14 Sethi S, Evans N, Grant BJ, Murphy TF. New strains of bacteria and exacerbations of chronic obstructive pulmonary disease. *N Engl J Med* 2002;**347**:465–71.

15 Stockley RA, Bayley D, Hill SL, Hill AT *et al.* Assessment of airway neutrophils by sputum colour: correlation with airways inflammation. *Thorax* 2001;**56**:366–72.

16 Stockley RA, O'Brien C, Pye A, Hill SL. Relationship of sputum color to nature and outpatient management of acute exacerbations of COPD. *Chest* 2000;**117**:1638–45.

17 White AJ, Gompertz S, Bayley DL, Hill SL *et al.* Resolution of bronchial inflammation is related to bacterial eradication following treatment of exacerbations of chronic bronchitis. *Thorax* 2003;**58**:680–5.

18 Anthonisen NR, Manfreda, Warren CP, Hershfield ES *et al.* Antibiotic therapy in exacerbations of chronic obstructive pulmonary disease. *Ann Intern Med* 1987;**106**:196–204.

19 Elmes PC, Fletcher CM, Dutton AA. Prophylactic use of oxytetracycline for exacerbations of chronic bronchitis. *BMJ* 1957;**3**:1272–5.

20 Rennard SI, Anderson W, ZuWallack R, Broughton J *et al.* Use of long-acting inhaled beta2-adrenergic agonist, salmeterol xinafoate, in patients with chronic obstructive pulmonary disease. *Am J Respir Crit Care Med* 2001;**163**:1087–92.

21 Brusasco V, Hodder R, Miravitlles M, Korducki L *et al.* Health outcomes following treatment for six months with once daily tiotropium compared with twice daily salmeterol in patients with COPD. *Thorax* 2003;**58**:399–404.

Pulmonary embolism: the difficult diagnosis

Paul Corris

□ INTRODUCTION

Pulmonary embolism (PE) would appear to be both under- and overdiagnosed in clinical practice, leading to one group of patients failing to receive treatment for a potentially life-threatening problem and another receiving potentially life-threatening treatment for a disease which is not present. In one audit, PE was not suspected clinically in 70% of patients in whom it was subsequently found to have been the major cause of death (although most patients had associated advanced other disease).[1] On the other hand, in 63% of patients previously diagnosed as having PE, this was not confirmed on autopsy.[2]

There is now a wealth of information that allows a rational approach to the management of suspected PE, but ignorance remains widespread and much current practice is unsatisfactory. Attempts to confirm the diagnosis are flawed as a result of difficulties in the local implementation of guidelines and the 'fear factor' causing physicians to decide that it is better to treat than not. Diagnostic strategies differ between acute presentations to the acute medical unit and patients already hospitalised.[3] In early studies most patients had moderate to severe embolism since the diagnosis of PE had to rely on clinical assessment and basic investigations.

Current evidence suggests that there is a much lower recurrence rate in untreated patients with either proven or probable small emboli and an identifiable point cause (eg recent lower limb surgery, air travel duration >6 hours). In a series of almost 8,000 hip replacements there were 83 postoperative deaths due to sudden PE; in the 308 patients who survived postoperative PE and were not anticoagulated there were only 10 recurrences, none fatal.[4] A review of the PIOPED pulmonary angiogram database found that in 20 patients not anticoagulated because smaller PEs had been overlooked there were only two recurrences, only one of which was fatal.[5]

The perceived danger of failing to treat a patient with a small PE may therefore be more than matched by the consequences of overdiagnosing the condition. The well recognised, but often overlooked, risks of oral anticoagulation should be considered. Other aspects to consider are:

- □ the inevitable worry and further unnecessary treatment should chest symptoms recur
- □ the inappropriate withdrawal of oral contraceptives
- □ mandatory anticoagulation during future pregnancies, and

- compromised insurance prospects if a diagnosis is made and treatment commenced inappropriately.

A further paradox of the 'fear factor' is the well recognised rate of recurrence (5–27%) 10-24 months after ceasing warfarin therapy for patients with idiopathic PE (no treatment risk factor). Physicians worry more about missing PE at initial presentation than about the duration of warfarin treatment to prevent further PEs.

The problem of both under- and overdiagnosis in the past has been in part due to overreliance on the ability of ventilation perfusion scanning to diagnose or exclude PE. The real value of accurate D-dimer testing is in the *exclusion* of PE in patients presenting with symptoms suggestive of this diagnosis rather than its widespread application to any patient presenting to hospital with respiratory symptoms leading to unwarranted protracted investigation to exclude PE if the D-dimer is positive.

CLINICAL FEATURES

A number of clinical scoring systems have been used to help decide about a clinical diagnosis of PE. In practice, their value is greatest when combined with the results of investigations which help to increase the probability of ruling in or ruling out PE. Nevertheless, in three situations clinical examination alone can be helpful.

Dyspnoea plus tachypnoea

Large studies have shown that dyspnoea plus tachypnoea (defined as respiratory rate >20 per min) is absent in only 10% of patients, and only 3% of patients with proven PE have neither tachypnoea nor pleuritic pain. The rest have either chest radiography changes or a low PaO_2. The absence of all these clinical features virtually excludes the diagnosis of PE.[6] Clinical investigation and direct investigations may make a positive diagnosis of other cardiac and respiratory conditions mimicking PE, including myocardial infarction (MI), left heart failure, pericarditis, dissecting aneurysm, pneumothorax or pneumonia.

Distinctive features

In practice, there are subgroups of patients with distinctive features indicating that PE presents in one of three main ways.

Pulmonary haemorrhage with pleuritic pain and/or haemoptysis

In patients with pulmonary haemorrhage, pleuritic pain and/or haemoptysis, chest radiographic changes are commonly located to the site of pleuritic pain but the ECG is often normal. This large group has the lowest severity, as assessed by pulmonary angiography which usually shows emboli to be peripheral rather than central; arterial gas tensions may be normal. Radiographic changes may clear rapidly in otherwise healthy patients, confirming that the commonest underlying pathology associated with PE is pulmonary haemorrhage without infarction.

Isolated dyspnoea

Acute breathlessness in the absence of other symptoms is termed 'isolated dyspnoea'. The thrombus is more likely to be central in such cases, leading to hypoxaemia.

Circulatory collapse

Patients presenting with hypotension and/or loss of consciousness with central chest tightness may have circulatory collapse. Common signs relate to faintness on sitting up and jugular vein engorgement. Suggestive ECG changes are common, but the chest radiograph may be unremarkable. Blood gas analysis commonly shows marked hypoxia, often accompanied by hypocapnia due to alveolar hyperventilation. This group of patients has the most extensive vascular occlusion and urgent echocardiography may confirm the presence of an acutely dilated and failing right ventricle.

Unexplained chest opacity, breathlessness and/or deep venous thrombosis

Most patients, including young adults and the elderly, have PE presenting with one of the patterns described above. The others may be diagnosed on the basis of an unexplained opacity on the chest radiograph accompanied by breathlessness and/or clinical deep venous thrombosis (DVT).

The most difficult diagnosis of PE is in patients with chronic symptomatic pre-existing cardiorespiratory disease. Diagnosis is difficult both because they can rapidly decompensate with a relatively small embolism and also because the clinical ECG and radiographic findings may mainly reflect underlying disease. The diagnosis is particularly problematic in patients with pre-existing severe chronic obstructive pulmonary disease (COPD) or interstitial fibrosis. Clues to the presence of PE may be a sudden deterioration associated with worsening hypoxaemia without evidence of significant changes in FEV_1 or vital capacity and in the absence of new radiographic changes. Table 1 indicates the main clinical presentations of PE.

It is essential for all clinicians to establish the clinical probability of PE prior to organising specific investigations because the specificity of their investigations is improved by the clinical probability. A useful assessment based on the Weils score can be found in the British Thoracic Society guidelines.[7]

☐ SPECIFIC INVESTIGATIONS FOR VENOUS THROMBOEMBOLISM

Plasma D-dimer

Venous thromboembolism (VTE) leads to activation of fibrin degradation, so there has been considerable interest in the development of blood assays to demonstrate this process. The most promising is the D-dimer, a breakdown product of cross-linked fibrin. Values are so rarely within the normal range in those with active VTE that this test can be used effectively to rule out PE in patients presenting with symptoms compatible with this diagnosis. The only false negatives reported in

Table 1 The main clinical presentations of pulmonary embolism.

	Collapse, previously well	**Pulmonary haemorrhage**	**Isolated dyspnoea**	**Collapse, poor reserve**
Frequency (%)	5	60	25	10
Pulmonary artery occlusion	Extensive	Small/moderate	Moderate/large	Small/moderate
Examination	Acute right heart strain	May have localising signs	Tachypnoea	Unhelpful
Chest radiograph	Usually normal	Often suggestive	Usually normal	May be suggestive
ECG	Often acute right heart strain	Normal	Non-specific changes	Unhelpful
Arterial gas exchange	Markedly abnormal	May be normal	Usually abnormal	Unhelpful

several large studies have been in patients with a high clinical suspicion of PE based on history and examination. D-dimer levels are commonly raised in other patients presenting to hospital with inflammatory diseases, so the great value of D-dimer assays is to exclude – but NOT confirm – VTE.

In practice, the test is of greatest value in non-hospitalised patients presenting acutely to hospital with chest pain. The demonstration of a normal D-dimer level in such a patient should mean no further investigation to try to find a diagnosis of PE.[8] However, investigations must then be continued to find a definitive diagnosis of the cause of such symptoms because the exclusion of PE does not indicate a satisfactory clinical end-point. The value of the test is less clear-cut in hospitalised patients because many of them will have raised levels as a consequence of their underlying disease process unrelated to VTE. A number of D-dimer assays are available and currently under assessment by the National Institute for Clinical Excellence:

- The SimpliRED test is simple and based on a qualitative red cell agglutination assay. It has a negative predictive valve of 85% of normal, rising to 95% if the clinical probability is low.
- The Vidus test is a rapid quantitative ELISA test of lower specificity than SimpliRED but with a high negative predictive value of 99%.
- The MDA-D-dimer latex test also has a negative predictive value of 99%.

All tests should be performed in the laboratory, and all trusts should establish local negative predictive values and set the normal level for their own assay.

Leg imaging

The logic of leg imaging lies in the fact that most patients with PE have proximal leg clots even in the absence of evidence of DVT. Leg vein imaging may be indicated in the assessment of PE as a first-line investigation in those with clinical DVT or in patients with chronic cardiorespiratory disease, particularly if the symptoms suggest small peripheral emboli with lung haemorrhage and pleural pain when spiral computed tomography (SPCT) may have a lower sensitivity. Compression ultrasound enhanced by the addition of colour Doppler imaging is now the optimal leg imaging technique. Such techniques allow demonstration of DVT affecting iliac, femoropopliteal and calf veins. The failure to identify thrombus in the lower limb in a patient suspected of having a PE may simply indicate that all pre-existing thrombus has passed to the lungs; proximal clot is seen in only 23–52% of patients with confirmed PE. Leg imaging for PE has become less well used with the advent of CT pulmonary angiography (see below).

Ventilation perfusion imaging

Ventilation perfusion imaging has the advantage of being non-invasive and widely available, but few hospitals offer a seven-day on-call service. Imaging is safe in pregnant women suspected of having PE. Ventilation scans are obtained using ^{81m}Kr, technegas, Tc-DTPA aerosol or xenon-133. Perfusion scanning is performed by the intravenous (iv) injection of ^{99m}Tc-labelled macroaggregates of albumin or human albumin microspheres, with the patient supine to reduce the gravitational effects of pulmonary circulation. After injection, scanning should be performed within 24 hours of clinical suspicion of PE since some scans revert to normal quickly (half do so within a week).

The problem with ventilation perfusion scanning is that many patients investigated for suspected PE have pre-existing conditions that result in an indeterminate scan. Such situations include:

- previous PE unless a follow-up scan has been performed
- left heart failure, which can cause regional variations in pulmonary perfusion
- COPD with non-homogeneous ventilation and areas in which the vascular bed may be constricted due to hypoxia
- fibrosis where there are patchy unmatched defects in both ventilation and perfusion
- proximal lung cancer causing vascular occlusion leading to a marked perfusion defect with preserved ventilation.

The limitation of ventilation perfusion scanning may be one reason why many physicians have previously been prepared to make management decisions without any specific imaging of PE. The previously noted problem of both under- and overdiagnosis may also in part be due to the previous overreliance on the potential ability of ventilation perfusion scanning to diagnose or exclude PE. In practice, as few as 11% of scans may confirm or exclude PE. However, a completely normal scan excludes PE with absolute confidence.

Spiral computed tomographic scanning

SPCT (or, more accurately described, helical or constant volume CT) scanning can detect intravascular clot in the pulmonary trunk to segmental arteries. Studies suggest good sensitivity and specificity for central or segmental thrombus, making SPCT scanning the investigation of choice in patients with isolated dyspnoea and in those with pre-existing cardiopulmonary disease. Emboli in small subsegmental pulmonary arteries may not be reliably visualised – although studies suggest sensitivity is increasing. It is essential to give high-volume contrast (150–200 ml) and to optimise the timing of the scan with respect to contrast injection to show the pulmonary circulation. The advent of the multiple slice scanner has improved sensitivity of this technique to demonstrate emboli in peripheral vessels.

Outcome studies have shown that negative scans are associated with recurrent PE over the subsequent three months in only 1% of patients. There has been widespread recognition of the value of SPCT to confirm or rule out suspected PE in patients. However, the logistical issues in terms of availability of scanning on an urgent basis in many hospitals still cause problems despite guidelines advocating SPCT as the investigation of first choice.

Pulmonary angiography

Pulmonary angiography may be considered in patients with suspected PE where other investigations have failed to give a firm diagnosis but where it is still strongly suspected on clinical grounds. However, there are practical problems in that the films should be inspected by a radiologist experienced in undertaking and reporting pulmonary angiography. This situation does not exist in the UK and studies show interobserver disagreements in 30% of cases.

Urgent echocardiography

In patients with suspected PE, echocardiography can both establish and exclude the diagnosis. The echocardiogram may demonstrate right ventricular dilatation and hypokinesis, pulmonary artery enlargement, normal septal movement and lack of inferior vena cava collapse during inspiration or tricuspid regurgitation. The clot may be demonstrated in the right heart or main pulmonary arteries.

The advantage of this investigation is that conditions which may mimic PE (eg MI, aortic dissection, pericardial tamponade) may easily be distinguished; thus, it not only helps confirm or exclude a diagnosis of PE but also offers an alternative diagnosis.

□ INITIAL TREATMENT

Low molecular weight heparin

PE remains a difficult diagnosis because once a diagnosis has been confirmed there are choices regarding the best options for therapy. There is clear evidence that subcutaneous (sc) low molecular weight heparin (LMWH) is at least as effective as continuous iv heparin for most patients. However, the iv route may still be preferable in some cases, including situations where the rapid onset of a heparinised state is required to help prevent further formation of new thrombi. This may be an issue in patients with pre-existing severe cardiorespiratory disease. Another relative indication for iv therapy is when it may be deemed necessary rapidly to reverse anticoagulation should bleeding occur; iv heparin has advantages here over sc LMWH.

A large PE is probably best treated by an initial iv dose of heparin (5,200 units), followed by sc LMWH.

Thrombolysis

Further consideration should be given to the role of thrombolytic therapy in patients who have a massive PE leading to haemodynamic upset or even right ventricular dysfunction on echocardiography.

There is still no clear consensus about the true role of thrombolytic therapy in patients with PE. Studies have demonstrated more rapid relief of symptoms and abnormal haemodynamics but clear, definitive survival advantage has not yet been consistently demonstrated. Nevertheless, current teaching supports the use of thrombolytic therapy administered via a peripheral vein in patients with haemodynamic compromise as a result of PE. Patients with PE with evidence of right ventricular dysfunction or raised troponin T as a result of right ventricular strain may also be candidates for thrombolysis. Thrombolysis is effective by iv recombinant tissue plasminogen activator (eg alteplase 100 mg over 90 min). The risk of major haemorrhage is approximately twice that for heparin.

☐ DURATION OF ANTICOAGULATION

How long to continue anticoagulation remains a difficult area in all but those who have an easily identifiable point cause for VTE. However, recurrence during and after treatment is unusual where there are temporary risk factors for VTE (eg surgery). Most studies on duration of anticoagulation suggest that treatment for 3–6 months is adequate in the absence of coexistent underlying risk factors or thrombotic disorder such as antithrombin 3 deficiency or factor V Leiden deficiency.[9,10]

The situation is not so clear-cut in patients without a temporary risk factor. In studies of large groups of patients presenting with VTE, the overall risk of recurrent emboli after discontinuing warfarin is relatively high (5–27%).[11-13] When stopping anticoagulation is considered in patients without a temporary risk factor they should have blood taken to exclude a prothrombotic disorder, the presence of which should indicate lifelong anticoagulation.[14] Patients without underlying prothrombotic disorder should be monitored and, if there is recurrent VTE, considered for lifelong anticoagulation aiming at a low target level of international normalised ratio (1.5–2).[13] There is a role for the use of D-dimer testing as part of the monitoring process.[15]

☐ CONCLUSIONS

Despite major advantages in imaging and other modalities, PE remains a difficult diagnosis. Not only are there problems in confirming a diagnosis in certain clinical situations but there are also uncertainties about the best initial therapeutic strategy and the duration of warfarin therapy. Finally, several new agents (including fondiparinux and ximelagatran) have been developed which have considerable advantages over the current anticoagulants. It is likely that these will ultimately replace existing therapies given that they do not require careful monitoring.

☐ TAKE-HOME MESSAGES

1. When in doubt, do not think it is better to treat than *not* – further investigation to confirm is mandatory.
2. V/Q imaging is *not* the best initial imaging modality for most cases; it must be avoided in established cardiopulmonary disease.
3. Patients with good quality negative SPCT do *not* need further investigation or treatment for PE. They do need a diagnosis.

4 Further work is needed to determine the optimum duration of anticoagulation in patients with idiopathic PE.

REFERENCES

1 Stein PD, Henry JW. Prevalence of acute pulmonary embolism among patients in a general hospital and at autopsy. *Chest* 1995;**108**:978–81.

2 Modan B, Sharon E, Jelin N. Factors contributing to the incorrect diagnosis of pulmonary embolic disease. *Chest* 1972;**62**:388–93.

3 Barritt DW, Jordan SC. Anticoagulant drugs in the treatment of pulmonary embolism. A controlled trial. *Lancet* 1960;**i**:1309–12.

4 Johnson R, Charnley J. Treatment of pulmonary embolism in total hip replacement. *Clin Orthop* 1997;**124**:149–54.

5 Stein PD, Hendry JW, Relyea B. Untreated patients with pulmonary embolism. Outcome, clinical and laboratory assessment. *Chest* 1995;**107**:931–5.

6 British Thoracic Society Standards of Care Committee Pulmonary Embolism Guideline Development Group. British Thoracic Society guidelines for the management of suspected acute pulmonary embolism. *Thorax* 2003;**58**:470–83.

7 Optimum duration of anticoagulation for deep-vein thrombosis and pulmonary embolism. Research Committee of the British Thoracic Society. *Lancet* 1992;**340**:873–6.

8 Perrier A, Bounameaux H, Morabia A, de Moerloose P *et al.* Diagnosis of pulmonary embolism by a decision analysis-based strategy including clinical probability, D-dimer levels, and ultrasonography: a management study. *Arch Intern Med* 1996;**156**:531–6.

9 ten Cate JW, Koopman MM, Prins MH, Buller HR. Treatment of venous thromboembolism. *Thromb Haemost* 1995;**74**:197–203.

10 Schulman S, Rhedin AS, Lindmarker P, Carlsson A *et al.* A comparison of six weeks with six months of oral anticoagulant therapy after a first episode of venous thromboembolism. Duration of Anticoagulation Trial Study Group. *N Engl J Med* 1995;**332**:1661–5.

11 Kearon C, Gent M, Hirsh J, Weitz J *et al.* A comparison of three months of anticoagulation with extended anticoagulation for a first episode of idiopathic venous thromboembolism. *N Engl J Med* 1999;**340**:901–7.

12 Agnelli G, Prandoni P, Santamaria MG, Bagatella P *et al.* Three months versus one year of oral anticoagulant therapy for idiopathic deep venous thrombosis. *N Engl J Med* 2001;**345**:165–9.

13 Ridker P, Goldhaber SZ, Danielson E, Rosenberg Y *et al.* Long-term, low-intensity warfarin therapy for the prevention of recurrent venous thromboembolism. Warfarin Optimal Duration Italian Trial Investigators. *N Engl J Med* 2003;**348**:1425–34.

14 Hyers TM. Duration of anticoagulation in venous thromboembolism. *Arch Intern Med* 2003;**163**:1256–66.

15 Palareti G, Legnani C, Cosmi B, Valdre L *et al.* Predictive value of D-dimer test for recurrent venous thromboembolism after anticoagulation withdrawal in subjects with a previous idiopathic event and in carriers of congenital thrombophilia. *Circulation* 2003;**108**:313–8.

Community-acquired pneumonia

Mark Woodhead

☐ INTRODUCTION

Community-acquired pneumonia (CAP) is one of many common types of respiratory infection, but especially important because it is associated with significant morbidity and mortality. It occurs in about one per 1,000 of the adult population per year but is more common in the very young and very old. Most cases are managed outside hospital, but data from 1998 through to 2003 suggest that, in England at least, the number admitted to hospital has increased by up to 30% in all age groups except those younger than 15 years (Fig 1).[1] Growth in the elderly population, reduced general practitioner (GP) out-of-hours work and changing public expectations are all possible contributors to this trend. The fall in GP consultations for respiratory tract infections demonstrates that it is not due to a general increase in the frequency of pneumonia. The importance of correct recognition and treatment is thus especially important for those working in hospital where mortality is 5–10%, rising to 50% in those admitted to the intensive care unit (ICU).

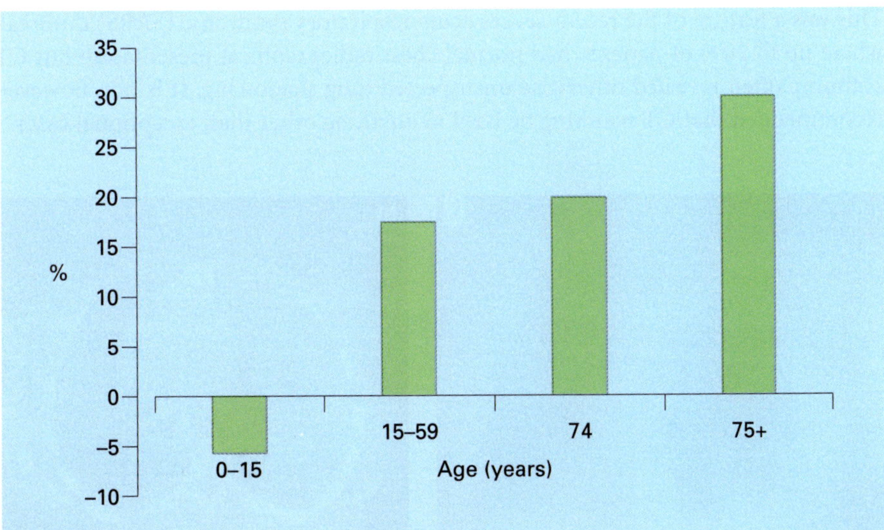

Fig 1 Change in hospital admission for pneumonia (ICD J10–J18) England between 1998–1999 and 2002–2003.[1]

□ DIAGNOSIS

Diagnosis in hospital is usually straightforward, based on the presence of acute respiratory symptoms, often accompanied by fever and focal chest clinical signs and confirmed by lung shadowing on a chest radiograph. The most common differential diagnosis is a non-pneumonic acute exacerbation of chronic obstructive pulmonary disease (COPD); this may share similar symptoms but radiographic lung shadowing is absent. This distinction is important as the clinical management of these two conditions is different (for further discussion on this, see the first chapter in this section).

In the elderly, the diagnosis may be less certain as symptoms may be non-specific (eg acute neurological deterioration, absence of fever) and the coexistence of other pathologies may make physical signs and radiographic changes less easy to interpret (eg lung shadowing in left ventricular failure). In these circumstances, raised peripheral blood white cell count or C-reactive protein (CRP) may point to the diagnosis of pneumonia. There remains a lack of consensus whether CRP can also be a marker of illness severity or of any individual causal pathogen.

It is important (particularly, but not exclusively, in younger patients) to seek pointers (eg intravenous (iv) drug use, sexual habits) to the presence of recognised or unrecognised immune compromise which might point to opportunist pathogens possibly requiring different diagnostic and therapeutic approaches.

Rarely, the chest radiograph may be normal, especially if a patient with pneumonia is seen very early in their illness. A repeat chest radiograph after an interval may be helpful, and computed tomography (CT) scanning of the thorax may show lung changes of pneumonia not visible on the chest radiograph (Fig 2). This was a feature of the recent severe acute respiratory syndrome (SARS) outbreak where up to 30% of patients had normal chest radiographs at presentation but CT scanning often revealed otherwise unsuspected lung shadowing. It is not, however, recommended that CT scanning be used in anything other than exceptional cases.

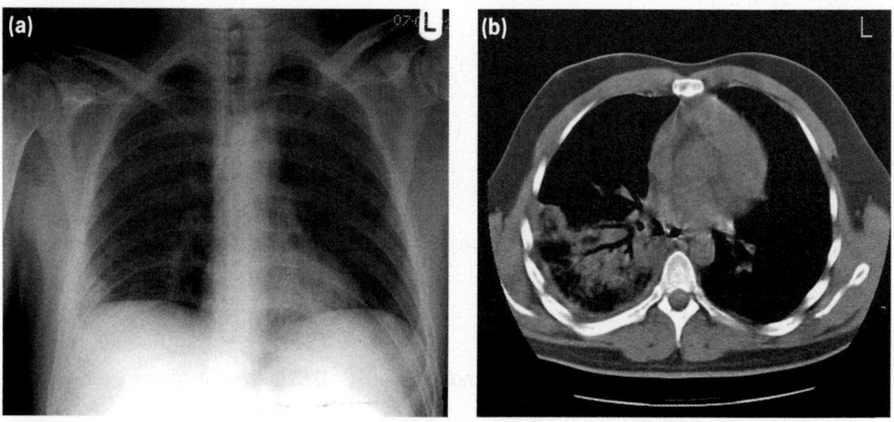

Fig 2 Patient with clinical presentation compatible with pneumonia: **(a)** chest X-ray shows only minimal shadowing in right costophrenic recess; **(b)** contemporary computed tomography scan shows extensive consolidation.

☐ SEVERITY ASSESSMENT

Most of those patients at risk of death can be identified from severity markers available at hospital admission. Similarly, those with non-severe illness, who could be managed at home can also be highlighted in the same way. There have been no prospective studies (which would probably be unethical) to show that severity assessment alters outcome, but retrospective studies suggest benefit. The consensus is that this approach is good clinical practice.

A multicentre study of adults admitted to hospital with CAP in the UK identified the presence of two or more of the following three features as markers of severe illness:

- respiratory rate
- diastolic blood pressure, and
- blood urea.

A New Zealand study improved the prognostic value of this approach by the addition of mental confusion. A limitation of this method is that it produces only two severity categories: severe and non-severe. In a more recent, large multinational study, the risk of death was related to the number of risk factors present when age (65 or above) was also included.[2] This allows patient stratification into three management groups according to risk (Fig 3). This approach uses readily available clinical and laboratory data and is simple to apply and is easily remembered as the **CURB65** score (**C**onfusion, **U**rea, **R**espiratory rate, **B**lood pressure and age **≥65**).

A pneumonia severity index (PSI) has been developed in North America which similarly links admission clinical and laboratory features with outcome, but uses

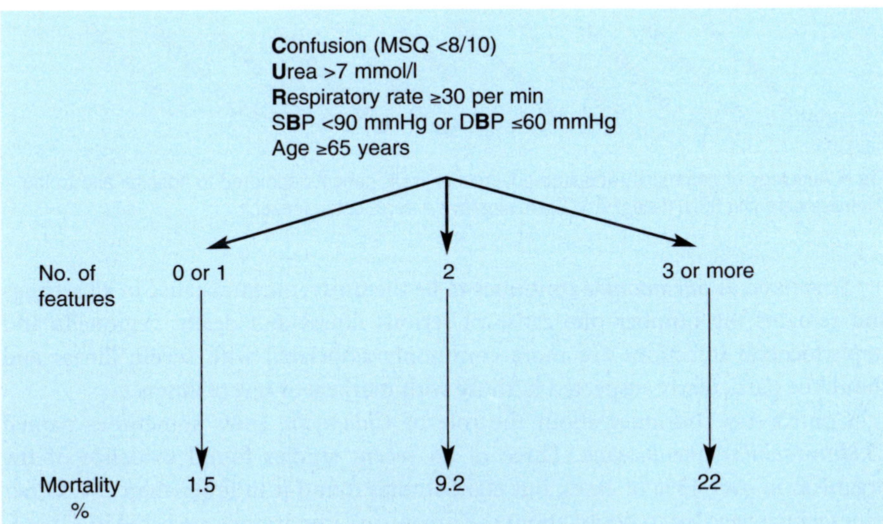

Fig 3 CURB65 score. Severity assessment in community-acquired pneumonia (DBP = diastolic blood pressure; MSQ = mental status questionnaire; SBP = systolic blood pressure).[3]

20 variables and is therefore more difficult to apply in clinical practice.[3] The stratification of patients into three management groups can be used to guide place of care (home, hospital, ICU), microbial investigation, clinical review strategy and antibiotic therapy (see section on treatment).

□ MICROBIAL AETIOLOGY

Knowledge of causative pathogens, based on prospective studies, is important as a guide to treatment, especially since the causative pathogen is not usually identified in an individual patient in routine practice.[4] The commonly identified microorganisms are well-known (Fig 4).

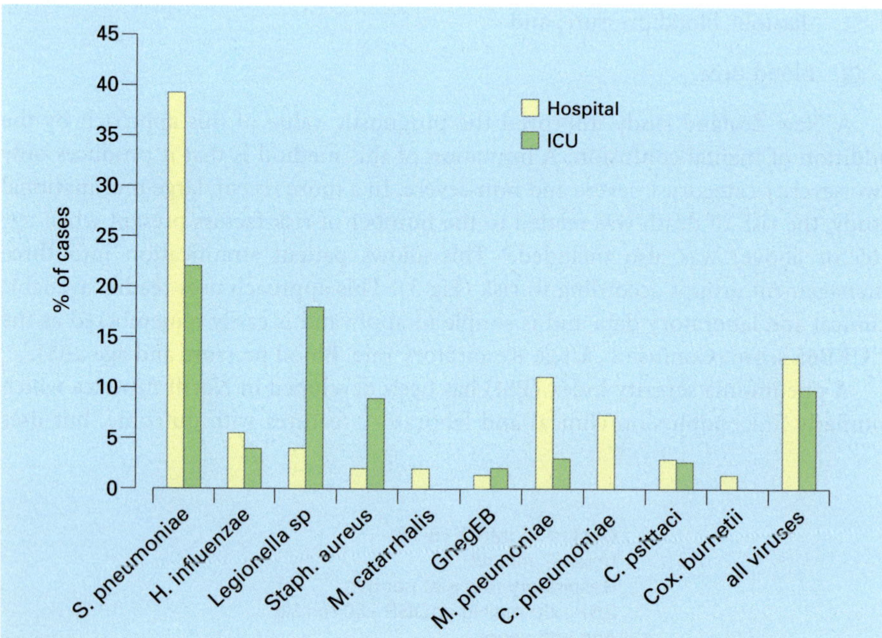

Fig 4 Aetiology of community-acquired pneumonia in UK patients admitted to hospital and to the intensive care unit (ICU) (GnegEB = Gram-negative enterobacteriaceae).[6]

Streptococcus pneumoniae continues to be the most common cause in all settings and remains the number one cause of serious illness and death. Legionella and staphylococcal infections are more commonly associated with severe illness and should be particularly suspected in those with markers of severe illness.

Controversy continues about the role of *Chlamydia* (now sometimes named *Chlamydophila*) *pneumoniae.* Three of 16 recent studies found evidence of the organism in over 15% of cases, but eight studies found it in fewer than 5%. Other issues which have led to doubt about the organism's importance are listed in Table 1. The current consensus is that its possible presence can probably be ignored other than in patients who are severely ill.

Table 1 Reasons to doubt the need for specific antibiotic therapy against *Chlamydia pneumoniae* in community-acquired pneumonia.

- Currently no satisfactory microbiological test
- Other bacterial pathogens (mainly *Streptococcus pneumoniae*) present in up to 74%
- Recovery common with antibiotics to which *C. pneumoniae* is not susceptible
- Organism may persist after clinical recovery

North American studies have generally included a higher proportion of nursing home residents than those from the UK and Europe. They suggest that different antibiotic therapy is required for such patients as Gram-negative enterobacteriaceae and *Staphylococcus aureus* form a significant portion of the spectrum of causative organisms. However, a recent UK study found no such difference in causative pathogens in nursing home residents.

Severe acute respiratory syndrome

The recent outbreak of pneumonic illness caused by the SARS coronavirus is a timely reminder that new or known, but uncommon, causes of CAP can occur at any time. This possibility needs to be considered if the clinical picture is unusual or the patient fails to respond to therapy. The principal problem with SARS is how to recognise a potentially fatal and transmissible lung infection presenting with features common to other common respiratory infections and for which there is no recognised curative therapy. At the time of writing, sporadic cases of SARS are occurring in Southern China but it is not currently known whether spread to other countries will occur as in the original outbreak.

☐ ANTIBIOTIC RESISTANCE

Acquired resistance to antibiotics in common pathogenic bacteria is a growing problem. Resistance to penicillins, macrolides and fluoroquinolones in *S. pneumoniae* is of great potential relevance to the management of CAP. Frequency of resistance in an individual bacterium varies according to its isolation source and few studies have sought such information in patients with CAP. Most available data on *S. pneumoniae* include a large number of childhood upper respiratory tract and eye isolates which appear to exhibit higher resistance rates than isolates from patients with CAP. In a recent study of isolates of *S. pneumoniae* from lower respiratory tract samples (ie including, but not exclusively, CAP) in Great Britain, only 0.3% showed clinically relevant penicillin resistance.[5] In a separate, recent UK study only one of 129 cases of pneumococcal CAP had a penicillin resistant organism.[4] Resistance to penicillins is a graded phenomenon and the frequency and levels currently encountered in the UK, with the exception of meningeal infections, are insufficient to lead to penicillin failure. Macrolide resistance in *S. pneumoniae* is more common than penicillin resistance and, like fluoroquinolone resistance (currently rare), has been associated with microbiological failures in CAP. For this and other reasons (see later) penicillins remain the preferred antibiotic choice in CAP.

☐ MICROBIOLOGICAL TESTS

Debate about the continued use of the common tests of sputum examination and blood culture is topical. Many studies have shown the insensitivity of such tests in routine clinical practice. Recent studies have confirmed that blood cultures are positive in 14% of patients at best, and 6% at worst, leading to few alterations in treatment. One study found a correlation between blood culture positivity and CAP severity, but another found no such relationship.

In patients who are severely ill, where correct choice of antibiotic might be more likely to influence outcome than in the non-severely ill, rigorous investigation, including blood cultures and sputum examination, is appropriate. In the non-severely ill patient, where the patient is at low risk of adverse outcome and pathogen identification is unlikely to alter therapy, blood culture and sputum examination may be omitted. Sputum samples should be examined only when sputum is purulent and prior antibiotics have not been given.

There is little or no evidence that microbiological tests alter outcome, but one recent study during an outbreak of Legionnaires' disease found that early diagnosis using the urine legionella antigen test led to early appropriate antibiotic therapy and significant reduction in mortality and use of intensive care compared with those diagnosed late. All hospital laboratories can do, or have access to, this test, which is therefore recommended for all those with CAP with signs of severe illness, where clusters of cases occur or during a known outbreak.

☐ TREATMENT

Non-antibiotic treatment

Non-invasive ventilation

Correction of fluid balance and gas exchange abnormalities, coupled with appropriate antimicrobial therapy, are the cornerstones of therapy for CAP. The principles of fluid balance and gas exchange management have not changed significantly, but a new approach to the correction of gas exchange, non-invasive ventilation (NIV), is now available in most hospitals. For most patients with CAP, the provision of an increased inspired oxygen fraction is sufficient to correct hypoxia. For those who remain hypoxic, but normo- or hypocapnic, the use of continuous positive airway pressure may be useful. However, in the presence of hypercapnia and respiratory acidosis, additional measures such as NIV may help.

NIV has been pioneered as an acute treatment for non-pneumonic exacerbations of COPD in the presence of hypercapnic respiratory failure and respiratory acidosis where the predominant problem is often simply inadequate ventilation. Inadequate ventilation does occur in severe CAP, but the condition is often more complex, with shunting due to failure of hypoxic vasoconstriction in the consolidated lung as well as the additional systemic effects of severe sepsis. Studies in adults with CAP have shown that NIV may be associated with reduced tracheal intubation and death rates compared with conventional therapy.[6] However, the intubation rate appears to be higher (up to 66%) than in non-pneumonic exacerbations of COPD. While NIV may prevent intubation in some patients, it should be used with the knowledge that intubation remains likely. Thus, it should be used only where facilities for intubation are immediately available.

Antibiotic treatment

Antibiotic management is based principally on assessment of illness severity and knowledge both of the likely causative pathogens and of antibiotic sensitivities (as discussed above). Until recently, a combination of antibiotics was needed to cover all possible causative pathogens as no single antibiotic had the necessary spectrum of activity. Two new fluoroquinolones, levofloxacin and moxifloxacin, are now available with the potential to be used as monotherapy because they have activity against all common causative organisms. The appropriate place for these new agents continues to be debated. Currently, they are recommended only when other first-line antibiotics are contraindicated (eg hypersensitivity) or where institutional issues (eg prevalence of *Clostridium difficile*-related illness) exclude the use of first-line antibiotics. There are several reasons for this:

- lack of randomised controlled trial (RCT) data showing clear advantage
- lack of clinical experience with their use (compared with older well-known agents)
- potential for development of resistant *S. pneumoniae* during treatment (levofloxacin)
- lack of an iv formulation (moxifloxacin)
- lack of a licence for severe CAP (moxifloxacin), and
- potential for promotion of colonisation with methicillin-resistant *S. aureus* (MRSA).

Non-severely ill patients

Legionella and staphylococcal infections are unlikely in the non-severely ill patient. The main pathogens to be covered are therefore *S. pneumoniae* and possibly mycoplasma in younger adults. There continues to be debate about the adequacy of narrow spectrum therapy focused on *S. pneumoniae* (eg penicillin) in this group and whether broader cover to include atypical organisms is necessary. No adequately powered RCTs are available to answer this question, so the antibiotic choice has to be based on weaker evidence. In some countries such as Sweden patients are mostly managed with antibiotic monotherapy (mainly penicillin and cephalosporins), with no evidence that outcome is any worse than in the UK. On the other hand, a number of retrospective studies have shown higher mortality in those treated with monotherapy (usually a beta-lactam) than when this is combined, for example, with a macrolide.

British guidelines suggest that for non-severely ill patients, suitable for home management, a beta-lactam or macrolide alone is adequate (Table 2), but for those admitted to hospital a combination of the two is recommended unless the admission is for non-clinical reasons or the patient has not received prior antibiotics. North American guidelines favour a macrolide or fluoroquinolone as first choice, based largely on a higher rate of penicillin resistance and different perceptions of the importance of atypical infections and potential adverse effects of overuse of fluoroquinolones.

Table 2 Antibiotic recommendations for community-acquired pneumonia from the British Thoracic Society guidelines.[7]

Severity of illness	Treatment
Home treated, not severe*	Amoxicillin 500 mg-1 g tds po
Hospital treated, not severe* (admitted for non-clinical reasons or previously untreated)	Amoxicillin 500 mg-1 g tds po
Hospital treated, not severe**	Oral: Amoxicillin 500 mg-1 g tds *plus* Erythromycin 500 mg qds *or* Clarithromycin 500 mg bd
***	If intravenous: Ampicillin 500 mg qds *or* Benzylpenicillin 1.2 g qds *plus* Erythromycin 500 mg qds *or* Clarithromycin 500 mg bd
Hospital treated, severe ****	Co-amoxiclav 1.2 g qds *or* 2nd/3rd generation Cephalosporin *plus* Erythromycin 500 mg qds *or* Clarithromycin 500 mg bd *plus or minus* Rifampicin

Alternatives:
* Erythromycin 500 mg qds *or* clarithromycin 500 mg bd
** Fluoroquinolone with enhanced pneumococcal activity (eg levofloxacin, moxifloxacin)
*** Levofloxacin 500 mg od iv
**** Levofloxacin 500 mg od iv *plus* benzylpenicillin 1.2 g qds

Severely ill patients

In more severely ill patients, where risk of death is higher, antibiotic cover must be broader to include all possible pathogens. In this situation, the combination of a beta-lactam and a macrolide remains the treatment of choice.

Treatment duration

Duration of antibiotic therapy should be guided by clinical progress. In a number of studies, usually in countries where a longer duration of parenteral therapy has been the norm, switching patients from iv to oral therapy has been found to be safe using a variety of clinical parameters. The non-severely ill patient, even in hospital, may not need more than oral therapy. Therapy for 5–7 days is usually adequate, but longer may be necessary for the more severely ill patient.

☐ CONCLUSIONS

There are many aspects to the management of patients with this common condition, some of which have been discussed in this chapter. These and other issues are usefully captured in national and international guidelines, to which the reader is referred for further information.[7-9] The frequency, morbidity and mortality of CAP mean that careful attention must continue to be paid to its correct diagnosis and management.

REFERENCES

1 http://www.doh.gov.uk/hes/free_data/index.html

2 Lim WS, van der Eerden MM, Laing R, Boersma WG *et al.* Defining community acquired pneumonia severity on presentation to hospital: an international derivation and validation study. *Thorax* 2003;**58**:377–82.

3 Fine MJ, Auble TE, Yealy DM, Hanusa BH *et al.* A prediction rule to identify low-risk patients with community-acquired pneumonia. *N Engl J Med* 1997;**336**:243–50.

4 Lim WS, Macfarlane JT, Boswell TC, Harrison TG *et al.* Study of community acquired pneumonia aetiology (SCAPA) in adults admitted to hospital: implications for management guidelines. *Thorax* 2001;**56**:296–301.

5 Reynolds R, Shackcloth J, Felmingham D, MacGowan A. Antimicrobial susceptibility of lower respiratory tract pathogens in Great Britain and Ireland 1999–2001 related to demographic and geographical factors: the BSAC Respiratory Resistance Surveillance Programme. *J Antimicrob Chemother* 2003;**52**:931–43.

6 Confalonieri M, Potena A, Carbone G, Porta RD *et al.* Acute respiratory failure in patients with severe community-acquired pneumonia. A prospective randomized evaluation of noninvasive ventilation. *Am J Respir Crit Care Med* 1999;**160**:1585–91.

7 BTS Guidelines for the Management of Community Acquired Pneumonia in Adults. *Thorax* 2001;**56**(Suppl 4):IV1–64. *Note*: updated 2004, see http://www.brit-thoracic.org.uk/docs/MACAPrevisedApr04.pdf

8 Niederman MS, Mandell LA, Anzueto A, Bass JB *et al.* Guidelines for the management of adults with community-acquired pneumonia. Diagnosis, assessment of severity, antimicrobial therapy, and prevention. *Am J Respir Crit Care Med* 2001;**163**:1730–54.

9 Mandell LA, Bartlett JG, Dowell SF, File TM Jr *et al.* Update of practice guidelines for the management of community-acquired pneumonia in immunocompetent adults. *Clin Infect Dis* 2003;**37**:1405–33.

☐ RESPIRATORY SELF ASSESSMENT QUESTIONS

Asthma or chronic obstructive pulmonary disease? Managing the acute exacerbation

1 Bacteria:
(a) Cause 50% of exacerbations in chronic obstructive pulmonary disease (COPD)
(b) Colonisation is present in 40% of COPD patients
(c) Positive culture requires antibiotic therapy
(d) Lead to exacerbations of asthma
(e) Are a contraindication for steroid therapy

2 Exacerbations:
(a) Of COPD influence disease progression
(b) Of COPD usually reflect bacterial or viral infection
(c) Of COPD may be associated with eosinophils
(d) Of COPD are prevented by inhaled anticholinergic therapy
(e) Of asthma are prevented by inhaled anticholinergic therapy

3 COPD:
(a) Is airflow obstruction that is non-reversible
(b) Is improved by long-acting beta2-agonists
(c) Exacerbations are associated with increased airflow obstruction
(d) Air trapping can be improved with no change in FEV_1
(e) Inhaled beta2-agonists reduce bacterial exacerbations

Pulmonary embolism: the difficult diagnosis

1 A 68-year-old smoker with chronic obstructive pulmonary disease (COPD) presents with acute shortness of breath associated with pleuritic pain, worsening hypoxia and no change in FEV_1. A V/Q scan shows an indeterminate result:
(a) The scan should not have been carried out
(b) The result excludes pulmonary embolism (PE)
(c) PE is clinically likely and a spiral computed tomography with contrast is appropriate
(d) Acute exacerbation of COPD is most likely

2 D-dimer test:
(a) All D-dimer tests have the same sensitivity and specificity for PE
(b) If raised in a patient presenting with clinical features of pneumonia, should provoke a series of investigations to exclude coexistent PE
(c) Should be used as a bedside test
(d) If normal, effectively excludes PE

3 Thrombolysis for PE:
(a) Should be given to patients with PE whose respiratory rate is over 25 per minute

(b) Should not be considered in patients over 65 years
(c) Increases the rate of recovery in hypotensive patients
(d) Has approximately a fourfold higher rate of haemorrhage than warfarin

4 Idiopathic PE with no reversible cause:
(a) Has a low risk of recurrence after three months' treatment with warfarin
(b) Does not require a thorough search for a thrombotic tendency
(c) Indicates the need for an inferior vena cava filter
(d) Should be treated acutely by thrombolysis rather than by low molecular weight heparin (LMWH)

5 In the acute investigation and management of PE:
(a) Patients presenting with significant breathlessness should receive a loading dose of intravenous heparin prior to LMWH
(b) Tropinin T may indicate the presence of right ventricular strain
(c) A clinical estimate of probability should be formally made prior to arranging investigations
(d) V/Q scan is contraindicated in pregnancy

Community-acquired pneumonia

1 Severe community-acquired pneumonia (CAP) is commonly caused by:
(a) *Streptococcus pneumoniae*
(b) *Streptococcus pyogenes*
(c) *Staphylococcus aureus*
(d) *Haemophilus influenzae*
(e) *Moraxella catarrhalis*

2 The following are markers of illness severity used in the CURB65 score:
(a) Hypoxia
(b) Hyponatraemia
(c) Confusion
(d) Blood urea >7 mmol/l
(e) Respiratory rate >25 per min

3 The following are statements about antibiotic resistance:
(a) *In vivo* resistance always translates into clinical antibiotic failure
(b) Penicillin resistance is present in over 50% of *S. pneumoniae* isolates in the UK
(c) Penicillins cannot be used in the presence of penicillin resistance in *S. pneumoniae*
(d) Resistance is more common in bacteria isolated from the upper respiratory tract of children
(e) Fluoroquinolone resistance in *S. pneumoniae* has not been recorded

4 Concerning antibiotic therapy in CAP:
(a) Oral therapy is preferred where appropriate
(b) Amoxicillin is the therapy of choice for the patient managed at home
(c) An antibiotic combination is essential for all admitted to hospital
(d) A beta-lactam plus a macrolide is the treatment of choice for the severely ill patient
(e) Fluoroquinolones offer an alternative for those unable to take first choice antibiotics

Gastroenterology

Management of dyspepsia

John Atherton

□ INTRODUCTION

The management of dyspepsia, especially for patients presenting to general practitioners (GPs) or pharmacists, is a fast-evolving topic, for several reasons:

- the recognition of *Helicobacter pylori* as the cause of most peptic ulceration and much gastric adenocarcinoma
- the rapidly changing prevalence of diseases causing dyspepsia (increase in gastro-oesophageal reflux (GORD) and related diseases and decrease in *H. pylori* and related diseases)
- the realisation that treatable gastric cancer rarely presents with dyspepsia alone, and
- the economic drive to avoid investigations such as upper gastrointestinal (GI) endoscopy when clear evidence of benefit is lacking.

These issues have led practice away from the traditional approach of making a diagnosis (in this case usually by upper GI endoscopy) and treating the condition, towards a new approach of investigating patients only if they have 'alarm symptoms'. This approach is encapsulated in recent management guidelines from several countries, including those from the Scottish Intercollegiate Guideline Network (SIGN) in 2003.[1] The National Institute for Clinical Excellence (NICE) will publish UK guidelines on the management of dyspepsia in the community in the summer of 2004.

□ DEFINITIONS, PREVALENCE AND ECONOMIC IMPORTANCE

Unfortunately, dyspepsia is defined differently in different clinical studies and by different guideline writers and epidemiologists. The broadest definition is 'any group of symptoms alerting doctors to consider disease of the upper GI tract' and includes symptoms such as epigastric pain, heartburn, bloating, eructation, nausea, vomiting and dysphagia. Many guidelines, including previous British Society for Gastroenterology (BSG)[2] and future NICE guidelines have adopted this pragmatic definition. Clinical trials have used a variety of definitions, leading to difficulties in comparing results; this led in 1999 to a consensus panel developing a tighter definition, referred to as Rome II.[3] This definition is 'pain or discomfort centred predominantly in the upper abdomen for at least 12 weeks in the last year'. The

Rome II definition is used in the SIGN guidelines, although without the time element.

Differences in dyspepsia definition not only make application to guidelines of results from clinical trials difficult but also affect the measured prevalence of dyspepsia. Using the pragmatic definition, the community prevalence of dyspepsia is 25–50%, while with the Rome II definition it is 15–30%, the main difference being due to exclusion of predominant heartburn in the latter. About 50% of people with dyspepsia self-medicate, 25% consult their GPs, 5% of the latter being primarily for dyspepsia by its wider definition. Dyspepsia is also a huge cost to the nation: in 2000, prescribed drugs and investigations (including endoscopy) cost £600 million, and in the year 2002 £100 million-worth of remedies were sold over-the-counter for indigestion. Given these figures, it is clear why dyspepsia should be a target for national guidelines.

□ CAUSES OF DYSPEPSIA AND PREDICTIVE VALUE OF SYMPTOMS

The causes of dyspepsia can broadly be divided into three groups (Table 1):

- □ diseases outside the upper GI tract
- □ structural diseases of the upper GI tract (where endoscopy can identify the cause), and
- □ diseases where endoscopy is normal.

One of the central tenets of dyspepsia management is that individual symptoms have repeatedly been shown to be poor predictors of the underlying cause.[4] An exception is heartburn, which has fairly good predictive value for GORD, whether erosive or non-erosive. However, heartburn is also a common presenting symptom of peptic ulceration and modern management of the two conditions is different. Other patient characteristics, such as age, body habitus and response to starting or stopping acid-suppressing drugs, can make one or other diagnosis more or less likely – but, ultimately, without investigation the diagnosis is an informed guess.

Table 1 Common causes of dyspepsia.

Location	Cause
Outside the upper GI tract	Numerous, including pathology affecting the heart, lung, liver, gall bladder, pancreas and lower GI tract Some systemic illnesses
Upper GI tract, diagnosed at upper GI endoscopy	Reflux oesophagitis Duodenal ulceration Gastric ulceration Oesophageal carcinoma Gastric carcinoma
Upper GI tract with normal upper GI endoscopy	Non-erosive gastro-oesophageal reflux disease Functional dyspepsia

GI = gastrointestinal.

Using alarm symptoms to select patients for endoscopy

One way in which guidelines seek to limit upper GI endoscopy use is to confine it to patients with 'alarm symptoms' (Table 2).[1] There have been mixed findings from several studies that have addressed the value of alarm symptoms in predicting severe underlying causes of dyspepsia, but there is agreement that most symptomatic patients with upper GI cancer have one or more alarm symptoms.

Table 2 Alarm symptoms/signs prompting urgent referral for upper gastrointestinal (GI) endoscopy.

- Haematemesis or malaena*
- Dysphagia**
- Weight loss
- Persistent vomiting
- Abdominal mass
- Anaemia due to possible GI blood loss

* Requires same day referral and usually urgent hospital admission.
** Many endoscopists consider barium swallow safer for high dysphagia.

The best evidence comes from retrospective studies. For example, a study from Glasgow of 169 patients with gastric cancer showed that only five presented without alarm symptoms and that all these five had metastatic disease.[5] Several prospective population-based studies have shown that even alarm symptoms are poorly predictive of cancer, although their sensitivity is good. However, investigating people with alarm symptoms does not help diagnose early (curable) cancer. Indeed, there is no good evidence that early gastric cancer presents with dyspepsia. This should not be surprising because a small lesion in a large hollow organ such as the stomach might be predicted not to cause symptoms. Thus, the presence of symptoms, whether simple dyspepsia or alarm symptoms, appears not to be able to identify patients with curable gastric cancer.

A logical extension to this argument is that there is no rationale for upper GI endoscopy for patients at any age presenting with simple dyspepsia. Older people are more likely to have gastric cancer as the condition is age-related, but there is no clear evidence that endoscopy for older patients with simple dyspepsia will pick up more curable gastric cancer than endoscopy of the asymptomatic population. Further research is urgently required in this area.

□ UPPER GASTROINTESTINAL ENDOSCOPY

The presence of alarm symptoms with dyspepsia increases, at least modestly, the chance of endoscopy yielding a positive finding. However, even in the absence of a positive finding, endoscopy provides reassurance to a patient with worrying symptoms and to his physician and other carers. Endoscopy is often also of value to hospital inpatients requiring investigation for dyspepsia. Such patients will often have alarm symptoms, but even in their absence endoscopy may be valuable to exclude or make diagnoses based on other symptoms or to guide management of unrelated conditions, for example whether to anticoagulate for various thromboses in borderline cases.

Preparation for endoscopy

When endoscopy is planned, it is important to maximise the information that can be obtained.

Acid suppression

Acid-suppressing drugs should preferably be withheld for two weeks before endoscopy, if possible for longer, because they may heal ulcers and oesophagitis and result in false-negative findings. If it is not feasible to withhold treatment, it is better to give antacids or, if necessary, H_2-receptor antagonists (H_2RAs) as these drugs have no anti-*H. pylori* activity.

Drugs that affect Helicobacter pylori testing

Antibiotics and bismuth compounds should not be given for four weeks before endoscopy if *H. pylori* tests are to be accurate. Proton-pump inhibitors (PPIs) should be used only if absolutely necessary because they too can render biopsy-based tests for *H. pylori* false-negative. They should be omitted for at least two weeks before endoscopy and four weeks may be even better. If *H. pylori* status is needed for a patient on PPIs, it is still worth taking gastric biopsies but these should be from corpus as well as antrum. In this situation, a positive test is helpful but a negative test less so. One option in this situation is to use serology if previous specific treatment for *H. pylori* has not been given. A second option is to decide from the endoscopy results whether knowledge of *H. pylori* status is necessary; if it is thought necessary, PPIs should be withdrawn and replaced with H_2RAs with a urea breath test (UBT) performed at least four weeks later.

Management of patients after endoscopy is straightforward.

□ MANAGEMENT OF CONDITIONS CAUSING DYSPEPSIA DIAGNOSED AT ENDOSCOPY

Duodenal ulceration

Up to 90% of duodenal ulcers are secondary to *H. pylori* infection, so *H. pylori* should be treated and successful eradication confirmed by UBT four weeks later. There is no further need for acid suppression after *H. pylori* treatment, although many physicians give acid suppression for a month for large chronic ulcers or those that have bled. The management of ulcers caused by aspirin or non-steroidal anti-inflammatory drugs (NSAIDs) is discussed later.

Gastric ulceration

More gastric ulcers than duodenal ulcers are caused by aspirin/NSAIDs. Some are caused by gastric malignancies, although the main cause is *H. pylori* which should be sought and treated. Gastric ulcers sometimes heal more slowly and most physicians prescribe acid-suppressing drugs until the ulcer has healed. Gastric ulcer healing should be confirmed by endoscopy to exclude malignancy, and biopsy specimens taken for histological examination.

Gastric or oesophageal adenocarcinoma

Adenomas, both gastric and oesophageal, are managed by surgery, chemotherapy, radiotherapy and/or palliative measures where appropriate.

Reflux oesophagitis

Management of reflux oesophagitis is with PPIs at a healing dose and lifestyle advice, followed by reduction of the PPI dose to that needed to control symptoms. Although PPIs currently appear safe for long-term use, many physicians prefer to substitute H_2RAs or even antacids if symptoms are well controlled.

Normal endoscopy

If endoscopy is normal, it is useful to divide patients into those with predominant reflux symptoms and those with other symptoms. Many of the former group will have abnormal acid reflux on 24-hour pH monitoring, although this is rarely performed. A pragmatic approach is to manage such patients (assumed to have GORD) with PPIs. Symptoms usually respond well.

Functional dyspepsia

Patients fulfilling Rome II criteria for dyspepsia but with a normal upper GI endoscopy are difficult to manage. The 'diagnosis' of functional dyspepsia has a benign prognosis although many patients are still symptomatic after 10 years. Because of its benign course and frequent resistance to treatment, the mainstay of management is reassurance. Lifestyle advice is often given to avoid smoking, reduce alcohol intake, avoid precipitating foods (especially fatty foods) and to lose weight, although there is no hard evidence that these changes help symptoms.

A few patients respond to specific treatments, but the disadvantage is that these treatments do not work for most of them. Thus, the costs for the successful treatment of a few cases are unnecessary side effects for the majority of patients, financial costs (in terms of drugs and consultations) and, if managed poorly, loss of confidence in physicians and erosion of the doctor-patient relationship.

Treatment studies

Four large studies of patients with functional dyspepsia who were colonised with *H. pylori* compared *H. pylori* eradication with PPIs (using PPIs and antibiotics) with no eradication (using PPIs and placebos).[6-9] Only one, in a population with a high background prevalence of peptic ulcer disease, showed a significant benefit of treatment.[6]

Three meta-analyses from these and other studies have produced conflicting conclusions. The most recent calculated a one-year 43% response (defined as minor symptoms or none) compared with 36% in control groups, giving a 7% advantage over PPIs alone (95% confidence interval 4–10%) and a number-needed-to-treat of 14 to get one response. The prevalence of *H. pylori* in patients with functional dyspepsia in the UK is approximately 50%, so the number needed to screen for *H. pylori* for one success is approximately 28. Despite this, some physicians believe that treatment is worthwhile because, if successful, a week of antibiotics will potentially abolish long-term symptoms as well as the associated drug and health service costs. Longer-term follow-up of the best studies will determine whether this is true. In the meantime, research is needed to try to identify which patients will respond, so that treatment can be more effectively targeted. One possibility is that responders are patients with the ulcer diathesis whose ulcers have remitted or were missed at endoscopy.

Proton pump inhibitors

The good response of the PPI group in the *H. pylori* eradication studies reinforces an older approach of using acid suppression for functional dyspepsia. However, four recent large, high quality studies found mixed results on the effectiveness of PPIs in functional dyspepsia: two showed overall benefit[10,11] and two no benefit.[11,12] One study showed benefit only in *H. pylori* colonised patients,[10] reinforcing the possibility that some of the response may be from treatment of the ulcer diathesis. A second, community-based study showed an advantage of treatment, but a hospital-based study with the same first author showed no significant benefit.[11] The difference between these studies may have been due to the inclusion of more patients with reflux symptoms in the community study. In support of this, the fourth study, from Hong Kong, where GORD is uncommon, showed no benefit of treatment.[12] Thus, one possibility is that the success of PPIs in the treatment of functional dyspepsia is in patients with GORD or with *H. pylori* and the ulcer diathesis. Taking the trials together, a recent meta-analysis showed benefit over placebo for PPIs of 11% and a number-needed-to-treat of 9.

Many physicians embark on a trial of PPI treatment arguing that it is simple with few side effects and may be effective. However, it is important to recognise that many responses may be due to the placebo effect. Long-term follow-up data are lacking.

Other treatments

Several studies have addressed the place of other treatments in functional dyspepsia, notably prokinetic drugs, cytoprotective agents and antidepressants, all of which show benefit in some cases. Further research is required to separate functional dyspepsia into pathophysiologically relevant groups which will respond more reliably to specific treatment modalities. In the meantime, a good pragmatic approach is to reassure and educate patients and perhaps advise on lifestyle as first-line management. For persistent cases with significant disturbance of lifestyle it may be worth trying treatment in the context of appropriate informed patient information, possibly starting with a PPI trial. A few patients with functional dyspepsia have persistent and troubling symptoms, occasionally including weight loss. Such patients should be referred to a gastroenterologist for further investigation; some of them will have an identifiable and treatable cause such as gastroparesis.

□ MODERN APPROACH TO MANAGEMENT OF DYSPEPSIA IN THE COMMUNITY

Avoiding unnecessary endoscopy

The approach to a patient with dyspepsia in the community starts with assessing whether symptoms may be caused by pathology outside the upper GI tract, then identifying and, if possible, stopping precipitating drugs (Table 3). Patients with alarm symptoms (Table 2) require urgent upper GI endoscopy. The rest can be managed with the knowledge that:

- □ *H. pylori* treatment is effective in curing non-NSAID ulcers
- □ PPIs are effective treatment for GORD, and
- □ treatable gastric adenocarcinoma rarely, if ever, presents with simple dyspepsia.

SIGN, BSG and future NICE guidelines are largely based on these premises. One possible algorithm is presented in Fig 1.

Table 3 Drugs commonly causing dyspepsia.

- Aspirin/NSAIDs
- Calcium antagonists
- Nitrates
- Theophyllines
- Etidronate
- Steroids

NSAID = non-steroidal anti-inflammatory drug.

'Test and treat' approach

Three large studies have addressed the issue of whether testing for *H. pylori* and treating those who are positive ('test and treat') or initial endoscopy has a better patient outcome for previously uninvestigated dyspepsia.[13-15] Endoscopies were reduced by about 75% in the test and treat group, but there was no significant difference in patient outcome between the strategies. It seems unlikely that these studies would have missed a benefit for endoscopy large enough to offset the financial advantages of the test and treat approach, although again long-term follow-up is lacking.

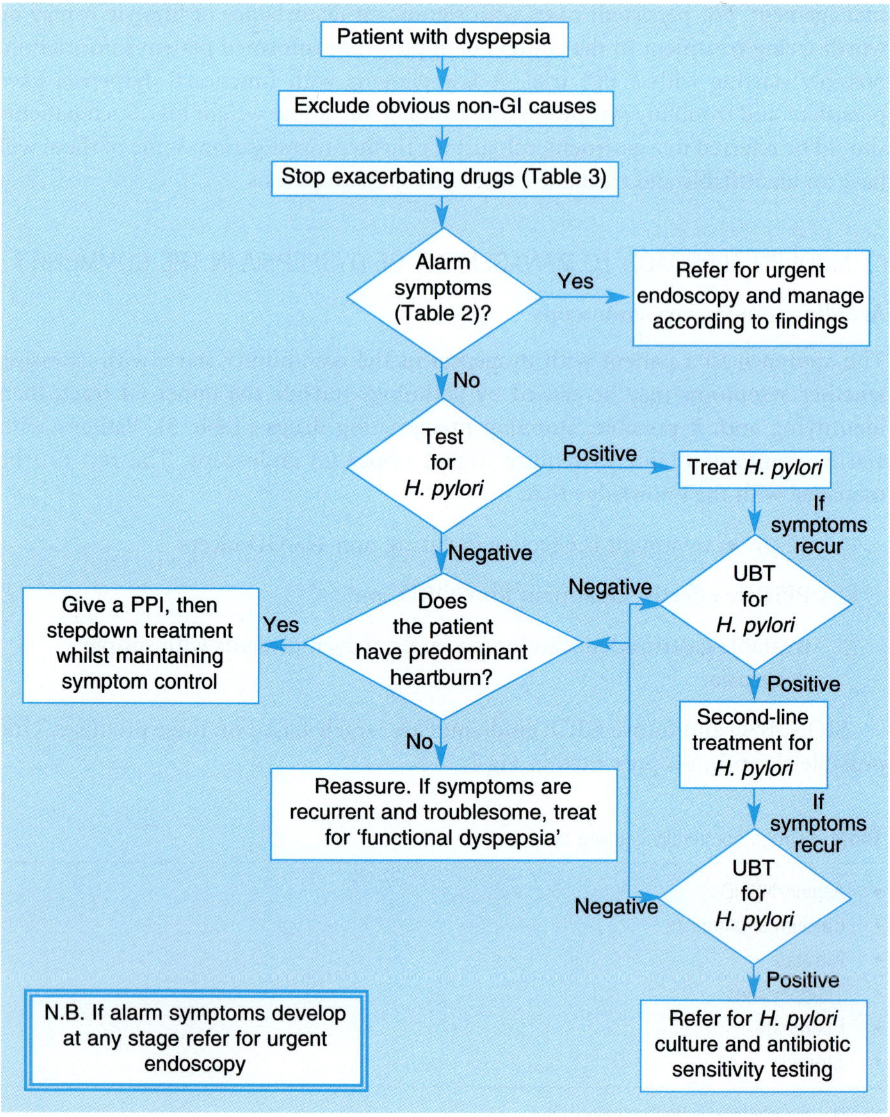

Fig 1 Simplified algorithm for one possible community management protocol for dyspepsia (GI = gastrointestinal; PPI = proton pump inhibitor). (For alternatives, see Refs 1 and 2, and NICE guidelines to be published summer 2004.)

An unanswered question is whether the test for *H. pylori* and treat strategy or a strategy of empirical acid suppression is better for the management of newly presenting dyspepsia in the community. For *H. pylori*-positive patients, two recent large trials show that *H. pylori* treatment is more effective.[16,17] However, modelling suggests that PPI treatment may be a more effective first approach where *H. pylori* prevalence is low. A large Medical Research Council (MRC) funded trial is now addressing this question in the community.

Management of *Helicobacter pylori* in the community

Identification

The UBT is the most accurate non-invasive test for *H. pylori* but also the most costly. A new stool antigen test is nearly as accurate but may not find acceptance in UK practice. Serology is accurate if the best hospital-based ELISAs are used and these are locally validated. Blood and serum tests which give near-immediate results and are designed for use in GP surgeries (near patient tests) are not accurate and should not be used. Antibiotics, PPIs and bismuth compounds should be avoided for four weeks before UBTs and stool tests, although these tests are usually accurate two weeks after finishing PPI treatment. Stopping drugs is not necessary for serum-based ELISAs, but these tests may be false-positive if the patient has recently had specific anti-*H. pylori* treatment or PPIs and concurrent antibiotics active against *H. pylori*. Properly validated serology is probably the most practical test in most situations.

Treatment

Treatment of *H. pylori* is now simple, with a one-week course of antibiotics taken twice a day (Table 4). The patient should be warned that close compliance is necessary for treatment success and that antibiotics should be continued in the face of mild side effects. These include a metallic taste from clarithromycin, bowel disturbance from amoxicillin and occasional nausea and the need to avoid alcohol for metronidazole. If severe diarrhoea develops, the drugs should be stopped. With good compliance, treatment is successful in about 90% of patients.

Most physicians do not check for eradication success unless symptoms recur or the patient has previously demonstrated duodenal ulceration. The UBT should then

Table 4 Recommended treatment regimens for *Helicobacter pylori*.

Treatment	Drugs	Duration
First-line		
Regimen 1[a]	Omeprazole 20 mg bd[b] Clarithromycin 500 mg bd Amoxicillin 1 g bd	7 days
Regimen 2	Omeprazole 20 mg bd[b] Clarithromycin 500 mg bd Metronidazole 400 mg bd	7 days
Second-line[c]	Omeprazole 20 mg bd[b] Bismuth subcitrate 120 mg qds Tetracycline hydrochloride 500 mg qds Metronidazole 400 mg tds	14 days

a Regimen 1 is preferable to regimen 2 for first-line therapy as it avoids the use of metronidazole, an important constituent of second-line therapy. Regimen 2 should be used if the patient is allergic to penicillins.
b Omeprazole may be replaced with any proton pump inhibitor at equivalent dose or, in regimens 1 and 2, with ranitidine bismuth citrate 400 mg.
c Various combinations based on ranitidine plus bismuth citrate are also effective second-line therapies. An alternative to 'blind' second-line therapy is to culture *H. pylori* and be guided by antibiotic sensitivities. Patients failing second-line therapy should be referred for consideration of endoscopy, *H. pylori* culture and antibiotic sensitivity.

be used because antibody titres drop too slowly for ELISAs to have any practical place in assessing therapeutic success.

Following treatment failure, a second-line drug regimen can be used (Table 4). Two failures should prompt referral for endoscopy, *H. pylori* culture, antibiotic sensitivity testing and appropriate guided therapy.

☐ ASPIRIN/NSAID ASSOCIATED DYSPEPSIA AND PEPTIC ULCERATION

NSAID-associated dyspepsia and ulceration should be minimised by a sensible prescribing policy. NSAIDs should be avoided if there is a sensible alternative; if they are necessary, those with low gastric toxicity such as ibuprofen should be prescribed at the lowest effective dose. In patients with dyspepsia or diagnosed peptic ulceration, NSAIDs should be stopped and a course of PPIs given. Immediate *H. pylori* eradication is not helpful, and may even marginally slow ulcer healing with PPIs, but *H. pylori* should be sought and at some stage usually eradicated.

There is good evidence that *H. pylori*-negative people are less likely to get peptic ulceration if they are started on NSAIDs; the same probably applies to restarting these drugs.[18,19]

H. pylori increases the risk of aspirin-induced ulceration and may increase the risk of ulceration for patients taking a specific selective cyclo-oxygenase-2 (COX-2) inhibiting NSAID. Whether patients requiring chronic NSAIDs and taking PPIs for ulcer protection should also have *H. pylori* eradicated remains controversial. For patients with successfully treated ulcers, the chance of future relapse if further NSAIDs are needed can be reduced by using a COX-2 inhibitor or co-prescribing a PPI.

☐ THE FUTURE OF DYSPEPSIA MANAGEMENT IN THE UK

Optimal dyspepsia management will change rapidly. The prevalence of dyspepsia is increasing and the prevalence of underlying diseases is changing: GORD and associated diseases, including oesophageal adenocarcinoma, are fast increasing in prevalence as is functional dyspepsia. The prevalence of peptic ulceration and gastric adenocarcinoma is decreasing with the falling prevalence of *H. pylori*. *H. pylori* antibiotic resistance is an increasing problem which requires central and local monitoring and may require future changes in treatment regimens. Changes in public health are needed to reduce GORD, and community management strategies are needed to reverse the rapid increase in oesophageal adenocarcinoma. NSAID- and aspirin-associated disease should be reduced by rational prescribing and perhaps primary prescription of COX-2 inhibitors in high-risk groups including the elderly.

Functional dyspepsia requires research to characterise the underlying pathophysiological mechanisms and allow subdivision into groups which will respond to specific treatment strategies. A wider and more effective range of management options is also needed.

Dyspepsia management is likely to remain a challenge in the UK. It is to be hoped that current and future guidelines do not encourage lazy thinking by clinicians and discourage badly needed research.

Acknowledgements

John Atherton is funded by a Senior Clinical Fellowship from the MRC UK.

REFERENCES

1 Dyspepsia. A national clinical guideline. Edinburgh: Scottish Intercollegiate Guideline Network, 2003. http://www.sign.uk

2 Dyspepsia management guidelines. London: British Society for Gastroenterology, 2002. http://www.bsg.org.uk/clinical_prac/guidelines/dyspepsia.htm

3 Talley NJ, Stanghellini V, Heading RC, Koch KL *et al.* Functional gastroduodenal disorders. Review. *Gut* 1999;**45**(Suppl 2):II37–42.

4 Talley NJ, Weaver AL, Tesmer DL, Zinsmeister AR. Lack of discriminant value of dyspepsia subgroups in patients referred for upper endoscopy. *Gastroenterology* 1993;**105**:1378–86.

5 Gillen D, McColl KE. Does concern about missing malignancy justify endoscopy in uncomplicated dyspepsia in patients aged less than 55? *Am J Gastroenterol* 1999;**94**:75–9.

6 McColl K, Murray L, El-Omar E, Dickson A *et al.* Symptomatic benefit from eradicating *Helicobacter pylori* infection in patients with nonulcer dyspepsia. *N Engl J Med* 1998;**339**:1869–74.

7 Blum AL, Talley NJ, O'Morain C, van Zanten SV *et al.* Lack of effect of treating *Helicobacter pylori* infection in patients with nonulcer dyspepsia. Omeprazole plus Clarithromycin and Amoxicillin Effect One Year after Treatment (OCAY) Study Group. *N Engl J Med* 1998;**339**:1875–81.

8 Talley NJ, Vakil N, Ballard ED 2nd, Fennerty MB. Absence of benefit of eradicating *Helicobacter pylori* in patients with nonulcer dyspepsia. *N Engl J Med* 1999;**341**:1106–11.

9 Talley NJ, Janssens J, Lauritsen K, Racz I, Bolling-Sternevald E. Eradication of *Helicobacter pylori* in functional dyspepsia: randomised double blind placebo controlled trial with 12 months' follow up. The Optimal Regimen Cures Helicobacter Induced Dyspepsia (ORCHID) Study Group. *BMJ* 1999;**318**:833–7.

10 Blum AL, Arnold R, Stolte M, Fischer M, Koelz HR. Short course acid suppressive treatment for patients with functional dyspepsia: results depend on *Helicobacter pylori* status. The Frosch Study Group. *Gut* 2000;**47**:473–80.

11 Talley NJ, Meineche-Schmidt V, Pare P, Duckworth M *et al.* Efficacy of omeprazole in functional dyspepsia: double-blind, randomized, placebo-controlled trials (the Bond and Opera studies). *Aliment Pharmacol Ther* 1998;**12**:1055–65.

12 Wong WM, Wong BC, Hung WK, Yee YK *et al.* Double blind, randomised, placebo controlled study of four weeks of lansoprazole for the treatment of functional dyspepsia in Chinese patients. *Gut* 2002;**51**:502–6.

13 Heaney A, Collins JS, Watson RG, McFarland RJ *et al.* A prospective randomised trial of a 'test and treat' policy versus endoscopy based management in young *Helicobacter pylori* positive patients with ulcer-like dyspepsia, referred to a hospital clinic. *Gut* 1999;**45**:186–90.

14 Lassen AT, Pedersen FM, Bytzer P, Schaffalitzky de Muckadell OB. *Helicobacter pylori* test-and-eradicate versus prompt endoscopy for management of dyspeptic patients: a randomised trial. *Lancet* 2000;**356**:455–60.

15 McColl KE, Murray LS, Gillen D, Walker A *et al.* Randomised trial of endoscopy with testing for *Helicobacter pylori* compared with non-invasive *H. pylori* testing alone in the management of dyspepsia. *BMJ* 2002;**324**:999–1002.

16 Chiba N, Van Zanten SJ, Sinclair P, Ferguson RA *et al.* Treating *Helicobacter pylori* infection in primary care patients with uninvestigated dyspepsia: the Canadian adult dyspepsia empiric treatment–*Helicobacter pylori* positive (CADET-*Hp*) randomised controlled trial. *BMJ* 2002;**324**:1012–6.

17 Manes G, Menchise A, de Nucci C, Balzano A. Empirical prescribing for dyspepsia: randomised controlled trial of test and treat versus omeprazole treatment. *BMJ* 2003;**326**:1118.

18 Chan FK, Sung JJ, Chung SC, To KF *et al.* Randomised trial of eradication of *Helicobacter pylori* before non-steroidal anti-inflammatory drug therapy to prevent peptic ulcers. *Lancet* 1997;**350**:975–9.

19 Chan FK, To KF, Wu JC, Yung MY *et al.* Eradication of *Helicobacter pylori* and risk of peptic ulcers in patients starting long-term treatment with non-steroidal anti-inflammatory drugs: a randomised trial. *Lancet* 2002;**359**:9–13.

Advances in gastrointestinal bleed management

Kelvin Palmer

□ INTRODUCTION

Acute upper gastrointestinal (GI) haemorrhage is responsible for about 25,000 hospital admissions each year in the UK, with an incidence of 50–150 cases per 10,000 per year and highest in areas of social deprivation. There is approximately 10% mortality among patients admitted to hospital because of acute GI haemorrhage; this has not changed over a half a century. In mitigation, case mix has markedly changed over this time: patients are now older and have more medical disability than 50 years ago.

□ CAUSES (TABLE 1)

Peptic ulcer

The most important cause of major life-threatening acute GI bleeding is peptic ulcer. Significant haemorrhage is due to erosion of an underlying artery, with the magnitude related to the size of the arterial defect and the arterial diameter. Thus, bleeding can be particularly severe from either a large posterior duodenal ulcer which may erode the gastroduodenal artery or from a high, lesser curve gastric ulcer involving branches of the left gastric artery. Most cases present with little or no history of dyspepsia, whilst a history of aspirin or non-steroidal anti-inflammatory drug (NSAID) consumption is common.

Table 1 Causes of acute upper gastrointestinal bleeding.

Cause	Frequency (%)
Peptic ulcer	35–50
Varices	5–12
Mallory-Weiss tear	2–5
Oesophagitis	20–30
Gastritis/Duodenitis/Erosions	10–20
Vascular anomalies	2–3
Tumours	2–5
Aorto-duodenal fistula	<1

Oesophago-gastric varices

A less common cause of GI bleeding is oesophago-gastric varices. The impact on hospital resources is high both because the patient often has other features of decompensated cirrhosis and because bleeding is often high volume. Prognosis is related to the severity of liver disease rather than to the magnitude of bleeding.

Mallory-Weiss tears

Mallory-Weiss tears are usually associated with retching from alcohol abuse, but other causes of vomiting including drugs (chemotherapy, digoxin toxicity etc), renal failure or advanced malignancy may be responsible. Bleeding usually stops spontaneously and endoscopic therapy required only in rare severe cases.

Oesophagitis

A common finding in elderly patients who present with 'coffee ground' haematemesis is oesophagitis. Bleeding is never life-threatening; conservative supportive therapy combined with the use of proton-pump acid inhibitor (PPI) drugs is all that is necessary.

Gastritis, duodenitis and gastroduodenal erosions

Other conditions often linked to NSAID use and *Helicobacter pylori* infection are gastritis, duodenitis and gastroduodenal erosions. Circulatory support, stopping NSAIDs and *H. pylori* eradication are required.

Vascular anomalies

A range of vascular anomalies may be responsible for GI bleeding:

- *Large or multiple arteriovenous malformations* (AVMs) usually present with iron deficiency anaemia but occasionally cause major acute haemorrhage. Most AVMs have no obvious cause and are more common in elderly patients; in younger patients they are sometimes due to hereditary haemorrhagic telangiectasia. Other patients have valvular heart disease or artificial heart valves, and bleeding may be exacerbated by anticoagulant drugs.
- *Gastric antral vascular ectasia* (GAVE) is an uncommon vascular anomaly characterised by linear, readily bleeding red streaks radiating from the pyloris into the gastric antrum. It is sometimes associated with liver disease.
- *Portal hypertensive gastropathy* is due to venous congestion of the gastric mucosa from portal hypertension.

- *Dieulafoy's lesion* is an unusual cause of severe and recurrent bleeding in which a superficial submucosal artery is eroded by a small strategic ulcer. The commonest site is the gastric fundus, although it can occur in the duodenum and other parts of the stomach.

Oesophago-gastric tumours

A relatively uncommon cause of acute upper GI haemorrhage is oesophago-gastric tumour. The most important benign type is GI stromal cell tumour. Carcinomas and lymphomas of the stomach tend to present with other upper GI symptoms and iron deficiency anaemia rather than with acute bleeding.

Aorto-duodenal fistula

The possibility of aorto-duodenal fistula should be considered in patients who present with major upper GI bleeding after aortic graft insertion. Bleeding occurs from the second part of the duodenum, is massive and may recur over hours or days.

Bowel diseases

Small bowel or right-sided colonic diseases sometimes present as melaena and rarely as haematemesis. Colonoscopy, barium radiology and enteroscopy may identify the underlying tumour or vascular anomaly when upper GI endoscopy fails to identify a bleeding source. In young patients, a bleeding Meckel's diverticulum should be considered.

RISK ASSESSMENT

Risk assessment is based both on the severity of haemorrhage and on the general health of the patient. The best risk assessment tool is the Rockall score,[1] developed from a large prospective audit in England of patients managed for acute upper GI bleeding. Multivariant analysis identified age, shock, medical comorbidity and specific endoscopic findings as independent variables which predicted rebleeding and death (Tables 2 and 3). The Rockall score has been validated by other groups and is useful in both clinical practice and clinical trials.

Endoscopy provides important prognostic information. The presence of blood within the upper GI tract, active spurting haemorrhage and a 'non-bleeding visible vessel' are signs of poor prognosis. Active ulcer bleeding implies an 80–90% risk of continuing haemorrhage or rebleeding, whilst the visible vessel (representing adherent blood clot or a pseudo-aneurysm over the arterial defect) is associated with a 50% chance of rebleeding during the hospital admission. Rebleeding is associated with a tenfold increase in hospital mortality.

The mortality of patients who bleed during the course of an admission for other serious disease is particularly high, approaching 40% in published series, compared with 10–12% in patients admitted to hospital because of GI bleeding.[1]

Table 2 The Rockall scoring system.[1]

	Score			
Variable	**0**	**1**	**2**	**3**
Age (years)	<60	60–79	>80	
Shock	None	Pulse >100 Normal BP	Pulse >100 Systolic BP <100 mmHg	
Comorbidity	None		Cardiac GI cancer Other major comorbidity	Renal failure Liver failure Disseminated malignancy
Major SRH	None or dark spots		Blood in the upper GI tract Spurting vessel Non-bleeding visible vessel Adherent clot	

BP = blood pressure; GI = gastrointestinal; SRH = stigmata of recent haemorrhage.

Table 3 Rockall score, rebleeding and mortality.[1]

Risk score	**No. of patients**	**Rebleed (%)**	**Mortality (%)**
0	144	5	0
1	281	3	0
2	337	5	0.2
3	444	11	3
4	528	14	5
5	455	24	11
6	312	33	17
7	267	44	27
>8	190	42	41

□ MANAGEMENT

Resuscitation

The principles of 'airway, breathing and circulation' apply. Patients who present with major bleeding are frequently elderly and have significant cardiorespiratory, renal and cerebrovascular comorbidity. It is crucial that this is recognised and supported since most deaths are due to decompensation of general medical diseases, precipitated either by the bleed itself or by postoperative complications which are much more likely in the presence of medical comorbidity.

Central venous pressure (CVP) monitoring is useful in the elderly and in patients with cardiac disease to optimise decisions concerning fluid replacement. Intravenous fluids should be given through a large cannula inserted in an anti-cubital vein. Crystalloids (principally normal saline) are used to normalise blood pressure and urine output; colloids (such as gelefusin) are often employed in the presence of major hypotension. Saline should be used with care in patients with liver disease.

Patients who are shocked and actively bleeding are given a blood transfusion; this is also necessary when the haemoglobin concentration is less than 10 g/dl. The evidence base for this transfusion threshold is rather poor, but it is known in the intensive care setting that a haemoglobin concentration below 7 g/dl has significant adverse cardiac effects. It is therefore reasonable to pre-empt this by using a value of 10 g/dl in bleeding patients.

Appropriate monitoring includes measurement of pulse, blood pressure, urine output (through an indwelling catheter) and CVP. Actively bleeding, shocked patients are managed in a high dependency environment.

Endoscopy (Table 4)

Endoscopy is the primary diagnostic modality and is undertaken after optimum resuscitation has been achieved. Endoscopy has three purposes:

1. To establish an accurate diagnosis.
2. To obtain prognostic information which will influence transfer of the patient to the high dependency unit, general ward or, in some low risk patients, immediate hospital discharge.
3. Most importantly, endoscopic therapy is used to stop bleeding from specific disease processes (see below).

In most instances, endoscopy is best done within 24 hours of admission on the first available elective list. 'Out of hours' emergency endoscopy is necessary only in a small minority of cases.

Table 4 Stigmata of recent haemorrhage.

Endoscopic finding	Rebleeding (%)
Clean base	3
Flat spots	7
Oozing	10
Adherent blood clot	33
Non-bleeding visible vessel	50
Spurting vessel	80

Endoscopic therapy

At least 80% of patients admitted to hospital because of acute bleeding have an excellent prognosis; bleeding stops spontaneously and only circulatory supportive therapy is required. Endoscopic therapy is indicated in the following situations:

- bleeding oesophageal varices
- peptic ulcer with major stigmata of recent haemorrhage (active spurting bleeding, non-bleeding visible vessel or non-adherent blood clot) (Table 4)
- vascular malformations including actively bleeding AVMs, GAVE and Dieulafoy's malformation
- rarely, for active bleeding from a Mallory-Weiss tear.

The evidence base of endoscopic therapy for non-variceal causes comes principally from clinical trials for peptic ulcer haemorrhage.[2] Three types of direct endoscopic treatments have been evaluated, each of which is designed to seal the arterial defect created by the ulcer:

- injection
- heat energy
- mechanical devices.

Injection

Direct injection of fluids into the bleeding ulcer using disposable needles is technically straightforward and its efficacy has been demonstrated in several clinical trials. However, the mechanism of action is uncertain: tamponade, vasoconstriction from adrenaline, endarteritis after sclerosant or alcohol injection, and a direct effect upon blood clot formation from fibrin glue or thrombin may all be relevant.

The most widely used injection fluid is 1:10,000 adrenaline. This stops active bleeding in more than 90% of cases but 15–20% of patients will rebleed.[3] Sclerosants (polidocanol, sodium tetradecyl sulphate or ethanolamine) or alcohol should not be used; they do not reduce the risk of rebleeding[4] and may cause life-threatening necrosis of the injected area. Fibrin glue (a mixture of thrombin and fibrinogen) and human thrombin are probably the most effective injection materials and have few complications.[5,6]

Heat energy

Devices are applied directly to the bleeding point to cause coagulation and thrombosis. The heater probe is pushed firmly on to the bleeding lesion to apply tamponade and deliver defined pulses of heat energy. Clinical trials have shown that this approach is as effective and safe as injection therapy.[7] The argon plasma coagulator and multipolar coagulation, in which electrical energy is conducted between multiple probes on the tip of an endoscopically positioned catheter, have comparable efficacy.

Mechanical devices.

'Endoclips' can be applied to visible vessels. Although they may be difficult to deploy on to awkwardly positioned ulcers, they may represent the best option for major bleeding ulcers. Arterial defects greater than 1 mm in diameter do not usually respond to injection or thermal therapies but an adequately positioned clip can stop bleeding from relatively large arteries.

Endoscopic therapy combinations

The exact modes of action of the various endoscopic therapies are largely speculative, but clearly each achieves haemostasis by a different mechanism. Several groups have examined the hypothesis that combinations of endoscopic therapies are better than single modalities. Two large studies have compared the haemostatic effect of the heater probe plus injection with injection alone.[8,9] Neither study showed a significant advantage for combination treatment, although one showed a trend suggesting that the combination was more effective in the subgroup treated for extremely severe active ulcer bleeding (Table 5).[8]

Table 5 Adrenaline plus heater probe versus adrenaline alone for peptic ulcer bleeding.[8]

Outcome	Adrenaline plus heater probe (No. of patients)	Adrenaline alone (No. of patients)
All patients	**136**	**134**
Primary haemostasis	135	131
Rebleed	5	12
Transfusion (median units)	3	2
Surgery	8	14
Death	8	7
Subgroup with spurting haemorrhage	**32**	**25**
Primary haemostasis	31	25
Rebleed	2	6
Transfusion (median units)	4	5
Surgery	2	8*
Death	not stated	not stated

* $p = 0.03$.

Rebleeding after endoscopic therapy

Primary haemostasis can be achieved in the great majority of ulcer bleeding patients using endoscopic therapy but there is rebleeding in 15–20%, usually within the first 24 hours. This is most common when the initial bleeding episode is severe; thus, shocked patients presenting with active, spurting haemorrhage from large posterior duodenal ulcers are the most likely to rebleed.

Management following rebleeding is often difficult and, to a large extent, based upon clinical judgement and local expertise. Discussion between endoscopist and GI surgeons is vital. In most patients it is appropriate to repeat the endoscopy and retreat the bleeding lesion. An important trial from Hong Kong showed that the mortality and blood transfusion requirements of patients who rebled after initially successful endoscopic treatment were similar whether they were treated by urgent operative surgery or repeat endoscopic therapy (Table 6).[9,10] No further intervention is necessary if adequate haemostasis is achieved by endoscopic retreatment, but further bleeding is an absolute indication for operative intervention.

Table 6 Repeat endoscopic therapy versus surgery for patients rebleeding after successful initial endoscopic treatment.[9]

Outcome	Endoscopic therapy (n = 48)	Surgery (n = 44)
Transfusion (median units)	8	7
No. developing complications	7	17*
Death (30 days)	5	8

* $p < 0.05$.

Drug therapy

Three groups of drugs have been used in an attempt to reduce the risk of further bleeding in high risk patients:

- acid suppressing drugs
- somatostatin and its analogue octreotide
- tranexamic acid.

Gastric acid lowering drugs

A blood clot is not stable in an acid environment; powerful gastric acid suppressing drugs therefore have the potential to optimise clot formation, thereby reducing the rebleeding risk. It is crucial that the gastric pH does not fall below 6; the only practical way to achieve this is by constant infusion of a PPI. However, only patients at high risk of rebleeding should receive a PPI infusion since the prognosis of the remainder (the majority) is good without its use. It follows that patients with major stigmata of recent haemorrhage who have undergone endoscopic therapy should be treated by PPIs. Clinical trials have shown that an 80 mg bolus of omeprazole followed by a 72-hour infusion at a flow rate of 8 mg/hour significantly reduces the risk of rebleeding and the need for emergency surgery. A trend for reduction in mortality just fails to achieve statistical significance (Table 7).[11]

Table 7 Omeprazole versus placebo for endoscopically treated bleeding peptic ulcers.[11]

	Omeprazole (n = 120)		Placebo (n = 120)		
Outcome	**No.**	**%**	**No.**	**%**	***p* value**
Rebleeding	8	7	27	23	<0.001
Surgery	3	3	9	18	0.14
Transfusion (mean/SD)	2.7	2.5	3.5	3.8	0.04

SD = standard deviation.

Somatostatin

Somatostatin and its analogue octreotide are theoretically attractive because they reduce mesenteric arterial flow and suppress gastric acid secretion. A meta-analysis showed significant reduction in rebleeding and need for emergency surgery in bleeding ulcer patients treated with somatostatin compared with those receiving placebo infusions.[12] However, the quality of some of the trials is relatively weak, and octreotide appears ineffective. The efficacy of somatostatin in endoscopically treated patients has not been evaluated and the drug is not widely used in clinical practice.

Tranexamic acid

The antifibrinolytic agent tranexamic acid has the potential to improve clot stability and reduce the risk of rebleeding. One trial showed benefit in treated patients, but tranexamic acid is not often used possibly because of a fear that it could lead to the development of venous thrombosis.

Surgical intervention

Emergency surgery is required in situations in which endoscopic therapy combined with pharmacological intervention fails to secure permanent haemostasis:

- When there is active bleeding which cannot be controlled by endoscopic therapy, either because torrential haemorrhage obscures the bleeding point or when it continues despite successful application of endoscopic therapy.
- If there is rebleeding following initially successful endoscopic treatment. As previously discussed, it is reasonable to repeat endoscopic therapy on one occasion after rebleeding provided that local expertise is available and only after discussion between endoscopist and surgeon.

The type of operation depends upon the site of the ulcer. Bleeding duodenal ulcers are treated by under-running the ulcer, sometimes with pyloroplasty. Gastric ulcers are treated by partial gastrectomy or simple ulcer excision. Vagotomy is no longer undertaken since PPIs abolish acid secretion.

Secondary prophylaxis

After haemostasis has been achieved it is important to prevent late recurrent ulcer haemorrhage. *H. pylori* eradication virtually abolishes the risk of late rebleeding. If a patient has good reason to continue NSAID therapy, the following should be considered:

- ☐ use the least toxic NSAID which controls the arthritic symptoms
- ☐ co-prescribe a PPI with the NSAID
- ☐ consider use of a cytochrome C oxidase-2 (COX2)-specific anti-inflammatory drug; these are associated with significantly less recurrent ulcer-related adverse events than non-selective NSAIDs.

Treatment in patients who have *H. pylori* and need to continue an NSAID remains controversial. Gastritis, an inevitable consequence of *H. pylori* infection, induces prostaglandin production which may protect the gastroduodenal mucosa from the harmful effects of NSAIDs. Current studies suggest, however, that the magnitude of prostaglandin production is unlikely to outweigh the deleterious effects of *H. pylori* and that eradication therapy is indicated in patients who have developed ulcer bleeding, are *H. pylori* positive and require long-term NSAID therapy.

REFERENCES

1 Rockall TA, Logan RF, Devlin HB, Northfield TC. Risk assessment after acute upper gastrointestinal haemorrhage. *Gut* 1996;**38**:316–21.

2 Cook DJ, Guyatt GH, Salena BJ, Laine LA. Endoscopic therapy for acute nonvariceal upper gastrointestinal hemorrhage: a meta-analysis. *Gastroenterology* 1992;**102**:139–148.

3 Chung SC, Leung JW, Steele RJ, Crofts TJ, Li AK. Endoscopic injection of adrenaline for actively bleeding ulcers: a randomised trial. *BMJ (Clin Res Ed)* 1988;**296**:1631–3.

4 Choudari CP, Palmer KR. Endoscopic injection therapy for bleeding peptic ulcer: a comparison of adrenaline alone with adrenaline plus ethanolamine oleate. *Gut* 1994;**35**:608–10.

5 Rutgeerts P, Rauws E, Wara P, Swain P *et al.* Randomised trial of single and repeated fibrin glue compared with injection of polidocanol in treatment of bleeding peptic ulcer. *Lancet* 1997;**350**:692–6.

6 Kubba AK, Murphy W, Palmer KR. Endoscopic injection for bleeding peptic ulcer: a comparison of adrenaline alone with adrenaline plus human thrombin. *Gastroenterology* 1996;**111**:623–8.

7 Fullarton GM, Birnie GG, Macdonald A, Murray WR. Controlled trial of heater probe treatment in bleeding peptic ulcers. *Br J Surg* 1989;**76**:541–4.

8 Chung SS, Lau JY, Sung JJ, Chan AC *et al.* Randomised comparison between adrenaline injection alone and adrenaline injection plus heat probe treatment for actively bleeding ulcers. *BMJ* 1997;**314**:1307–11.

9 Church NI, Dallal HJ, Masson J, Mowat NA *et al.* A randomized trial comparing heater probe plus thrombin with heater probe plus placebo for bleeding peptic ulcer. *Gastroenterology* 2003;**125**:396–403.

10 Lau JY, Sung JJ, Lam YH, Chan AC *et al.* Endoscopic retreatment compared with surgery in patients with recurrent bleeding after initial endoscopic control of bleeding ulcers. *N Engl J Med* 1999;**340**:751–6.

11 Lau JY, Sung JJ, Lee KK, Yung MY *et al.* Effect of intravenous omeprazole on recurrent bleeding after endoscopic treatment of bleeding peptic ulcers. *N Engl J Med* 2000;**343**:310–6.

12 Jenkins SA, Poulianos G, Coraggio F, Rotondano G. Somatostatin in the treatment of non-variceal upper gastrointestinal bleeding. Review. *Dig Dis* 1998;**16**:214–24.

Biological therapies for inflammatory bowel disease

Chris Hawkey

□ INTRODUCTION

The cause of inflammatory bowel disease (IBD) is not known but current data support the notion of abnormal interactions between the environment and the host genotype. A family history has long been recognised as a strong predisposition to IBD and recent data point to polymorphisms on a number of chromosomes. Most notably, mutations of the NOD-2 (caspase activating and recruitment domain (CARD) 15) gene, located on chromosome 16, have been shown to increase substantially the risk of ileocolonic or colonic Crohn's disease.[1,2] NOD-2/CARD 15 consists of an intracellular Toll-like receptor responding to the bacterial lipopolysaccharide and peptidoglycan motif muramyl dipeptide; this results in a number of responses including activation of NFκB. Thus, NOD-2 is a central component of the innate immune system.

Crohn's disease

NOD-2 is expressed in monocytes, macrophages and lymphocytes, making it plausible that abnormalities in the handling of bacterial antigens and cell wall lipopolysaccharide could account for the T helper (Th)-1 skewed immunological response that is fairly well recognised in Crohn's disease. This response is associated with increased production by inflammatory cells of interleukins (IL)-18, IL-1 and IL-2, interferon gamma and tumour necrosis factor (TNF) alpha and reduced production of IL-10.

The most impressive natural experiment implicating NOD-2 in Crohn's disease comes from a case report in which the disease developed in a patient who received an allogeneic stem cell transplant for Hodgkin's disease. The transplanted stem cells contained the NOD-2 mutation and the patient developed Crohn's disease. NOD-2 is also expressed in Paneth cells, suggesting an alternative explanation about how NOD-2 could lead to Crohn's disease. Paneth cells elaborate endogenous antibiotic molecules such as defensin and there is some evidence that this is depressed in Crohn's disease.[3] Therefore, there could be an excessive Th-1 response because inadequate endogenous antibiotic defences would lead to prolonged immune stimulation.

Other environmental factors that contribute to Crohn's disease are:

- □ smoking, which increases the risk and severity of the disease

- □ consumption of a low carbohydrate diet (whether this is primary or secondary is debated), and
- □ a history compatible with reduced early exposure to bacteria.

Ulcerative colitis

Ulcerative colitis is in many ways less well understood than Crohn's disease. In the former, smoking has an exactly converse effect in that ulcerative colitis is extremely rare in patients who smoke. However, there is little direct evidence that smoking simply determines whether those with an inherited susceptibility to IBD develop the phenotype of Crohn's disease or of ulcerative colitis. Also, in contrast to Crohn's disease, ulcerative colitis is more characterised by a partial Th-2/humoral response associated with increased production of IL-8.

□ INFLAMMATORY MEDIATORS AND TARGETS FOR TREATMENT

Regardless of the precise pathogenesis, both ulcerative colitis and Crohn's disease are associated with enhanced production of multiple cytokines (as mentioned above) and increased expression in active disease of adhesion molecules on endothelial cells and leukocytes. These are now targets for the bioengineering of new treatments.

Tumour necrosis factor alpha

The central role played by TNF alpha as an accessory signal and mediator of increased adhesion molecule expression, together with some early evidence for significant increases in its production in Crohn's disease, made this the first target chosen for monoclonal antibody (MAb) technology. Two fundamental approaches were initially made:

1. Infliximab (Remicade) was made by grafting the variable portion of antibodies generated from mice immunised with human TNF alpha on to a human immunoglobulin (Ig) G-4 (complement-fixing) FAb fragment.[4] This resulted in reduced, but not absent, immunogenicity in humans.
2. The MAb CDP-571 was based on the principle of engraftment of mouse MAb on to a human IgG-1 FAb fragment, taking it further by 3-dimensional re-engineering of the variable portion with a view to maintaining antibody responsiveness but with humanised elements.[5]

Infliximab and CDP-571 have not been compared in terms of immunogenicity, but indirect evidence suggests a lower, but not absent, level of immunogenicity for CDP-571. Most evidence comes from infliximab. Because infliximab can bind activated complement and lyse cells such as macrophages via expressed TNF alpha on the cell surface, the possibility of this effect rather than specific 'mopping up' of TNF alpha could be the predominant mechanism of action.

□ CLINICAL DATA

Treatment of active non-fistulating Crohn's disease

Infliximab

The first controlled study of infliximab compared the effect of single infusions of infliximab 5 mg/kg, 10 mg/kg or 20 mg/kg and placebo (Fig 1).[4] The primary end-point was the proportion of patients achieving response or remission on any dose of infliximab compared with placebo at four weeks. On the lowest dose of infliximab, 81% responded and 48% went into remission, but there was a curious reverse dose-dependence on the higher doses with fewer patients appearing to achieve remission. The effectiveness of infliximab 5 mg/kg infusions as initial therapy has been confirmed in two trials (ACCENT 1 and 2) which were designed principally to investigate maintenance treatment with infliximab (see below).[6] These latter trials have used a three-infusion induction regimen.

CDP-571

In the first controlled study of anti-TNF antibody treatment in Crohn's disease, a pilot Phase 2 study, patients were randomised to receive either 5 mg/kg CDP-571

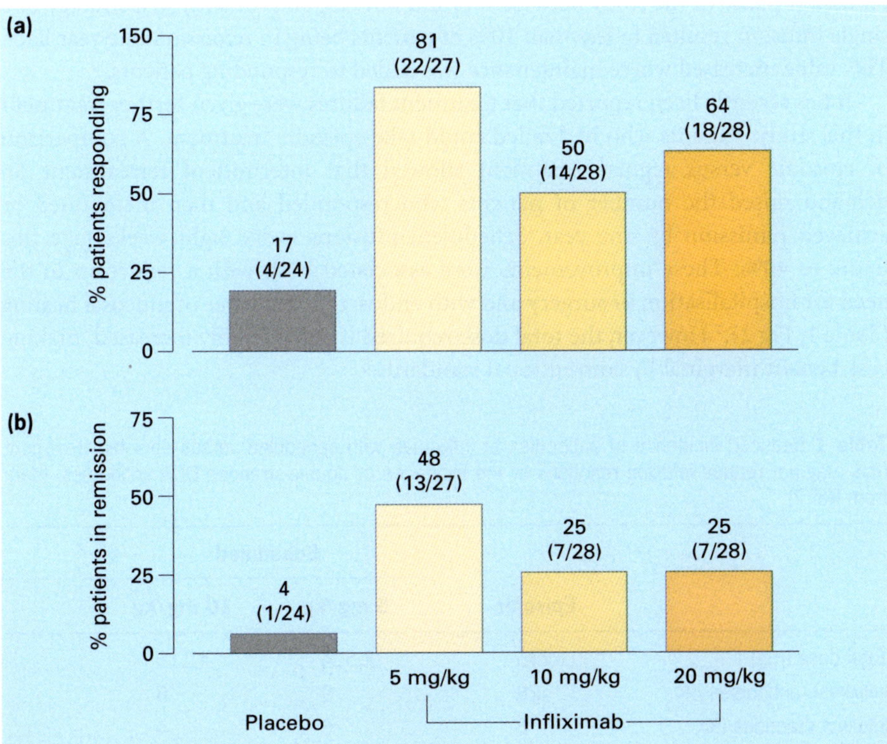

Fig 1 Responses to infliximab, showing percentages of patients **(a)** responding and **(b)** in remission (reproduced, with permission, from Ref 4).

(20 patients) or placebo (10).[5] The purpose of the placebo was not to provide a comparator but to minimise placebo responses. The primary end-point was suppression of the Crohn's disease activity index (CDAI) at two weeks. There was a mean CDAI reduction from 264 to 167 at two weeks, but the CDAI scores and other indices of activity returned towards normal over the following six weeks of the study. Commercial considerations delayed, and ultimately prevented, development of CDP-571 as treatment for Crohn's disease.

Non-fistulating Crohn's Disease

Maintenance treatment

Relapse occurred soon after cessation of treatment with both infliximab and CDP-571. The ACCENT trials investigated whether regular injections of infliximab (5 mg/kg or 10 mg/kg) over one year could maintain remission compared with placebo. In ACCENT 1, placebo (group 1) or infliximab injections at 5 mg/kg were given to patients with non-fistulating disease at baseline, two and six weeks, then eight weekly at 5 mg/kg (group 2) or 10 mg/kg (group 3) up to 52 weeks.[6] The primary end-point was remission, based on the CDAI at 30 weeks. After an initial response to infliximab, 21% of group 1 were in remission compared with 38% and 44% of groups 2 and 3, respectively, with somewhat lower values at 54 weeks. Not all patients entered the remission phase of the study because they did not respond initially, so a strategy of a single infusion resulted in less than 10% of patients being in remission one year later. This value increased where maintenance was added to responding patients.

It has recently been reported that treatment failures were given further treatment in this study. Patients who had failed could take episodic treatment. A comparison of episodic versus regular treatment showed that intermittent retreatment on demand raised the number of patients who responded and then maintained or achieved remission by one year. Scheduled infusions every eight weeks take this figure to 40%. These improvements were associated both with a reduction in the need for hospitalisation or surgery and with endoscopic evidence of mucosal healing (Table 1, Fig 2).[7] However, the total dose required is considerably increased, making cost-benefit marginal by conventional standards.[8]

Table 1 Reduced incidence of antibodies to infliximab with scheduled versus episodic treatment (this may not reduce infusion reactions or the incidence of double-stranded DNA antibodies) (data from Ref 7).

		Scheduled	
	Episodic	**5 mg/kg**	**10 mg/kg**
Total dose (mg)	795	2,524	4,119
Infliximab antibodies (%)	28	9	6
Infusion reactions (%)	3	6	4
Double-stranded DNA antibodies (%)	11	34	

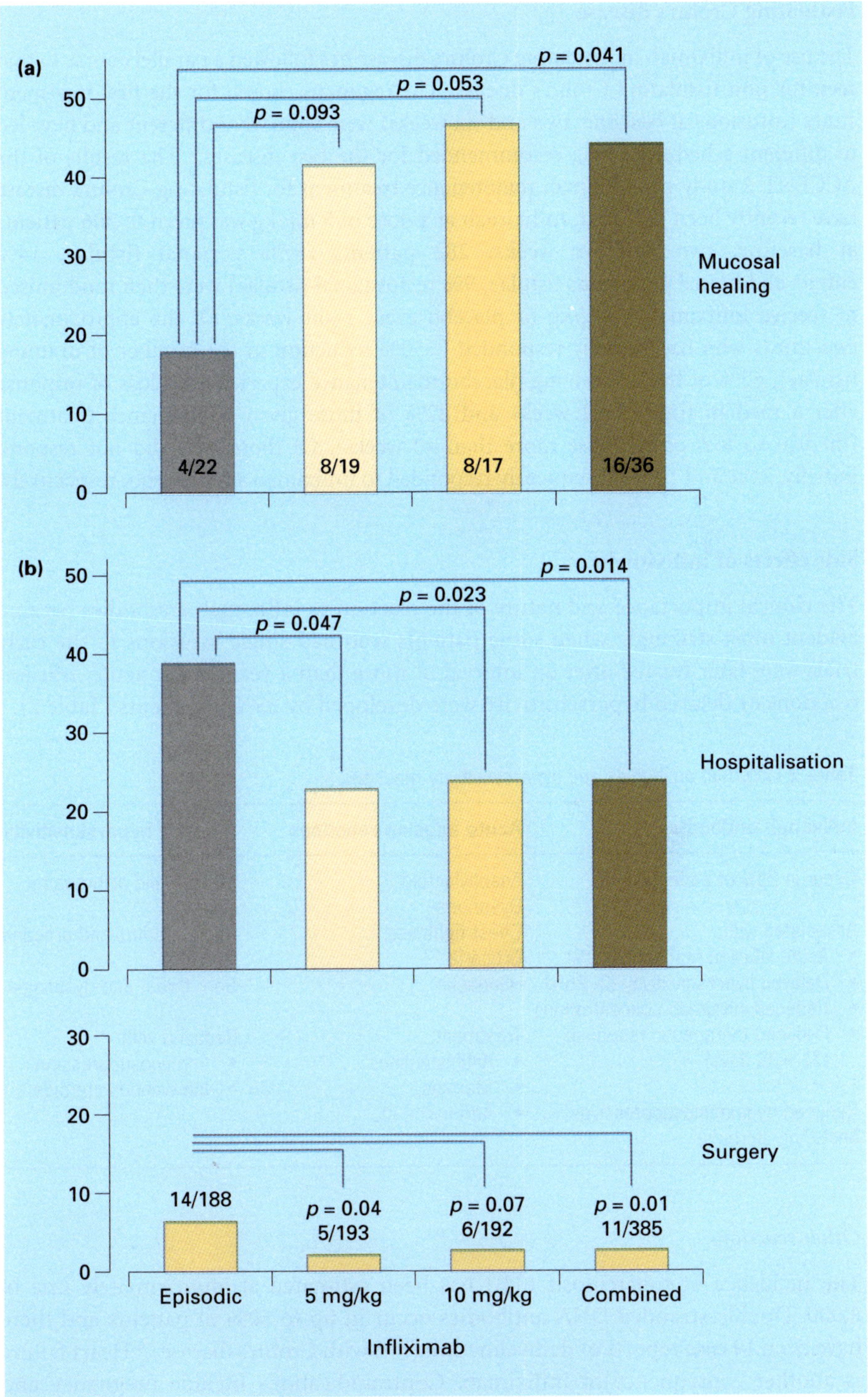

Fig 2 (a) Improvement in mucosal healing and **(b)** reduction in hospitalisation following surgery with maintenance infliximab (reproduced, with permission, from Ref 7).

Fistulating Crohn's disease

The use of infliximab in fistulating Crohn's disease has followed a parallel course to that seen for non-fistulating Crohn's disease. The regimens chosen for the first treatment study (infusions at baseline, two and six weeks) were somewhat different and have led to different schedules being recommended for the two diseases.[9] The results of the ACCENT 2 study of infliximab maintenance treatment for fistulating Crohn's disease have recently been reported. Infliximab at a dose of 5 mg/kg was given to 306 patients at baseline, two and six weeks; 282 patients (87% perianal fistulae, 14% entero-abdominal cutaneous fistulae, 9% rectovaginal fistulae) were then randomised to receive infliximab 5 mg/kg or placebo every eight weeks. Of the approximately two-thirds who had initially responded (>50% reduction in the number of draining fistulae), 62% of those receiving placebo maintenance experienced a loss of response after a median time of 14 weeks and 42% of those given maintenance treatment (median to loss of response more than 40 weeks). Of those who did not respond initially, 21% and 16% subsequently responded to infliximab and placebo, respectively.

Side effects of infliximab

The clinical importance and nature of the reaction to infliximab antibodies became evident most strikingly when some patients who had single infusions in the early trials were later treated after an interval of more than a year. Either acute infusion reactions or delayed hypersensitivity were developed by 25% of patients (Table 2).

Table 2 Infliximab antibodies and hypersensitivity reactions.

Infliximab antibodies	Acute infusion reactions	Delayed hypersensitivity
Occur in 25% of patients	Anaphylactoid	Myalgia and arthropathy
	Dyspnoea	Fever
Associated with:	Chest tightness	Rash, pruritus and urticaria
• Acute infusion reactions (10%)	Urticaria	Oedema
• Delayed hypersensitivity (2–25%)	Headache	Sore throat and dysphagia
• Reduced infliximab concentrations		
• Reduced therapeutic response (71→35 days)	Treatment:	Reduced with:
	• Antihistamines	• Immunosuppression
	• Steroids	• Intravenous steroids
Reduced by immunosuppressives (including steroids)	• Adrenaline etc	

Other reactions

The incidence of tuberculosis (TB) has been estimated at approximately one in 2,000. Double-stranded DNA antibodies occur in up to 50% of patients and there have been 19 case reports of demyelination (not with Crohn's disease).[9] Heart failure is another consequence of infliximab. Contraindications include pregnancy and lactation, infection and abscess, heart failure and malignancy, while care should be exerted in patients with multiple sclerosis.

Acute infusion reactions

Anaphylactic reactions may occur, accompanied by dyspnoea, chest tightness, urticaria and headache. They should be treated with antihistamines, steroids or adrenaline, and can be reduced in patients known to suffer anaphylactic reactions or to be at risk of them by prior use of immunosuppressives, including steroids.

Delayed hypersensitivity

Delayed hypersensitivity usually occurs several days after the infusion in a patient who typically has not had infliximab for at least a year. Symptoms are of myalgia and atrophy, fever, rash, pruritus and urticaria, oedema, sore throat and dysphagia. These problems can also be reduced with immunosuppression and intravenous steroids.

□ PRESCRIBING INFLIXIMAB

Guidance on infliximab for Crohn's disease

The data on infliximab have led the National Institute for Clinical Excellence (NICE) to recommend infliximab for patients with severe active Crohn's disease (with or without fistulae) (Table 3).[10] Primary care trusts are required to make funds available to prescribe drugs approved by NICE within three months of approval, without caveats or the need to have negotiated additional funding. Nevertheless, difficulties are found in some areas of the country. (Prescribers experiencing such difficulties should contact the Department of Health where specific individuals deal with problems of activating NICE guidelines.)

Table 3 National Institute for Clinical Guidance on the use of infliximab in Crohn's disease (2002).[10]

Recommended for severe active (± fistulating) Crohn's disease:

- Poor health, weight loss, fever, pain, diarrhoea, ± fistulae, extra-intestinal manifestations
- Refractory to, intolerant of, or side effects from corticosteroids and/or immunosuppressives
- Surgery inappropriate

Repeat infusion for patients relapsing

Should be prescribed by experienced gastroenterologist

A practical strategy

There is some confusion about the ideal induction dose for active Crohn's disease. Many advocate single infusions for non-fistulating disease and three infusions at baseline, two and six weeks for fistulating Crohn's disease. More recently, on the basis of the ACCENT trials, it is now recommended that all patients receive the latter regimen. This recommendation is regarded as evidence-based – but only because these are the only regimens to have been assessed. In fact, only a facile view of evidence-based medicine would embrace such a rigid approach.

The available evidence allows the following practical prescribing recommendations:

1. Induction with three infusions at baseline, two and six weeks gives good response rates and may result in lower antibody levels and therefore reduced incidence of infusion reactions. It is the preferred regimen if money is no object.
2. Those on tighter budgets should realise that some patients respond to continued infliximab even when there is no response to the first infusion. If infliximab is employed, prescribers should give at least two infusions separated by not more than eight weeks before abandoning the approach.
3. Treatment with infliximab should be initiated only by an individual with expertise in its use. Ideally, hospitals should work through one individual gastroenterologist specialising in IBD. Patients should receive infliximab only if they are established on long-term immunosuppression unless there are compelling reasons (eg drug toxicity) making this impossible. This approach will reduce antibody formation and probably infusion reactions.
4. Antibody formation and probably infusion reactions are also minimised by regular use of infliximab as maintenance (every eight weeks). This is expensive, but the alternative (stopping infliximab and restarting when major relapse occurs) is associated with a high incidence of infusion reactions, especially if there has been an interval of one year before restarting infliximab. A single intravenous infusion of hydrocortisone should be given prior to infliximab to avoid acute anaphylactic reactions, and patients warned about the possibility of late reactions (also requiring steroids) 2–3 days later.
5. Infliximab is profoundly immunosuppressive and renders patients more susceptible to infections, of which TB is the most important. Some recommend screening by Mantoux testing. I do not agree because this delays treatment and is often misleading and hard to interpret because active Crohn's disease patients on immunosuppressive drugs may be rendered anergic. It is more important to search vigilantly for TB before and during infliximab infusions, including baseline and on-treatment chest X-rays and appropriate response to any development of fever.

Infliximab in children

The use of infliximab in children has been limited, but two studies suggest likely benefit.[11]

□ OTHER TUMOUR NECROSIS FACTOR ALPHA MODULATORS

TNF alpha receptor proteins have been successful in the treatment of rheumatoid, but there is limited experience in Crohn's disease. No benefit was shown for etanercept in a 12-patient open patient study, a 43-patient blind study versus placebo and another unpublished 49-patient study. Onercept has been studied in very small numbers of patients, although a dose-dependent therapeutic effect has not been excluded.[10]

☐ OTHER MONOCLONAL ANTIBODIES

Natalizumab is a humanised MAb directed against the alpha-4 integrin molecules. In a Phase 2 study of 248 patients with moderate to severe Crohn's disease, natalizumab 6 mg/kg gave higher remission rates than placebo and produced significant improvements in response, although the differences failed to reach statistical significance.[12] Natalizumab led to significant reductions in C-reactive protein (CRP) (Fig 3), suggesting objective evidence of an effect. This agent is not yet available for clinical use and is currently undergoing Phase 3 studies.

Several other monoclonal antibodies directed against biological targets are under evaluation in clinical trials. These are listed in Table 4, overleaf.

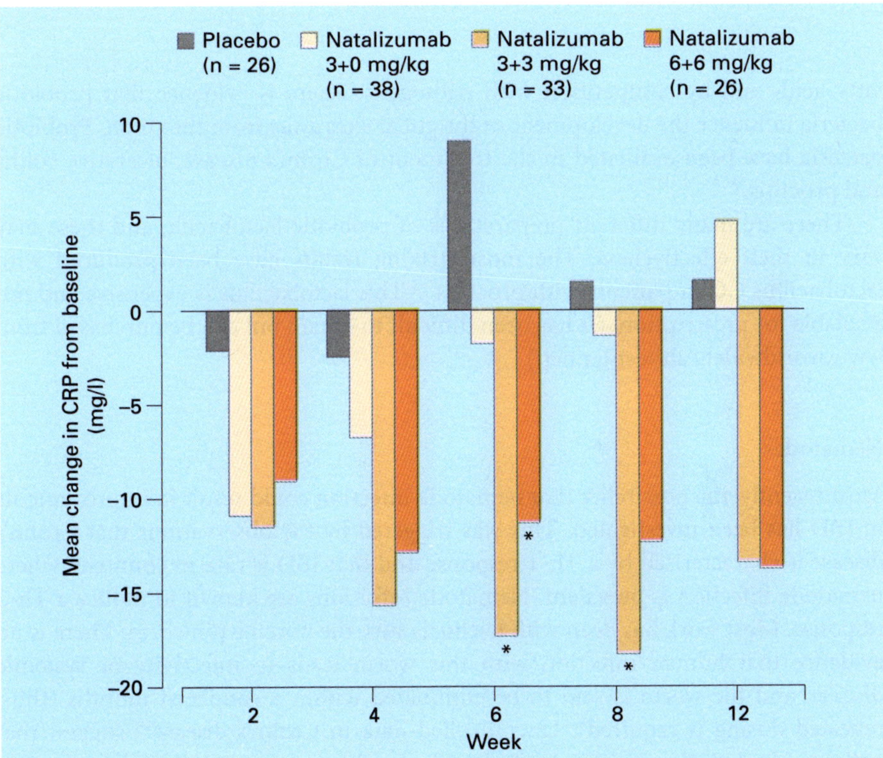

Fig 3 The effect of natalizumab on C-reactive protein (CRP) (* = significant) (reproduced, with permission, from Ref 6).

☐ OTHER BIOLOGICAL THERAPIES

Therapies that are biological in another sense are under current scrutiny in IBD.

Probiotic bacteria

Probiotic bacteria in the colon (eg lactobacilli) help to maintain mucosal health both by symbiotic digestion of non-absorbed carbohydrate with production of volatile

Table 4 Monoclonal antibodies (other than natalizumab) directed against biological targets.

Name	Property	Molecular target	Functional target
Adalimumab	Neutralising antibody	TNF alpha	Immune activation
Visilisumab	Neutralising antibody	CD3	Immune initiation
Basiliximab	Neutralising antibody	CD25	Steroid resistance[13]
Sargromostin	GM-CSF analogue	*	Mucosal barrier

* uncertain
For information on drugs in development:
http://www.abpi.org.uk/publications/publication_details/targetCrohns/marketing.asp
GM-CSF = granulocyte-macrophage colony stimulating factor; TNF = tumour necrosis factor.

fatty acids and by competition with pathogens. There is evidence that probiotic bacteria influence the development of the gut at sites away from the colon. Probiotic bacteria have been evaluated in the treatment of Crohn's disease, ulcerative colitis and proctitis.

There are many different preparations of probiotic lactobacilli, and these may vary in their effectiveness. The most striking results have been produced with lactobacillus GG in patients with proctitis.[14] This lactobacillus is expensive and not available for prescription. (It has been difficult to obtain but can be purchased from www.worldwidehealthcenter.net.)

Nematodes

Most recently, the possibility that nematode infection could result in improvements in IBD has been investigated. This was triggered by the observations that Crohn's disease is characterised by a Th-1 response and that IBD is rare in countries where nematode infection is prevalent. Nematode infections are known to induce a Th-2 response. Most work has been with trichuris suis, the porcine pinworm. There is no evidence that human infection with this worm leads to infectivity or systemic disease, and the worm is said to be eliminated within a couple of months (thus, repeated dosing is required). Uncontrolled data in Crohn's disease[15] suggest that patients given trichuris suis respond with a reduction in disease activity but no objective changes in CRP. Although ulcerative colitis is not characterised by a Th-2 response, trichuris suis has also been evaluated as a treatment for ulcerative colitis. There were positive results in a placebo-controlled trial.

□ CONCLUSIONS

Biological therapies are difficult to make and administer, and they are expensive. They may ultimately be replaced by small molecules that target the processes they inhibit, possibly depending on the speed of onset of these alternatives compared with biological therapies.

REFERENCES

1 Hugot JP, Chamaillard M, Zouali H, Lesage S *et al.* Association of NOD2 leucine-rich repeat variants with susceptibility to Crohn's disease. *Nature* 2001;**411**:599–603.

2 Louis E, Michel V, Hugot JP, Reenaers C *et al.* Early development of stricturing or penetrating pattern in Crohn's disease is influenced by disease location, number of flares, and smoking but not by NOD2/CARD15 genotype. *Gut* 2003;**52**:522–57.

3 Lala S, Ogura Y, Osborne C, Hor SY *et al.* Crohn's disease and the NOD2 gene: a role for paneth cells. *Gastroenterology* 2003;**125**:47–57.

4 Targan SR, Hanauer SB, van Deventer SJ, Mayer L *et al.* A short-term study of chimeric monoclonal antibody cA2 to tumor necrosis factor alpha for Crohn's disease. Crohn's Disease cA2 Study Group. *N Engl J Med* 1997;**337**:1029–35.

5 Stack WA, Mann SD, Roy AJ, Heath P *et al.* Randomised controlled trial of CDP571 antibody to tumour necrosis factor-alpha in Crohn's disease. *Lancet* 1997;**349**:521–4.

6 Hanauer SB, Feagan BG, Lichtenstein GR, Mayer LF *et al.* Maintenance infliximab for Crohn's disease: the ACCENT I randomised trial. *Lancet* 2002;**359**:1541–9.

7 Rutgeerts P, Feagan BG, Lichtenstein GR, Mayer LF *et al.* Comparison of scheduled and episodic treatment strategies of infliximab in Crohn's disease. *Gastroenterology* 2004;**126**:402–13.

8 Feagan BG, Yan S, Bala M, Bao W, Lichtenstein GR. The effects of infliximab maintenance therapy on health-related quality of life. *Am J Gastroenterol* 2003;**98**:2232–8.

9 Present DH, Rutgeerts P, Targan S, Hanauer SB *et al.* Infliximab for the treatment of fistulas in patients with Crohn's disease. *N Engl J Med* 1999;**340**:1398–405.

10 www.**nice**.org.uk

11 Sandborn WJ, Hanauer SB. Infliximab in the treatment of Crohn's disease: a user's guide for clinicians. *Am J Gastroenterol* 2002;**97**:2962–72.

12 Ghosh S, Goldin E, Gordon FH, Malchow HA *et al.* Natalizumab for active Crohn's disease. *N Engl J Med* 2003;**348**:24–32.

13 Creed TJ, Norman MR, Probert CS, Harvey RF *et al.* Basiliximab (anti-CD25) in combination with steroids may be an effective new treatment for steroid-resistant ulcerative colitis. *Aliment Pharmacol Ther* 2003;**18**:65–75.

14 Tamboli CP, Caucheteux C, Cortot A, Colombel JF, Desreumaux P. Probiotics in inflammatory bowel disease: a critical review. *Best Pract Res Clin Gastroenterol* 2003;**17**:805–20.

15 Summers RW, Elliott DE, Qadir K, Urban JF Jr *et al.* Trichuris suis seems to be safe and possibly effective in the treatment of inflammatory bowel disease. *Am J Gastroenterol* 2003;**98**:2034–41.

☐ GASTROENTEROLOGY SELF ASSESSMENT QUESTIONS

Management of dyspepsia

1 The following are considered indications for urgent referral for endoscopy in recent Scottish Intercollegiate Guideline Network and future National Institute for Clinical Excellence guidelines:
(a) New onset dyspepsia in a 70-year-old
(b) Weight loss of any extent
(c) Nausea
(d) Dysphagia
(e) Dyspepsia in a patient with recent demonstrated duodenal ulceration

2 Proton pump inhibitors (PPIs) should be stopped at least two weeks before the following tests for *Helicobacter pylori*:
(a) Urea breath test
(b) Serology by hospital-based ELISA
(c) Stool antigen test
(d) Biopsy urease test on endoscopic biopsy specimen
(e) Histological analysis of endoscopic biopsy specimen

3 The following treatments will help a proportion of patients with functional dyspepsia:
(a) *H. pylori* eradication
(b) PPI therapy
(c) Prokinetic agents
(d) Antidepressants
(e) Any drug, through a placebo effect

4 The following are important determinants of *H. pylori* treatment success:
(a) Sensitivity of the *H. pylori* strain to the antibiotics used
(b) Close compliance with treatment
(c) Younger age
(d) Female sex
(e) High titre of anti-*H. pylori* antibodies on serology

5 Gastric ulcers:
(a) Are more common than duodenal ulcers in the UK
(b) May sometimes be caused by underlying adenocarcinoma or lymphoma
(c) Have aspirin or non-steroidal anti-inflammatory drugs as a cause more frequently than do duodenal ulcers
(d) Can reliably be distinguished from duodenal ulcers by careful analysis of the patient's symptoms
(e) Are rarely caused by *H. pylori*

Advances in gastrointestinal bleed management

1 A 75-year-old man taking warfarin following aortic valve replacement presents with melaena. His systolic blood pressure is 105 mmHg, pulse 104, haemoglobin 9 g/dl and international normalised ratio 9. The following is appropriate management:
(a) Vitamin K, fresh frozen plasma and observe
(b) Emergency endoscopy, with treatment if major stigmata are present
(c) Fresh frozen plasma to optimise prothrombin time, followed by elective endoscopy but avoidance of endoscopic therapy
(d) Fresh frozen plasma and vitamin K, followed by endoscopic therapy
(e) Fresh frozen plasma, followed by endoscopy on the next elective list; endoscopic therapy if major stigmata present

2 Patients presenting with major upper gastrointestinal haemorrhage:
(a) Should be routinely started on a proton pump inhibitor (PPI) drug infusion
(b) Are best managed in a high dependency unit
(c) May benefit from octreotide infusion
(d) Should have a nasogastric tube
(e) Are referred to a vascular surgeon if aortic grafting has previously been undertaken

3 Appropriate endoscopic therapy for peptic ulcer bleeding may involve:
(a) Injection of dilute adrenaline to stop acute bleeding, followed by ethanolamine or alcohol to prevent rebleeding
(b) Application of thermal energy using diathermy
(c) Vigorously removing blood clot which has adhered to an underlying bleeding ulcer
(d) Routine repeat endoscopy within 24 hours to ensure haemostasis
(e) Application of clips

4 Rebleeding after initially successful endoscopic therapy for peptic ulcer bleeding:
(a) Is an indication for further endoscopy, and it may be reasonable to repeat endoscopic treatment
(b) Is more likely in the case of posterior duodenal ulcers than those at other sites
(c) Is indicated by the continued presence of black stool at day 5
(d) Is less likely in the presence of an intravenous PPI drug infusion
(e) Is associated with a tenfold increased mortality

Hepatology

Viral hepatitis and medical risks

David Mutimer and Douglas Thorburn

□ INTRODUCTION

In the course of their duties, doctors are repeatedly exposed to patients who have viral hepatitis. Thus, there is the potential for acquisition of hepatitis B virus (HBV) and/or hepatitis C virus (HCV) infection from their patients. This risk is perceived as an occupational hazard, to some extent unavoidable. During the performance of medical interventions, needle-stick injury to the doctor frequently occurs and may be associated with transmission of blood-borne infection from the healthcare worker (HcW) to the patient. Outbreaks of hepatitis transmission have occasionally been linked to hepatitis-positive HcWs. Such outbreaks often achieve notoriety in the press, followed by scrutiny of existing guidelines for practice by infected HcWs and then by tightening of the regulations.

The risk of transmission from HcW to patient is greatest during the performance of so-called 'exposure prone procedures' (EPP).[1] EPPs are those involving a risk that injury to the HcW may result in exposure of the patient's open tissues to the blood of the HcW. They include procedures where the gloved hands may be in contact with sharp instruments, needle-tips or sharp tissues (bone or teeth) inside a body cavity and where the fingertips may not be completely visible at all times. Thus, the key question when assessing whether or not a procedure is an EPP is 'Are the fingertips visible at all times?'. Useful specialty-specific examples are provided with the Health Service Circular (HSC) guidance.[1]

What is the risk that an HcW will be infected with hepatitis by a patient, and what is the risk that a patient will be infected by an HcW? This review will focus on the risks to and from doctors rather than more generally with the practice of other HcWs.

□ HEPATITIS B VIRUS INFECTION

The HBV immune status of every doctor should be known to both the doctor and the doctor's Occupational Health Service (OHS). Those not immune to HBV should receive vaccination, and non-responders screened for chronic HBV infection (an important possible cause of vaccine non-response). Most doctors will be either HBV immune or HBV carriers; a small number will be non-infected vaccine non-responders, a population at risk for HBV acquisition.

Hepatitis B virus transmission from doctor to patient

The risk of transmission of HBV from doctor to patient is proportional to the doctor's serum HBV titre at the time of the inoculation. It is not surprising, therefore, that early reports of HBV transmission involved doctors who were serum HBV e antigen (HBeAg)-positive. Serum HBeAg-positivity is usually associated with high serum titres. Most HBeAg-negative HBV carriers have low serum virus titres[2] and only a minority have high serum titres (this will be discussed later).

Hepatitis B e antigen-positive doctors

In 1993, as a consequence of reported cases of transmission from HBeAg-positive doctors, the Department of Health (DH) excluded HBeAg-positive doctors from performing EPPs. Unfortunately, doctors with high serum titres, despite serum HBeAg-negativity, continued to infect patients. Four UK single source outbreaks reported in 1997[3] found that the four surgeons involved had serum HBV titres greater than 10^5 copies/ml despite serum HBeAg-negativity (the same order of magnitude as observed for HBeAg-positive carriers). Because of this finding, the DH published a further HSC (2000/020) to address the problem of high titre HBeAg-negative HcWs.[4] It became the employer's obligation to measure the serum HBV titre of HBeAg-negative HcWs and to exclude from performance of EPPs those with titres above 10^3 copies/ml. Those with titres below that threshold could continue EPPs, but would be retested annually and excluded if the titres were found to exceed that threshold.

Antiviral therapy

In addition, HSC 2000/020 gave guidance on the role of antiviral therapy for those with serum titres greater than 10^3 copies/ml. The circular demanded that HcWs who have received antiviral therapy must be HBeAg-negative and have serum titres less than 10^3 copies/ml one year *after* cessation of treatment before being permitted to resume EPPs.

The rationale for this is illustrated in Fig 1. Until recently, lamivudine was probably the most popular candidate drug for use as long-term HBV suppressive therapy. Unfortunately, lamivudine selects drug-resistant species at a rate of approximately 20% of treated patients per annum.[5] Thus, after initial effective suppression by lamivudine (possibly to levels below 10^3 copies/ml) there is likely to be a secondary rise in viral titre as drug-resistant HBV emerges. In this circumstance, an infected HcW might find him/herself excluded from EPPs, reinstated when titres are suppressed by treatment, then suspended again when drug-resistant HBV emerges. It does not seem realistic to expect HcWs (or employers) to provide an effective and reliable clinical service when the threat of suspension looms unpredictably and possibly inevitably. Furthermore, serum titres may rise quite quickly as resistance emerges, so a doctor might be cleared to perform EPPs on one occasion, but then be excluded if the subsequent test showed titres above the critical threshold. The doctor will therefore have performed EPPs for a brief period with high serum titres. This would potentially place patients at risk for acquisition of HBV.

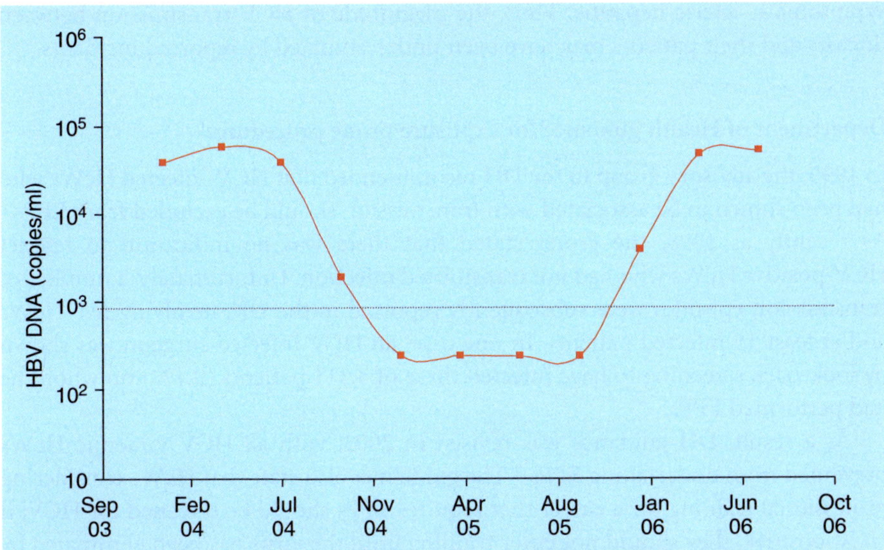

Fig 1 Suppression of hepatitis B virus (HBV) replication by antiviral therapy (lamivudine). The serum titre is initially reduced below the threshold of 10^3 copies/ml, but during prolonged therapy lamivudine-resistant virus will almost invariably emerge.

New antivirals

The existing policy that excludes the performance of EPPs during antiviral therapy may change. New antiviral agents have now been licensed, and a number of others are quite advanced in clinical development. For instance, the nucleotide analogue adefovir is a potent HBV antiviral effective against both wild-type and lamivudine-resistant virus. Prolonged treatment with adefovir is associated with a low rate of emergence of resistance. It seems likely that prolonged, possibly indefinite, suppression of HBV might be achieved with combination HBV antiviral treatment (akin to the application of highly active antiretroviral therapy for HIV infection). DH guidelines might then be revised and HcWs possibly be allowed to undertake EPPs during antiviral treatment.

For the present, however, serum titres greater than 10^3 copies/ml exclude the doctor from performing EPPs. In addition, in this risk-averse culture, employing trusts might find it undesirable to employ HcWs who may be required to perform EPPs even if their titre is below 10^3 copies/ml. Certainly, the young doctor with chronic HBV (regardless of serum HBV titre) is probably best advised to avoid any specialty that may involve EPPs.

□ HEPATITIS C VIRUS INFECTION

There is no effective vaccine against HCV infection. Doctors who treat HCV infected patients may acquire HCV after needle-stick injury. Good surgical training and practice may reduce the risk to medical staff. Conversely, HCV-positive HcWs who sustain needle-stick injury during the performance of EPPs may infect patients. Unlike acute HBV infection, acute HCV infection is rarely associated with symptomatic icteric hepatitis. Thus, the magnitude of HCV transmission between doctors and their patients may have been underestimated by reported incidents.

Department of Health guidance for exposure prone procedures

In 1995, the advisory group to the DH recommended that HCV-infected HcWs who had been shown to be associated with transmission should be excluded from EPPs.[6] As recently as 1998, the group stated that there was no indication to restrict HCV-positive HcWs who had not transmitted infection. Unfortunately, a number of transmission episodes were subsequently reported in the UK, involving five HcWs and at least 15 infected patients. In one case, an HCV infected surgeon was shown by look-back screening to have infected three of 3,311 patients (0.1%) on whom he had performed EPPs.

As a result, DH guidance was revised in 2002, with all HCV viraemic HcWs prevented from undertaking EPPs.[7] The guidelines also state that HcWs considering professional training for a career that requires EPPs should be screened for HCV; if HCV-positive, they should not enter training until the virus has been eliminated by antiviral therapy. The current DH guidance also permits re-entry to excluded doctors following successful antiviral treatment.

Doctors should probably be optimistic about this guidance. Current antiviral treatment for chronic HCV infection is successful and may eradicate the infection with therapy of finite duration in a large proportion of treated patients.[8] For instance, six months' treatment with pegylated interferon and ribavirin may cure as many as 80% of patients infected by genotype 2 or 3. For recently acquired infection, the results of treatment may be even better, with most treated patients cured, irrespective of genotype.[9] Doctors should be encouraged to submit themselves to their OHS for HCV testing after any potential exposure to HCV. The benefit would be that recently acquired infection would be detected, with the attendant excellent prognosis associated with early antiviral treatment.

The risks of hepatitis C virus transmission in the UK

What are the risks of HCV transmission between doctors and patients in the UK? The risk that an HCV-negative HcW would acquire HCV infection from an infected carrier patient and the risk that an HCV-negative patient would be infected by an HCV-positive HcW can be calculated as the product of:

- HCV prevalence in the source population
- the rate of transmission per exposure to infected blood, and
- the number of percutaneous injuries sustained.[10]

Cross-sectional anonymised serum studies suggest that the prevalence of HCV in the hospital patient population is about 1.4%.[11] The risk of HCV transmission in the surgical setting from an HCV-positive source is approximately 0.18% (assuming the injury is the result of needle-stick injury with a blunt needle to a gloved surgeon).

The number of percutaneous injuries sustained by a surgeon varies considerably at an individual, specialty and geographical level but is estimated to be 1–9 times per annum. On this basis, the estimated probability of HCV acquisition by a non-infected surgeon in the UK is 0.001–0.032% per annum, equivalent to a 0.035–1.12% risk for the surgeon over a 35-year surgical career.

Given that the estimated prevalence of HCV infection in UK surgeons is 0.23% – considerably lower than in the surgical patient population – nationally the risk of transmission of HCV from an HCV-positive source is reassuringly low for both patients and surgeons.

Of course, some specialist surgeons may be exposed to HCV more frequently and may be at a greater lifetime risk of acquiring HCV infection. The results of a recently undertaken anonymous survey of liver transplant surgeons may provide some reassurance. Thorburn and colleagues have examined the frequency of HCV carriage in a cohort of over 100 liver transplant surgeons, fewer than 1% of whom were HCV viraemic.[12]

☐ CONCLUSIONS

The prevalence of chronic HBV and chronic HCV in the UK population is quite low, so HcWs are only infrequently exposed to the risk of transmission. However, as the infected person is usually asymptomatic and unaware that he/she is a carrier of infection, HcWs are unlikely to be aware that a specific EPP is associated with a risk of hepatitis acquisition. Therefore, it is crucial that universal precautions and good surgical technique are observed at all times. As a consequence of vaccination of HcWs and exclusion of HBV-positive HcWs, the risks of HBV transmission to and from HcWs is very small.

Prevention of HCV transmission between patient and doctor remains the challenge. In the absence of an effective vaccine, good surgical technique remains the only preventive measure. It seems likely that those HcWs who undertake EPPs will be required to undertake frequent and regular blood testing for HCV. Acquired HCV would then be diagnosed at an early stage; early antiviral therapy should cure most infected HcWs, permitting the resumption of surgical practice.

REFERENCES

1 Department of Health. Guidance on the management of AIDS/HIV infected health care workers and patient notification. Health Service Circular 1998/226 (HSC 1998/226). London: DoH, 1998. www.open.gov.uk/doh/coinh.htm

2 Lindh M, Horal P, Dhillon AP, Norkrans G. Hepatitis B virus DNA levels, precore mutations, genotypes and histological activity in chronic hepatitis B. *J Viral Hepat* 2000;7:258–67.

3 Transmission of hepatitis B to patients from four infected surgeons without hepatitis B e antigen. The Incident Investigation Teams and others. *N Engl J Med* 1997;**336**:178–84.

4 Department of Health. Hepatitis B infected health workers. Health Service Circular 2000/020 (HSC 2000/020) 23 June 2000. London: DH, 2000. www.doh.gov.uk/nhsexec/hepatitisb.htm

5 Lai CL, Dienstag J, Schiff E, Leung NW *et al.* Prevalence and clinical correlates of YMDD variants during lamivudine therapy for patients with chronic hepatitis B. *Clin Infect Dis* 2003; **36**:687–96.

6 Public Health Laboratory Service. Hepatitis C virus transmission from health care worker to patient. Communicable Disease Report 30 June 1995;5:122. www.hpa.org.uk/cdr/CDR95/cdr2695.pdf

7 Department of Health. Hepatitis C infected health care workers. Health Service Circular 2002/010 (HSC 2002/010) 14 August 2002. London: DH, 2002. www.dh.gov.uk/assetRoot/04/01/22/17/04012217.pdf

8 Fried MW, Shiffman ML, Reddy KR, Smith C *et al.* Peginterferon alfa-2a plus ribavirin for chronic hepatitis C virus infection. *N Engl J Med* 2002;**347**:975–82.

9 Jaeckel E, Cornberg M, Wedemeyer H, Santantonio T *et al.* Treatment of acute hepatitis C with interferon alfa-2b. *N Engl J Med* 2001;**345**:1452–7.

10 Thorburn D, Roy K, Cameron SO, Johnston J *et al.* Risk of hepatitis C virus transmission from patients to surgeons: model based on an unlinked anonymous study of hepatitis C virus prevalence in hospital patients in Glasgow. *Gut* 2003;**52**:1333–8.

11 Thorburn D, Dundas D, McCruden EA, Cameron SO *et al.* A study of hepatitis C prevalence in healthcare workers in the west of Scotland. *Gut* 2001;**48**:116–20.

12 Thorburn D, Roy K, Wilson KS, Stell D *et al.* Anonymous study of HCV prevalence in liver transplant surgeons. *Gut* 2004;**53**(Suppl 1):A81.

Management of ascites

David Patch and Kevin Moore

□ INTRODUCTION

Ascites is a major complication of cirrhosis, occurring in 50% of patients during 10 years of follow-up. The development of ascites is an important landmark in the natural history of cirrhosis since it is associated with a 50% mortality over two years[1] and indicates the need to consider liver transplantation as a therapeutic option.[2] Most patients (75%) who present with ascites have underlying cirrhosis, with the rest due to malignancy (10%), heart failure (3%), tuberculosis (TB) (2%), pancreatitis (1%) and other rare causes. Isolated ascitic hydrothorax may be a presenting feature in 5% of patients. Management of these patients may be complex and should be performed by a gastroenterologist/haematologist.[3]

□ DEFINITIONS[4]

Uncomplicated ascites

Ascites is termed 'uncomplicated' when it is neither infected nor associated with the development of the hepatorenal syndrome. It can be graded as follows:

- *Grade 1* (mild): ascites detectable only by ultrasound examination
- *Grade 2* (moderate): ascites causing moderate symmetrical distension of abdomen
- *Grade 3* (large): ascites causing marked abdominal distension.

Refractory ascites

Ascites is refractory if either it cannot be mobilised or its early recurrence (ie after therapeutic paracentesis) cannot be satisfactorily prevented by medical therapy. There are two subgroups:

- *Diuretic-resistant ascites*: ascites refractory to dietary sodium restriction and intensive diuretic treatment (spironolactone 400 mg/day and furosemide 160 mg/day for at least one week, with a salt restricted diet below 90 mmol (5.2 g) salt/day).
- *Diuretic-intractable ascites*: ascites refractory to therapy due to the development of diuretic-induced complications that preclude the use of an effective diuretic dosage.

☐ PATHOGENESIS OF ASCITES FORMATION

Two factors are involved in the pathogenesis of ascites formation: portal (sinusoidal) hypertension and sodium and water retention.

Role of portal hypertension

Portal hypertension increases the hydrostatic pressure within the hepatic sinusoids and favours the transudation of fluid into the peritoneal cavity. Fluid is also lost from the splanchnic bed; this may not be as significant as loss from the liver because patients with presinusoidal portal hypertension (eg portal vein thrombosis or congenital hepatic fibrosis) rarely develop ascites, except following an insult to liver function such as gastrointestinal haemorrhage. Conversely, acute hepatic vein thrombosis, causing post-sinusoidal portal hypertension, is usually associated with ascites. In practice, plasma albumin concentrations probably have little influence on the rate of ascites formation.

Sodium and water retention

'Underfill' theory

When excess interstitial fluid is produced across the sinusoidal vascular bed it is initially drained by the regional lymphatics. Once the rate of lymph production exceeds that of removal, ascites begins to accumulate. The loss of intravascular volume activates the renin/angiotensin system and also results in salt and water retention – described as the 'underfill' theory.

'Overfill' theory

The situation is complicated because salt and water retention is seen *before* ascites formation ('overfill');[5] it is postulated that in sinusoidal portal hypertension a hepatorenal reflex results in primary renal activation and salt and water retention.

Renal vasoconstriction, a common feature of both theories, is partly a homeostatic response involving increased renal sympathetic activity and activation of the renin-angiotensin system in order to maintain blood pressure during the systemic vasodilatation seen in cirrhosis. There is also an imbalance of local vasoconstrictor substances such as endothelin 1 and thromboxane A2. Decreased renal blood flow decreases glomerular filtration rate and reduces fractional excretion of sodium.

☐ PROGNOSIS

The development of ascites is associated with a 50% mortality within two years of diagnosis. Once the ascites becomes refractory to medical therapy, up to 50% of patients die within six months.[6] Despite improving fluid management and patient quality of life while awaiting liver transplantation, treatments such as therapeutic paracentesis and transjugular intrahepatic portosystemic shunt (TIPS) do not improve long-term survival without transplantation for most patients.

Suitability for liver transplantation should be considered when any patient with cirrhosis develops ascites. The development of ascites should be seen as a state of markedly heightened renal sensitivity, and attention should always focus on renal function as opposed to abdominal distension.

□ DIAGNOSIS

Initial investigations

The underlying cause of ascites is frequently obvious from the history and physical examination, but it is important to exclude other causes of ascites. It should not be assumed that the alcoholic patient has alcoholic liver disease, so tests must be directed at diagnosing the cause of ascites. The essential investigations on admission include:

- diagnostic paracentesis with measurement of ascitic fluid albumin/protein
- ascitic fluid microscopy and culture, and
- ascitic fluid amylase ± cytology.

Other investigations should include abdominal ultrasound to evaluate the appearance of liver, pancreas and lymph nodes, as well as the presence of splenomegaly, which may signify portal hypertension. Blood tests should be taken for measurement of urea and electrolytes, liver function tests, prothrombin time and full blood count. Measurement of urinary sodium (preferably through a 24-hour urine collection) is also recommended. The presence of persistent ascites despite a urinary sodium of more than 90 mmol suggests the patient is not compliant with dietary advice or the original diagnosis is incorrect.

Abdominal paracentesis

The commonest site for an ascitic tap is about 15 cm lateral to the umbilicus usually in the left lower abdominal quadrant, with care taken to avoid an enlarged liver or spleen. The inferior and superior epigastric arteries run just lateral to the umbilicus towards the mid-inguinal point and should be avoided. For diagnostic purposes, 20–30 ml of ascitic fluid should be withdrawn for the inoculation of ascites into two blood culture bottles for the tests outlined below. (I use a blue 23 g needle, with a local anaesthetic in obese individuals, and do not replace/correct clotting factors for diagnostic paracentesis.)

Complications of ascitic taps (abdominal haematomas) occur in up to 1% of patients but are rarely serious or life-threatening. More serious complications such as haemoperitoneum or bowel perforation are rare (<1/1,000 procedures).

Ascitic fluid investigations

Microscopy and culture

All patients should be screened for the development of spontaneous bacterial peritonitis (SBP) which is present in approximately 15% of patients with cirrhosis and ascites admitted to hospital. An ascitic neutrophil count above 250 cells/mm^3 (0.25×10^9/l) is diagnostic of SBP in the absence of a known perforated viscus. (A culture with more than one organism should alert the clinician to the possibility of perforation.) Bloody ascitic fluid (>50,000 cells/mm^3) is present in about 2% of cirrhotics and may indicate an underlying hepatocellular carcinoma but no cause is found in 50% of these patients.

Gram-stain of ascitic fluid is not indicated as it is rarely helpful. The sensitivity of smear for mycobacteria is poor, while fluid culture for mycobacteria has a sensitivity of 50%.[7] If TB is suspected, a polymerase chain reaction test should also be requested. Several studies have shown that inoculation of ascitic fluid into blood culture bottles will identify an organism in 72–90% of cases of SBP, whereas ascitic fluid sent in a sterile container to the laboratory will do so in only about 40%.

Protein and ascitic fluid amylase

Conventionally, ascites is divided into exudates and transudates in which the ascitic protein concentration is above or below 30 g/l, respectively. This subdivision helps to identify the cause. Thus, malignancy classically causes an exudative ascites while cirrhosis causes a transudate. However, there are many misconceptions in clinical practice. For example, most clinicians believe that cardiac ascites is a transudate when this is rarely the case. In fact, ascitic protein is above 25 g/l in up to 30% of patients with otherwise uncomplicated cirrhosis whereas patients with cirrhosis and tuberculous ascites may have a low ascitic protein. The serum ascites-albumin gradient (SA–AG) is far superior in categorising ascites (97% accuracy) (Table 1).[8] Ascitic amylase should always be determined since a high ascitic amylase is diagnostic of pancreatic ascites.

Cytology

Only 7% of ascitic fluid cytologies are positive, but cytological examination is 60–90% accurate in the diagnosis of malignant ascites.

Table 1 Categorisation of ascites by the serum ascites-albumin gradient (SA–AG).

SA–AG (%)	Cause of ascites
>11	Cirrhosis Cardiac failure Nephrotic syndrome
<11	Malignancy Pancreatitis Tuberculosis

□ TREATMENT

Liver transplantation

It is worth reiterating that the development of ascites should trigger consideration of liver transplantation rather than waiting until the ascites has become problematic.

Dietary salt restriction

Dietary salt restriction alone can create a negative sodium balance in 10% of patients; it has been associated with lower diuretic requirement, faster resolution of ascites and shorter hospitalisation. In the past, dietary salt was often restricted to 20–50 mmol/day; this frequently led to protein malnutrition and is no longer recommended. The current recommendation is to restrict dietary salt to about 90 mmol/day (5.2 g) by adopting a no-added salt diet and avoidance of pre-prepared foodstuffs.

Role of water restriction

Water restriction is often (incorrectly) advised, particularly in patients with hyponatraemia. In most cases, hyponatraemia is a consequence of diuretic therapy; fluid restriction only exacerbates the state of intravascular volume depletion seen in patients with ascites. The correct approach is to stop diuretics and fluid challenge the patients. Fluid restriction should be employed only after these initial measures.

The role of new drugs such as specific vasopressin-2 receptor antagonists in the treatment of dilutional hyponatraemia is as yet unclear.

Diuretics

Diuretics have been the mainstay of treatment of ascites since the 1940s when they first became available. Many diuretic agents have been evaluated over the years, but in UK clinical practice diuretics have been mainly confined to spironolactone, amiloride, furosemide and bumetanide (see below). If a patient presents in hospital with tense ascites, my recommendation is that diuretics should *not* be the initial treatment as their use may cause dehydration and renal impairment.

Spironolactone

Spironolactone, an aldosterone antagonist, acts mainly on the distal tubules to increase natriuresis and conserve potassium. It is the drug of choice in the initial treatment of ascites due to cirrhosis. The initial daily dose of 100 mg may have to be progressively increased up to 400 mg to achieve adequate natriuresis. There is a lag of two days between starting spironolactone treatment and the onset of the natriuretic effect. In controlled studies spironolactone achieved better natriuresis and diuresis than a loop diuretic such as furosemide.[9]

Side effects. The most frequent side effects of spironolactone in cirrhotics are related to its anti-androgenic activity, such as decreased libido, impotence and gynaecomastia in men and menstrual irregularity in women (although most women with ascites do not menstruate). Gynaecomastia can be significantly reduced with the hydrophilic derivative potassium canrenoate, but this is not readily available in the UK. Hyperkalaemia is a significant complication that frequently limits the use of spironolactone in the treatment of ascites.

Furosemide

Furosemide, a loop diuretic, causes a marked natriuresis and diuresis in normal subjects. In the treatment of cirrhosis it is generally used as an adjunct to spironolactone because of its low efficacy when used alone. The simultaneous administration of furosemide and spironolactone increases the natriuretic effect. The initial dose of furosemide is 20 mg/day, usually increased every 2–3 days up to, but not exceeding, 160 mg/day. High doses of furosemide should be used cautiously because they are associated with severe electrolyte disturbance and metabolic alkalosis.

Other diuretics

Amiloride acts on the distal tubule and induces diuresis in 80% of patients at doses of 5–20 mg/day. It is less effective than spironolactone or potassium canrenoate but does not cause gynaecomastia. Bumetanide is similar to furosemide in its action and efficacy.

□ APPROACH TO MANAGEMENT

A 'stepped care' approach is usually taken in the management of ascites, starting with modest dietary salt restriction and an increasing dose of spironolactone. Furosemide is added when 200 mg spironolactone alone has proved ineffective. In patients with severe oedema there is less need to be too restrictive about the rate of daily weight loss. When the oedema has resolved but the ascites persists, the rate of weight loss should not exceed about 0.5 kg/day. Over-diuresis is associated with intravascular volume depletion (25%) leading to renal impairment, hepatic encephalopathy (26%) and hyponatraemia (28%).

About 10% of patients with cirrhosis and ascites have refractory ascites. In patients who fail to respond to treatment, a careful dietary and drug history should be obtained. It is important to ensure they are not consuming drugs rich in sodium or that inhibit salt and water excretion such as non-steroidal anti-inflammatory drugs.

□ THERAPEUTIC PARACENTESIS

Patients with large or refractory ascites are usually initially managed by repeated large volume paracentesis. Several controlled clinical studies have demonstrated that large-volume paracentesis with colloid replacement is rapid, safe and effective.[10]

Total paracentesis is safer than repeated paracentesis if volume expansion is administered post-paracentesis. Failure to give volume expansion can lead to post-paracentesis circulatory dysfunction with renal function impairment.

Ascites recurs in most patients (93%) following paracentesis if diuretic therapy is not reinstituted but in only 18% of patients treated with spironolactone. Reintroduction of diuretics after paracentesis does not appear to increase the risk of post-paracentesis circulatory dysfunction.

Haemodynamic changes following paracentesis

Total paracentesis is associated with significant haemodynamic effects[11] but does not lead to circulatory collapse. Large-volume paracentesis (average >10 litres over 2–4 hours) causes a marked reduction of intra-abdominal pressure and inferior vena cava pressure, leading to an immediate decrease in central venous pressure. This is accompanied by an increase in cardiac output and a decrease in systemic vascular resistance. These haemodynamic changes are maximal at three hours. Pulmonary capillary wedge pressure decreases at six hours and continues to fall further in the absence of colloid replacement. Blood pressure decreases by about 8 mmHg. The severity of post-paracentesis circulatory dysfunction correlates inversely with patient survival.

Plasma expansion post-paracentesis

Plasma expansion should always be used whenever five litres of ascites are removed. Serial paracentesis, with and without albumin replacement, has been evaluated in patients with tense ascites. For a single paracentesis of less than five litres, it is safe either to omit volume expansion or to use synthetic plasma expanders (I favour the latter approach).[12]

There is still some debate about whether volume expansion should be carried out with albumin or artificial plasma expanders. Randomised controlled trials (RCT) comparing dextran-70 or haemaccel with albumin suggest that artificial plasma expanders are clinically effective in the prevention of hyponatraemia and renal impairment but that their use is associated with a significantly greater activation of renin-angiotensin-aldosterone.[13] These data indicate that albumin would prove to be clinically superior to haemaccel, gelofusine or dextran if enough patients were studied. Analysis of data from all published studies also suggests that albumin is more effective in the prevention of hyponatraemia (8% of 482 patients developed hyponatraemia) than other plasma expanders (17% of 344 patients). Albumin (as a 20% or 25% solution) should be infused after completion of a paracentesis of over five litres at a dose of 8 g of albumin per litre of ascites removed.

Terlipressin

In the one pilot trial that compared terlipressin (3 doses of 1 mg) and albumin replacement in patients undergoing paracentesis there was no difference in markers of circulatory dysfunction.[14] I do not routinely use terlipressin, but only in patients who have previously had problems with paracentesis.

Procedure

Paracentesis should be carried out under strict sterile conditions. The cannula should have multiple side perforations, otherwise the end becomes blocked by bowel wall. The needle is usually inserted into the left or right lower abdominal quadrant. All ascitic fluid should be drained in a single session as rapidly as possible over 1–4 hours, assisted by turning the patient on to their side if necessary. It should *never* be left in overnight.

After the paracentesis, the patient should lie on the opposite side for two hours to prevent leakage of any remaining ascitic fluid and, if necessary, a suture inserted around the site of drainage. The author uses fresh frozen plasma pre-procedure when the prothrombin time exceeds 25 seconds.

□ TRANSJUGULAR INTRAHEPATIC PORTOSYSTEMIC SHUNT

Radiologically placed intrahepatic shunts have been used extensively in patients with uncontrolled variceal bleeding. Elevated portal pressure is one of the main factors contributing to the pathogenesis of ascites, so it is not surprising that TIPS is also a highly effective treatment for refractory ascites. This has been confirmed in numerous case reports and reflects the experience with surgical shunts. TIPS also improves the nutritional status of patients, though the mechanism is unclear.

However, RCTs comparing TIPS with large-volume paracentesis have not shown TIPS to be superior to intermittent paracentesis, with greater overall cost and the significant side effect of a much higher rate of encephalopathy.[15] There is some criticism of these trials (the shunts were large) but it is clear that TIPS is not the panacea for ascites and its role is limited to highly selected patients. It is particularly useful in patients with ascitic hydrothorax where the frequency of thoracocentesis may be high due to the inability of the thoracic cavity to expand to accommodate the ascitic fluid.

□ CONCLUSIONS

The development of ascites is an important landmark in the natural history of cirrhosis. Adequate management is important; not only does it improve quality of life in patients with cirrhosis but it also prevents serious complications such as SBP. However, treatment of ascites does not significantly improve survival, so development of ascites should be considered as an indication for liver transplantation – the ultimate treatment of ascites and its complications.

REFERENCES

1 Gines P, Quintero E, Arroyo V, Teres J *et al.* Compensated cirrhosis: natural history and prognostic factors. *Hepatology* 1987;7:122–8.

2 Powell WJ Jr, Klatskin G. Duration of survival in patients with Laennec's cirrhosis. Influence of alcohol withdrawal, and possible effects of recent changes in general management of the disease. *Am J Med* 1968;**44**:406–20.

3 Gines P, Cardenas A, Arroyo V, Rodes J. Management of cirrhosis and ascites. Review. *N Engl J Med* 2004;**350**:1646–54.

4 Moore KP, Wong F, Gines P, Bernardi M *et al.* The management of ascites in cirrhosis: report on the consensus conference of the International Ascites Club. Review. *Hepatology* 2003;**38**:258–66.

5 Wong F, Liu P, Blendis L. Sodium homeostasis with chronic sodium loading in preascitic cirrhosis. *Gut* 2001;**49**:847–51.

6 Bories P, Garcia-Compean D, Michel H, Bourel M *et al.* The treatment of refractory ascites by the LeVeen shunt. A multi-centre controlled trial (57 patients). *J Hepatol* 1986;**3**:212–8.

7 Manohar A, Simjee AA, Haffejee AA, Pettengell KE. Symptoms and investigative findings in 145 patients with tuberculous peritonitis diagnosed by peritoneoscopy and biopsy over a five year period. *Gut* 1990;**31**:1130–2.

8 Runyon BA, Montano AA, Akriviadis EA, Antillon MR *et al.* The serum-ascites albumin gradient is superior to the exudate-transudate concept in the differential diagnosis of ascites. *Ann Intern Med* 1992;**117**:215–20.

9 Perez-Ayuso RM, Arroyo V, Planas R, Gaya J *et al.* Randomized comparative study of efficacy of furosemide versus spironolactone in nonazotemic cirrhosis with ascites. Relationship between the diuretic response and the activity of the renin-aldosterone system. *Gastroenterology* 1983;**84**(5 Pt 1):961–8.

10 Gines P, Arroyo V, Quintero E, Planas R *et al.* Comparison of paracentesis and diuretics in the treatment of cirrhotics with tense ascites. Results of a randomized study. *Gastroenterology* 1987;**93**:234–41.

11 Panos MZ, Moore K, Vlavianos P, Chambers JB *et al.* Single, total paracentesis for tense ascites: sequential haemodynamic changes and right atrial size. Hepatology 1990;**11**:662–7.

12 Peltekian KM, Wong F, Liu PP, Logan AG *et al.* Cardiovascular, renal, and neurohumoral responses to single large-volume paracentesis in patients with cirrhosis and diuretic-resistant ascites. *Am J Gastroenterol* 1997;**92**:394–9.

13 Planas R, Gines P, Arroyo V, Llach J *et al.* Dextran-70 versus albumin as plasma expanders in cirrhotic patients with tense ascites treated with total paracentesis. Results of a randomized study. *Gastroenterology* 1990;**99**:1736–44.

14 Moreau R, Asselah T, Condat B, de Kerguenec C *et al.* Comparison of the effect of terlipressin and albumin on arterial blood volume in patients with cirrhosis and tense ascites treated by paracentesis: a randomised pilot study. *Gut* 2002;**50**:90–4.

15 Sanyal AJ, Genning C, Reddy KR, Wong F *et al.* The North American Study for the Treatment of Refractory Ascites. *Gastroenterology* 2003;**124**:634–41.

Non-alcoholic steatohepatitis and fatty liver disease

Oliver James

INTRODUCTION

The term non-alcoholic steatohepatitis (NASH) was coined as recently as 1980 by Ludwig *et al* at the Mayo clinic for the pathological and clinical features of non-alcoholic disease of the liver associated with the pathological features most commonly seen in alcoholic liver disease (ALD) itself.[1] Unfortunately, the appearance of simple fat without any of the features of steatohepatitis or fibrosis described in alcoholic hepatitis was not included in this original description. Consequently, the inelegant term of non-alcoholic fatty liver disease (NAFLD) was coined by Matteoni *et al* to describe the spectrum of pure fatty liver and NASH. NAFLD is now a widely accepted term describing this spectrum.[2]

HOW BIG IS THE PROBLEM?

The terms describing non-alcoholic fatty liver have been widely used only in the past few years but it is increasingly clear that a significant proportion of the population in westernised countries have fatty liver, many with concomitant elevation of liver enzymes. These patients are increasingly referred to liver clinics by primary care physicians. No prospective epidemiological studies of NAFLD have been carried out, but important evidence arises from two groups of studies:

1. The DIONYSOS study of liver disease in Northern Italy[3] carried out population surveys of abnormal liver blood tests and ultrasound examinations, with some longitudinal follow-up in two small towns. Up to 15% of non-heavy drinking (less than 21 drinks per week) and non-very obese (body mass index (BMI) <28) individuals in the general population were found to have the appearance of fatty liver on ultrasound.[3]

2. Studies arising from the US National Health and Nutrition Examination Survey (NHANES) have demonstrated that, depending upon the level at which the upper limit of normal is taken for serum alanine aminotransferase (ALT), 2.8–7.9% of the population have cryptogenic elevation of ALT after excluding known causes of liver disease (eg hepatitis B and C). This cryptogenic elevation of ALT is closely related to increases in BMI, waste-to-hip ratio, fasting insulin and serum leptin. Other features of the metabolic syndrome were found in 55% of those with raised ALT.[4,5]

NATURAL HISTORY

Most of the significant studies on the natural history of NAFLD have been cross-sectional. One of the first well conducted studies investigated 144 patients (97 female, median age 50) with NASH or simple fatty liver on liver biopsy from the histology archives of the Mayo clinic.[6] Rigorous case record review of these patients revealed those with alcohol consumption below 14 units per week and excluded other putative causes of liver disease or fatty liver (eg occasional drug reactions). Degree of fibrosis on liver biopsy was scored from 0 (simple fat alone) to 4 (severe fibrosis/cirrhosis). Clinical and biochemical variables were examined in the case records using univariate and multivariate analysis to search for independent predictors of increased fibrosis: 37 patients (26%) had fat alone. Obesity in this study was defined as BMI above 31.1 for men and above 32.3 for women – higher than in current conventional studies in which obesity is defined as BMI greater than 30. Interestingly, only two of 52 patients aged below 45 at the time of liver biopsy had any fibrosis. There were 59 individuals over age 45 with obesity and/or overt type 2 diabetes, 33 (60%) of whom had some degree of fibrosis. Age ($p < 0.001$), obesity ($p = 0.002$), diabetes ($p = 0.009$) and aspartate aminotransferase/ALT ratio greater than 1 ($p = 0.003$) were all independent predictors of fibrosis.

In another study, cirrhosis or marked fibrosis was found in 30% of 93 consecutive patients with abnormal liver blood tests and BMI over 25 in whom other liver disease had been rigorously excluded.[7] Multivariate analysis of clinical and biochemical variables was again examined to find independent predictors of the presence of fibrosis/cirrhosis. Age over 50 (odds ratio (OR) 14.1), BMI above 28 (OR 5.7), ALT more than twice normal (OR 4.6) and fasting triglyceride above 170 mg/dl (OR 5.0) were independently associated with marked fibrosis or cirrhosis in this study.

Possibly the best study of the spectrum and severity of NAFLD was by Matteoni *et al*[8] who reviewed all liver biopsies at the Cleveland Clinic with a histological diagnosis of fatty liver between 1979 and 1987. Exclusions were alcohol consumption over 30 g per day, some medications, previous jejuno-ileal bypass surgery or total parenteral nutrition (each known to produce NAFLD), other known liver disease and malignancy. Biochemical, demographic and clinical details were recorded and there was a mean follow-up of eight years after the original liver biopsy. Liver biopsies were classified from type 1 (simple fat alone) through to type 4 (significant fibrosis/cirrhosis), types 2 and 3 having features of alcoholic hepatitis. Two patients (4%) with type 1 on first biopsy had developed cirrhosis during follow-up, while five (9%) initially type 4 developed cirrhosis in addition to the nine who had cirrhosis on original biopsy (total 14 patients (25%)). There was no liver related mortality over eight years in type 1 and nine (12%) in types 2–4. In a subsequent analysis of individuals with type 2 diabetes, 44 patients had overt type 2 diabetes, 11 of whom developed cirrhosis and seven (15.6%) died of liver disease. In contrast, only nine (10%) of the 88 patients who did not have overt type 2 diabetes at presentation developed cirrhosis and there were only two (2.3%) liver related deaths.

Our group carried out a similar study to that at the Cleveland Clinic, but examined 50 patients found on initial liver biopsy to have simple fat alone, with no evidence of necrosis, inflammation or fibrosis and in whom alcohol had been rigorously excluded as a cause for the fatty liver.[9] At a median follow-up of 11 years following the original biopsy all the patients were traced: 15 had a further liver biopsy, 21 had clinical or laboratory follow-up but no biopsy, 14 had died but none of liver disease. There was no evidence of histological or clinical progression in any of those who had liver biopsy and on clinical/laboratory follow-up of the rest.

It should be noted that only two of the 49 comparable pure fatty liver alone patients described by Matteoni[8] had developed cirrhosis during a similar follow-up period. This implies that the likelihood or rate of progression of liver disease is low in individuals with simple fat alone and no features of steatonecrosis, inflammation or fibrosis.

A subsequent study from Newcastle carried out a fuller histological follow-up of 91 patients with NAFLD from the histology database (1985–1995) after exclusion of other liver disease and rigorous exclusion of significant alcohol consumption.[10] Of the 91 patients, 62 had fatty liver alone on initial biopsy and 29 features of NASH. At a median follow-up of 8.1 years, 42 (67%) of the 62 fatty liver patients had no clinical or histological progression and seven (11%) had worsening histology (six of them had developed fibrosis). Among the 29 NASH patients, 21 (72%) had no clinical or histological progression, three had worse fibrosis, there was one cirrhosis, 12 patients refused biopsy and three had died non-liver related deaths. The major factor predicting histological progression was increased severity of steatosis on the index liver biopsy.

It can now be concluded that at least 10% of those with simple fatty liver have a risk of developing liver fibrosis over about eight years, and that worsening fibrosis will occur in at least 10% over a subsequent eight years.

□ NON-ALCOHOLIC STEATOHEPATITIS, CRYPTOGENIC CIRRHOSIS AND HEPATOCELLULAR CANCER

In an important study, Caldwell and colleagues[11] compared the characteristics of 70 consecutive patients with cryptogenic cirrhosis with those of 50 patients with a histological diagnosis of NASH, 39 with cirrhosis from hepatitis C age over 50 at presentation, and 33 patients with primary biliary cirrhosis (PBC) who had cirrhosis. The term 'cryptogenic cirrhosis' is used for patients who have cirrhosis in whom there is no apparent clinical, laboratory or histological clue as to its possible underlying cause. A history of previous type 2 diabetes and/or obesity (BMI >31) was significantly more common in the cryptogenic patients than in the hepatitis C or PBC groups (73% vs 28% vs 33%).[11] In the NASH patients, 70% had diabetes and/or obesity. Interestingly, the median age of the NASH patients was 50 while that for patients with cryptogenic cirrhosis was 63.

A further possible final part of the natural history of fatty liver disease was suggested by Ratziu *et al.*[12] They identified 37 individuals from medical records in their Paris hospital between 1988 and 2000 with cryptogenic cirrhosis, 27 of whom were overweight (BMI >25) both 10 years before and at the time of diagnosis of cirrhosis and 10 had cryptogenic cirrhosis not associated with overweight. These patients were compared with 391 patients from the same institution over the same time period, diagnosed as having cirrhosis related to hepatitis C virus (HCV). The follow-up was 0–12 years. The features of the three groups are illustrated in Table 1.[12]

It is of interest that the age at development of cirrhosis in the overweight patients was 62 versus 45 in the lean cryptogenic cirrhosis group, there were more men in the overweight group and the mean BMI was considerably higher than in the other groups. At the time of presentation the complications of cirrhosis, as indicated by the Child-Pugh score, were worse in the overweight cryptogenic patients than in the lean or HCV groups. Finally, 30% of the cryptogenic overweight patients developed hepatocellular cancer (HCC) in the follow-up period compared with only 10% of the cryptogenic lean patients (more likely to be female) and 18% of the hepatitis C cirrhosis patients.

To support the idea that patients with cryptogenic cirrhosis, possibly associated with obesity and the metabolic syndrome – hence arising from NAFLD/NASH – may progress to HCC, a study from a single centre in the US[13] studied 105 consecutive patients with HCC. The commonest causes of the underlying liver disease were hepatitis C (51%) and cryptogenic cirrhosis (29%). Among the 30 individuals with HCC arising in cryptogenic cirrhosis, 58% had BMI over 30, 47% had type 2 diabetes and 29% elevated fasting lipids compared with 25%, 8% and 4%, respectively, in the other 75 patients with HCC.

Table 1 Comparison of patients with cryptogenic cirrhosis and hepatitis C virus infection.[12]

	Cryptogenic cirrhosis		
	Overweight	**Lean**	**Hepatitis C virus**
Age at cirrhosis	62	45	54
Male:female ratio	1.7	0.7	1.8
Mean BMI	31	22.6	25.1
Childs B/C (%)	30	10	18
HCC (%)	30	10	18

BMI = body mass index; HCC = hepatocellular cancer.

New profile of cryptogenic cirrhosis

The current best estimate is that about two-thirds of cryptogenic cirrhosis is probably attributable to preceding NAFLD. A proportion of the others may be associated with rather ill defined autoimmune chronic hepatitis, mainly found in women. The likelihood of developing HCC may be different in NASH related cirrhosis (with previous obesity, type 2 diabetes and other features of the metabolic syndrome) than in non-NASH cryptogenic cirrhosis. It appears possible that in NASH related cryptogenic cirrhosis the risk of developing HCC is similar to that in HCV related cirrhosis and other forms of cirrhosis (eg alcoholic cirrhosis). However, this is all speculation and requires further proof.

Figure 1 summarises the current concept of the natural history of fatty liver disease. Overweight individuals with the metabolic syndrome and insulin resistance,

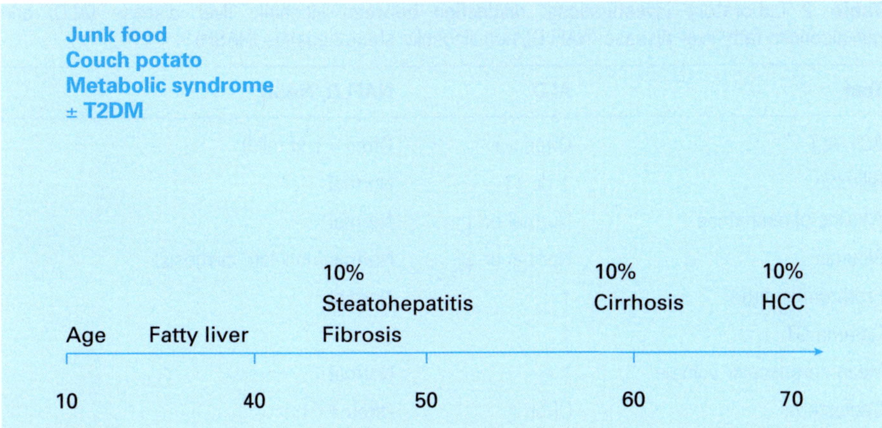

Fig 1 Natural history of non-alcoholic fatty liver disease (HCC = hepatocellular carcinoma; T2DM = type 2 diabetes mellitus).

possibly progressing to type 2 diabetes, have a high risk of developing simple fatty liver, often by the age of 40. Population estimates suggest that 3–10% of the population may have simple fatty liver. Over the next 8–10 years, 10–12% of these may progress to develop features of steatohepatitis and/or fibrosis, while a further 10–12% will go on to develop cirrhosis. The median age for development of cirrhosis is probably just over 60. A proportion of these individuals will progress to HCC. The 20–40 year time frame in this natural history in some ways parallels that seen in HCV.

□ DIAGNOSIS

The diagnosis of NAFLD rests upon the appropriate exclusion of other liver disease together with a strict history of alcohol consumption (more than 14 units of alcohol per week for women or 21 units for men take the 'N' out of NAFLD). It is increasingly clear that obesity and the features of the metabolic syndrome are additive in producing fatty liver, steatohepatitis, fibrosis and ultimately cirrhosis.[14]

Blood tests

Table 2 shows blood tests comparing NAFLD with ALD. Note that gamma-glutamyltransferase is elevated in both NAFLD and ALD. Both our observations and those of Ratziu *et al*[7] suggest that elevated red cell mean corpuscular volume (>100) is seldom found in NAFLD and may be the most discriminant blood test for NAFLD versus ALD.

Ultrasound

Apart from a diagnosis of exclusion, the second main pillar of diagnosis of NAFLD is ultrasound. Until the development of cirrhosis, when fat frequently disappears

Table 2 Laboratory investigations: distinction between alcoholic liver disease (ALD) and non-alcoholic fatty liver disease (NAFLD)/non-alcoholic steatohepatitis (NASH).

Test	ALD	NAFLD/NASH
AST/ALT	Often >1	Often <1 (if mild)
Bilirubin	↑ or ↑↑	Normal
Alkaline phosphatase	Normal or ↑	Normal
Albumin	Normal or ↓	Normal (until late cirrhosis)
Prothrombin time	↑	Normal
Gamma GT	↑	↑
Mean corpuscular volume	↑	Normal
Cholesterol	Often ↑	Often ↑
B1 ethanol	Present	Absent

ALT = alanine aminotransferase; AST = aspartate aminotransferase; gamma GT = gamma-glutamyltransferase.

from the liver, ultrasound shows a typical bright, usually homogeneous, appearance of fat which is easily distinguished. However, it is unwise to overinterpret the ultrasound appearance, so reports suggesting small degrees of liver fibrosis not amounting to cirrhosis are best ignored.[15]

Liver biopsy

Liver biopsy is often undertaken in patients with NAFLD. It may be carried out to stage the liver disease, for example to assess whether fibrosis has developed on a background of fatty liver. A histological staging and grading system has recently been proposed.[16] Liver biopsy should also form the basis for future controlled trials of putative new treatments for NAFLD.

In this, often indolent and relatively asymptomatic, disease the decision whether to carry out liver biopsy with its attendant discomforts and risks is difficult. However, the lessons being learnt from studies of the natural history of the disease should be borne in mind: although there is only a small likelihood of significant fibrosis or liver inflammation below age 40, there is a significant possibility that an obese individual with type 2 diabetes and/or hyperlipidaemia will develop silent cryptogenic cirrhosis by the age of 60. My current practice therefore is to carry out liver biopsies on all individuals with NAFLD (based on the other diagnostic criteria) aged 50 or over. Apart from the importance of staging the disease, and hence estimating the need for future surveillance, liver biopsy may indicate the relative urgency of need for treatment. At present, this approach is pragmatic and not evidence based.

☐ AETIOLOGY AND THE METABOLIC SYNDROME

It is becoming increasingly clear that fatty liver may be considered as part of the metabolic syndrome, which is defined as:[17]

- waist circumference greater than 102 cm (men) or 88 cm (women)
- fasting glucose equal to or greater than 100 mg/dl
- high-density lipoprotein cholesterol below 40 mg/dl (men) or below 50 mg/dl (women)
- triglycerides 150 mg/dl or above
- blood pressure 130/85 mmHg or above (untreated).

In addition to the observation that obesity and type 2 diabetes are frequently associated with fatty liver, the first of a number of observations of the close connection between NAFLD and insulin resistance was made by Marchesini's group in 1999.[18] Anthropometric and other clinical and biochemical indices were measured in 46 individuals with non-alcoholic fatty liver (defined by bright ultrasound and the usual exclusions) who did not have overt type 2 diabetes and in 92 controls. A standard glucose tolerance test (GTT) load was given, followed by measurement of serum glucose and insulin from which the index of insulin resistance was calculated. No difference was found in fasting glucose levels between patients and controls, but fasting insulins and average insulin during the GTT were almost twice as great in the fatty liver patients (index of insulin resistance 100% higher in the patients). Insulin resistance was the strongest predictor of fatty liver (*or* 15% increase in insulin resistance). Severity of insulin resistance was similar in overweight and normal weight fatty liver patients.

It can be hypothesised that peripheral insulin resistance and central obesity lead to increased delivery of fat to the liver, decreased hepatic oxidation of fat and possibly decreased hepatic export of fat – hence the appearance of fatty liver. A number of studies have suggested that increased insulin and glucose lead to raised connective tissue growth factor which is independently fibrogenic.[19]

Leptin

Not only is high plasma insulin associated with increased connective tissue growth factor but high insulin is associated with raised serum leptin – obese individuals have raised leptin possibly because they become 'leptin resistant'. Furthermore, leptin receptors are present on hepatic stellate cells.[20] A series of recent studies has shown, first, that *in vitro* addition of leptin to hepatic stellate cells leads to collagen deposition and, secondly, in the congenital Ob/Ob obese mouse which has no leptin there is gross fatty liver but never fibrosis. Addition of leptin to the Ob/Ob mouse leads to fibrosis.[20]

Diet

A proportion of NAFLD patients (perhaps about 10%) appear to have fatty liver although being neither grossly obese nor having insulin resistance. The explanation why these individuals develop fatty liver may conceivably lie in their diet. Recently Musso *et al*[21] carried out extremely careful dietary studies in 25 non-obese, non-diabetic subjects with NAFLD and 25 age-, sex- and BMI-matched controls. The dietary intake of the NASH patients was richer in saturated fats (13.7% vs 10%, $p = 0.001$) and cholesterol (506 mg/dl vs 405 mg/dl, $p = 0.002$). Saturated fat intake correlated with insulin resistance and other features of the metabolic syndrome and also with a rise in postprandial triglycerides.

These authors concluded that 'bad' diets may promote NASH both directly by modulating hepatic triglyceride accumulation and also indirectly by affecting insulin resistance. This may account for those NAFLD patients who have neither insulin resistance nor obesity.

Other risk factors

In addition to the mechanisms discussed above, there is evidence that lipid peroxidation/oxidative stress and also the presence of excess endotoxin – and consequently tumour necrosis factor and other cytokines – may, as in alcoholic steatohepatitis, play a significant role in converting innocent pure fatty liver to progressive steatohepatitis and steatonecrosis.

Finally, in terms of pathogenesis, genes associated both with the metabolic syndrome and with some of the possible processes involved in a tendency to steatohepatitis or fibrosis (eg polymorphisms in genes or gene promoters in lipid peroxidation/oxidative stress or the cytokine cascade) are certainly involved in determining which individuals develop the worst fatty liver, which go on to develop steatonecrosis, inflammation and fibrosis, and which ultimately develop cirrhosis and HCC. An amended paradigm of NASH natural history may now be considered.

□ MANAGEMENT

In view of its considerable indolence, the question might be asked why treat a patient aged, for example, 40 with transaminase of 100 and fatty liver on ultrasound? There are two powerful arguments.

1 First, a consideration of the natural history of the disease as it is now beginning to be understood. If patients with hepatitis C who may be relatively asymptomatic are increasingly being treated at earlier stages of their disease with lengthy, quite expensive and unpleasant interferon and antiviral agents, there is surely a justification to consider treatment for patients with NAFLD.

2 Although definite symptoms are not prominently reported in early NAFLD, about 30% of patients experience significant fatigue and perhaps 30% also experience persistent right upper abdominal discomfort possibly attributable to liver capsule distension. This can be improved with reversal of the fatty liver.

There is no clear definition at present of which NAFLD patients to treat. Based upon studies of natural history, my view is that treatment may be considered either on the basis of histological criteria (fibrosis and/or necroinflammation on biopsy) or of clinical and biochemical criteria (those with type 2 diabetes, older than 45, BMI >30 and ALT more than twice the upper limit of normal). All these criteria indicate a greater likelihood of fibrosis as far as is presently known.

□ CONCLUSIONS

In summary, management of NAFLD may be considered as follows:

1 Reduce alcohol: remember that NAFLD and alcoholic liver damage are not mutually exclusive but probably additive. In a patient with NAFLD, advise no more than seven units of alcohol per week.

2 Reduce weight if obese or overweight: aim to achieve a BMI below 25.

3 Reduce insulin resistance: exercise itself improves insulin sensitivity. Controlled trials are currently ongoing in a number of centres on the use of metformin or various thioglitazones. At present, no large good controlled trials have shown that any treatment is very effective.

4 An extraordinary epidemic of overweight/obesity, metabolic syndrome and type 2 diabetes is sweeping the western world. With the lag time between causative factors, the development of fatty liver and the subsequent development of significant further liver damage in NAFLD, an extremely steep increase in this disease may be expected over the next 10–20 years — with a spectrum from simple fat in the liver to HCC.

REFERENCES

1 Ludwig J, Viggiano TR, McGill DB, Oh BJ. Nonalcoholic steatohepatitis: Mayo Clinic experiences with a hitherto unnamed disease. *Mayo Clin Proc* 1980;**55**:434–8.

2 McCullough AJ. Non alcoholic liver disease: natural history in steatohepatitis. In: Leuschner U, James O (eds). *Steatohepatitis (NASH and ASH) Falk Symposium 121*. Dordrecht: Kluwer, 2001:11–20.

3 Bellentani S, Saccoccio G, Masutti F, Croce LS *et al.* Prevalence of and risk factors for hepatic steatosis in Northern Italy. *Ann Intern Med* 2000;**132**:112–7.

4 Ruhl CE, Everhart JE. Determinants of the association of overweight with elevated serum alanine aminotransferase activity in the United States. *Gastroenterology* 2003;**124**:71–9.

5 Clark JM, Diehl AM. Defining nonalcoholic fatty liver disease: implications for epidemiologic studies. Review. *Gastroenterology* 2003;**124**:248–50.

6 Angulo P, Keach JC, Batts KP, Lindor KD. Independent predictors of liver fibrosis in patients with nonalcoholic steatohepatitis. *Hepatology* 1999;**30**:1356–62.

7 Ratziu V, Giral P, Charlotte F, Bruckert E *et al.* Liver fibrosis in overweight patients. *Gastroenterology* 2000;**118**:1117–23.

8 Matteoni CA, Younossi ZM, Gramlich T, Boparai N *et al.* Nonalcoholic fatty liver disease: a spectrum of clinical and pathological severity. *Gastroenterology* 1999;**116**:1413–9.

9 Teli MR, James OF, Burt AD, Bennett MK, Day CP. The natural history of nonalcoholic fatty liver: a follow-up study. *Hepatology* 1995;**22**:1714–9.

10 Saksena S, James O, Craig W, Day CP. Clinical and laboratory parameters predicting presence of NASH in unselected patients with NAFLD. *Hepatology* 2002;**36**:222a.

11 Caldwell SH, Oelsner DH, Iezzoni JC, Hespenheide EE *et al.* Cryptogenic cirrhosis: clinical characterization and risk factors for underlying disease. *Hepatology* 1999;**29**:664–9.

12 Ratziu V, Bonyhay L, Di Martino V, Charlotte F *et al.* Survival, liver failure, and hepatocellular carcinoma in obesity-related cryptogenic cirrhosis. *Hepatology* 2002;**35**:1485–93.

13 Marrero JA, Fontana RJ, Su GL, Conjeevaram HS *et al.* NAFLD may be a common underlying liver disease in patients with hepatocellular carcinoma in the United States. *Hepatology* 2002;**36**:1349–54.

14 Bugianesi E, Leone N, Vanni E, Marchesini G *et al.* Expanding the natural history of nonalcoholic steatohepatitis: from cryptogenic cirrhosis to hepatocellular carcinoma. *Gastroenterology* 2002;**123**:134–40.

15 Siegelman ES, Rosen MA. Imaging of hepatic steatosis. Review. *Semin Liv Dis* 2001;**21**:71–80.

16 Brunt EM. Nonalcoholic steatohepatitis: definition and pathology. Review. *Semin Liv Dis* 2001;**21**:3–16.

17 Alberti KG, Zimmet PZ. Definition, diagnosis and classification of diabetes mellitus and its complications. Part 1: diagnosis and classification of diabetes mellitus provisional report of a WHO consultation. *Diabet Med* 1998;**15**:539–53.

18 Pagano G, Pacini G, Musso G, Gambino R *et al.* Nonalcoholic steatohepatitis, insulin resistance, and metabolic syndrome: further evidence for an etiologic association. *Hepatology* 2002;**35**:367–72.

19 Paradis V, Perlemuter G, Bonvoust F, Dargere D *et al.* High glucose and hyperinsulinemia stimulate connective tissue growth factor expression: a potential mechanism involved in progression to fibrosis in nonalcoholic steatohepatitis. *Hepatology* 2001;**34**:738–44.

20 Saxena NK, Ikeda K, Rockey DC, Friedman SL, Anania FA. Leptin in hepatic fibrosis: evidence for increased collagen production in stellate cells and lean littermates of ob/ob mice. *Hepatology* 2002;**35**:762–71.

21 Musso G, Gambino R, De Michieli F, Cassader M *et al.* Dietary habits and their relations to insulin resistance and postprandial lipemia in nonalcoholic steatohepatitis. *Hepatology* 2003;**37**:909–16.

☐ HEPATOLOGY SELF ASSESSMENT QUESTIONS

Viral hepatitis and medical risks

1 Exposure prone procedures (EPPs) include:
 (a) Phlebotomy
 (b) Dental extraction
 (c) Colonoscopy
 (d) Central venous line insertion
 (e) Open cholecystectomy

2 With regard to hepatitis B virus (HBV), infected healthcare workers (HcWs) performing EPPs:
 (a) All hepatitis B surface antigen-positive individuals are excluded
 (b) Individuals with HBV titres above 10^3 copies/ml are excluded regardless of their hepatitis B e antigen (HBeAg) status
 (c) Individuals may perform EPPs if HBV titres are maintained below 10^3 copies/ml on treatment
 (d) Individuals with HBV titres less than 10^3 copies/ml do not require regular follow-up
 (e) HBeAg-negative HcWs with titres persistently below 10^3 copies/ml who are not receiving antiviral therapy may perform EPPs

3 Hepatitis C virus infection:
 (a) Causes symptoms around the time of acquisition in most of those infected
 (b) Must be excluded by screening before HcWs can commence training in specialties performing EPPs
 (c) Must be excluded through annual screening in all surgeons practising in the UK
 (d) Associated with a low level of viraemia does not prohibit the performance of EPPs
 (e) Is more successfully treated in patients receiving interferon therapy early in the natural history of the infection

Management of ascites

1 Ascites due to cirrhosis:
 (a) Is characterised by sodium retention
 (b) May be confined to the thorax in 5% of patients
 (c) May be a presenting feature of hepatocellular carcinoma
 (d) Is sterile when the white cell count of neutrophils is below 500 per mm^3
 (e) Is best treated by transjugular intrahepatic portosystemic shunt

2 Treatment of ascites:
 (a) Ideally should be with diuretics
 (b) Paracentesis should be avoided

(c) Renal dysfunction occurs when more than two litres of ascites are removed
(d) Should routinely include prophylaxis against spontaneous bacterial peritonitis
(e) Should include dietary protein restriction

3 Renal failure in cirrhosis:
(a) Is often precipitated by sepsis
(b) Is characterised by renal vascular vasodilatation
(c) Aldosterone levels are characteristically low
(d) Vasoconstrictor therapy is of little benefit
(e) Responds to diuretic therapy

Non-alcoholic steatohepatitis and fatty liver disease

1 New estimates of the putative causes of 'cryptogenic cirrhosis' suggest:
(a) 50% undiagnosed alcoholic cirrhosis, 25% arising from non-alcoholic fatty liver, 25% from autoimmune liver disease
(b) 50% undiagnosed (and unknown) viral aetiology, 25% undiagnosed 'burnt out' alcoholic cirrhosis, 25% unrecognised autoimmune liver disease
(c) 65% arising from previous non-alcoholic fatty liver disease (NAFLD) and 30% from unrecognised autoimmune liver disease
(d) No real clues
(e) Cryptogenic cirrhosis will become more common as the prevalence of metabolic syndrome increases

2 The distinction between alcoholic (ASH) and non-alcoholic steatohepatitis (NASH) is helped by:
(a) Liver biopsy
(b) Gamma-glutamyltransferase raised in ASH but seldom in NASH
(c) Mean corpuscular volume raised in ASH but seldom in NASH
(d) Alanine aminotransferase/aspartate aminotransferase ratio often greater than 1 in NASH but seldom in ASH
(e) Raised bilirubin more frequent in NASH than in ASH

3 In the patho-aetiology of fatty liver disease:
(a) Even in the absence of diabetes, insulin resistance is the rule rather than the exception
(b) Central obesity is closely associated with development of NAFLD
(c) Alcohol consumption and obesity may be additive in development of fatty liver
(d) It is unlikely that genetic predisposition plays a role in development of NAFLD
(e) Drugs that reduce plasma cholesterol (eg statins) may worsen NAFLD

Transplantation

Bone marrow stem cells: from development to therapy

Tzung-Hai Yen, Nicholas Wright and Richard Poulsom

☐ INTRODUCTION

Since the world's first kidney transplant by Joseph Murray and David Hume in 1954 at Brigham Hospital, Boston, the replacement of faulty organs is no longer an experimental technique but a life-saving procedure for thousands of patients every year. However, the routine implementation of transplantation as a reparative therapy faces two major hurdles:

1. The recipients must endure lifelong immunosuppression in order to prevent graft rejection, despite the common association of chronic administration of calcineurin inhibitors and other immunosuppressants with serious side effects such as severe sepsis, hepatic failure, renal failure and secondary malignancy.
2. The current availability of organs and tissues for transplantation is insufficient to meet the demand. According to recent statistics (February 2004) from the UK Transplant Registry, 5,717 patients are on the waiting list for organ transplantation.

Stem cell therapies, using either embryonic or adult stem cells, may be the solution to the long waiting lists worldwide. A substantial number of reports of adult stem cell plasticity have been published over the last five years, challenging the long-held belief that adult mammalian stem cells are lineage-restricted. In most of the these studies, genetically marked cells from one organ of an adult mouse apparently gave rise to cell types characteristic of other organs following transplantation, suggesting that the cells were more plastic in their developmental potential than previously thought. Adult stem cells may offer therapeutic options to those who do not wish embryonic tissue to be used and would avoid many ethical and political problems. There are additional advantages in that the use of autologous adult stem cells would both reduce the problem of immunological rejection and also the risk of tumour formation found with embryonic stem cell transplantation.

Definitions of terms used in this chapter are listed in Table 1.

☐ THE COHNHEIM HYPOTHESIS

In 1867, Julius Cohnheim, a German pathologist, presented a pioneering hypothesis on tissue repair in mammals.[1] He studied wound repair by injecting an insoluble

Table 1 Definitions of terms.

Stem cell	Cell with the ability to give rise both to a large number of descendants and to specialised cells
Embryonic stem cell	Primitive (or undifferentiated) cell from the embryo with the potential to contribute to a wide variety of specialised cell types in the adult
Adult stem cell (tissue stem cell or somatic stem cell)	Relatively undifferentiated cell found in a differentiated tissue that can renew itself and (with certain limitations) differentiate to yield all the specialised cell types of the tissue from which it originated
Haematopoietic stem cell	Adult stem cell from which all red and white blood cells develop
Marrow stromal cell	Adult stem cell found in bone marrow that generates bone, cartilage, fat and fibrous connective tissue
Plasticity	Ability of stem cells from one adult tissue to generate the differentiated cell types of another tissue

aniline dye into the veins of animals and looked for the appearance of dye-containing cells in wounds created at a distal site. He concluded that most, if not all, of the cells appearing in the wounds came from the bloodstream and, by implication, from bone marrow. The stained cells included not only inflammatory cells but also cells with a fibroblast-like morphology and associated with thin fibrils. Cohnheim's work therefore raised the possibility that bone marrow may be the source of fibroblasts that deposit collagen fibres as part of the normal process of wound repair. This hypothesis has been the subject of much debate and experimentation for decades.

□ BONE MARROW STEM CELLS

Traditionally, adult tissue-derived stem cells of mammalian adults have been viewed as pluripotent precursors capable of lifelong maintenance of cellular compartments typical of the tissue in which they reside. Stem cells have been found in various tissues, including brain, muscle, liver, skin and bone marrow, where they play an important role in healing and regeneration of the tissue they occupy.

Stem cells are referred to as multi- or pluripotent because of their ability to differentiate to a variety of cell types present in a given tissue. Until recently, the differentiation potential of stem cells into tissues of adults has been thought to be limited to cell lineages in the organ from which they were derived. Bone marrow stem cells (BMSCs) are unique among stem cells with regard to their abundance and role in the continuous lifelong physiological replenishment of blood cells. By definition, BMSCs have been grouped into haematopoietic stem cells (HSCs) and non-haematopoietic stem cells or marrow stromal cells (MSCs), which are the progenitors of skeletal tissue components such as bone, cartilage and adipose tissues.

□ MORE STRICT CRITERIA IN DEFINING STEM CELL PLASTICITY

There are large variations in the definition of stem cell plasticity in the literature. Anderson *et al*[2] proposed that there should be a higher standard of experimental proof before it can be accepted that cells indeed cross such lineage boundaries. The following criteria are suggested:

1 The donor population should prospectively be isolated and transplanted without intervening manipulations in culture.

2 The transplanted stem cells should give rise to robust and sustained regeneration of the target tissues.

3 The phenotype of the converted cells needs to be demonstrated, not only anatomically and molecularly but also functionally.

4 The transdifferentiation should also be demonstrated to occur naturally – that is, in the absence of damage in the target organ.

Three lines of evidence are needed to establish the contribution that transplanted adult stem cells can become another organ:[3,4]

1 The detection of donor-derived cells in an inappropriate location.

2 The identification of the phenotype of the resultant cells.

3 The need for proof of functionality of these new cells.

To date, the most commonly used donor-specific markers are the Y chromosome (in sex-mismatched transplantations) and transgenes. Another approach to identify donor-derived cells is to use normal mice with genetic polymorphisms that can be detected in all daughter cells.

For transgenic markers, cells from transgenic donor mice that express β-galactosidase or green fluorescence protein are transplanted into recipients lacking the transgene. Alternatively, retroviral infection of donor cells can be used to mark individual donor cells. Retroviruses stably insert into the genomic DNA of infected cells so can be used to identify and track cell clones that will have the same insertion site. The phenotypes of target cells are usually assessed by immunohistochemistry or immunofluorescence for organ-specific proteins.

A further refinement on the transgenic and retroviral approaches is that the transgene can be expressed on a cell-type specific promoter so that its expression not only marks the cells as donor-derived but also indicates that this gene is being expressed in a cell-type specific manner. This approach, however, also limits observation of the hoped for engraftment.

Functional assays of individual donor-derived cells have been more difficult to perform. The studies that have most successfully demonstrated their functionality have used recipient animals mutant for normal cell function in the target organs so that the transplanted cells restore function to the recipients.

☐ POSSIBLE MECHANISMS UNDERLYING PLASTICITY OF ADULT STEM CELLS

Four possible mechanisms have been proposed to account for BMSC plasticity, but proof of one mechanism does not necessarily preclude other possibilities.[4]

Differentiation of pluripotent stem cells

One possible mechanism is that bone marrow cells that differentiate into these diverse cell types represent a previously unsuspected population of pluripotent stem cells located in the bone marrow that have not committed to becoming blood.

Direct transdifferentiation

Secondly, that BMSCs are committed HSCs that can transdifferentiate directly. An HSC may be able directly to change its gene expression pattern to that of an alternative cell type.

Indirect transdifferentiation

In the third possible mechanism, indirect transdifferentiation, an HSC changes its gene expression pattern to that of an alternative cell type through a dedifferentiation/redifferentiation pathway that presumably passes through an as yet unidentified intermediate cell type.

Cell fusion

Lastly, cell fusion could be the mechanism by which BMSCs acquire a non-haematopoietic phenotype. A marrow-derived cell, perhaps a macrophage, fuses with a non-haematopoietic cell and the nucleus of the marrow-derived cell takes on the gene expression pattern of the non-haematopoietic cell type.

☐ CLAIMS FOR TRANSDIFFERENTIATION

The claims for stem cell transdifferentiation began in 1998 when Ferrari *et al*[5] reported that mouse bone marrow cells could give rise to skeletal muscle cells when transplanted into a mouse muscle damaged by an injection of a muscle toxin. Earlier, Eglitis and Mezey[6] reported that transplanted mouse bone marrow cells could give rise to brain astrocytes in adult mice – but this received relatively little attention. These papers, however, were just the beginning and it was soon reported by our group and others[7-10] that transplanted BMSCs could produce either parenchymal or supportive cells, or both, in many solid organs such as liver, central nervous system, cardiac and skeletal muscle, lung, kidney, bone, cartilage, gastrointestinal tract, pancreas, skin and so on.[4,11–13] Figure 1 demonstrates the evidence for transdifferentiation of pericryptal sheath myofibroblasts of bone marrow origin.

The number of publications on stem cell plasticity is now too large to be summarised here. Furthermore, this topic has been extensively reviewed, written about and published by our group and others in the past few years.[4,11-13]

In a subsequent study, our group has tried to test experimentally the proposal that the bone marrow can contribute to myofibroblast and fibroblast populations in a variety of injured tissues.[10] Female mice were transplanted with male bone marrow, then the male cells were tracked throughout the body and identified as

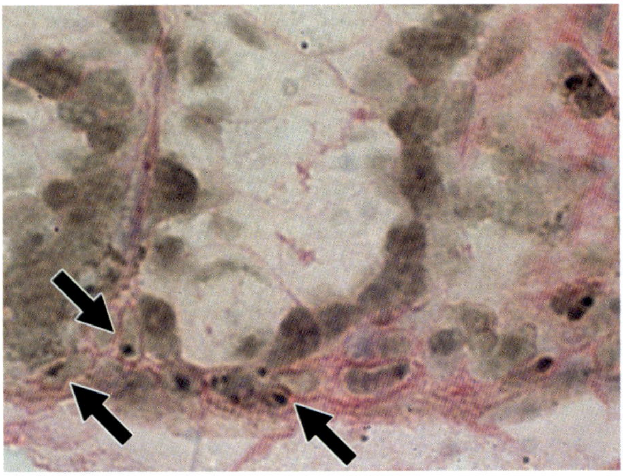

Fig 1 Evidence for the bone marrow origin of pericryptal sheath myofibroblasts. Combined Y chromosome *in situ* hybridisation (brown nuclear dot) and α-smooth muscle actin immunohistochemistry (Vector Red) reveal the presence of male myofibroblastic cells (arrowed) in the colon of a female mouse that received a male bone marrow transplant.

myofibroblasts. Skin wounding and paracetamol administration were used to assess whether myofibroblast engraftment was modulated by damage. Following radiation injury, a proportion of myofibroblasts in the lung, stomach, oesophagus, skin, kidney and adrenal capsule were found to be bone marrow derived. In the lung, there was significantly greater engraftment following paracetamol administration (41% vs 17%, $p < 0.005$), and bone marrow-derived fibroblasts were also found. These results suggest that bone marrow contributes to a circulating population of cells and, in the context of injury, these cells are recruited and contribute to tissue repair.

□ CLAIMS FOR CELL FUSION

The picture of Prometheus chained to Caucasus with an eagle eating his liver demonstrates the extraordinary regenerative capacity of the mammalian liver. However, stem cells are not required for liver regeneration, but rather the proliferation of mature liver cells. This Greek myth may provide the first opposition to those who hold strong beliefs in transdifferentiation.

Two independent studies by Wang *et al* and Vassilopoulos *et al* in 2003 claimed that cell fusion rather than transdifferentiation explained this liver regeneration in mammals (reviewed in Ref 12). These studies confirmed that stem cells derived from adult bone marrow can repair damaged liver tissue in mice. This was not achieved by direct conversion into liver cells, as might be expected if the stem cells could change their developmental 'destiny', but by cell fusion with host liver cells thought to be responsible for bringing down the barriers between bone marrow and liver. In this work, the contribution of the hybrid cells seemed to depend both on this liver regenerative capacity and on the space created by death of the diseased host liver cells.

Cell fusion between a marked donor cell and a resident cell could mimic the appearance of adult stem cell plasticity. Through cell fusion, molecules from one fusion partner could reprogramme gene expression in the genome of the other partner. Fusion might occur either between a donor cell with stem cell properties and a resident cell or between a transdifferentiated cell and a resident cell.

Thus, the astonishing clusters of 'wild type' hepatocytes that help normalise the liver of FAH null mice rescued by 'wild type' bone marrow appear mostly, if not exclusively, derived from fusion events. Transplantation with as few as 50 sorted HSCs and cycles of selection pressure can rescue the mouse and restore the missing biochemical function of its liver. However, the nodules of therapeutically successful cells are abnormal, expressing genes of both donor and recipient and with cytogenetic evidence indicating a high proportion of fused cells: 80,XXXY (diploid to diploid fusion) and 120,XXXXYY (diploid to tetraploid fusion). Irregular heterokaryons produced in the liver might subsequently die, shed a nucleus or proliferate. In mouse liver they could be involved in polyploidisation that normally results in over 80% of hepatocytes being binucleate, with nuclei containing substantially more than 2N chromosomes, especially in older mice.

Cell fusion followed by nuclear shedding or deletion may also account for the presence of mononucleate XY-Purkinje cells in the brains of female recipients of male bone marrow.[14] These cells have incredibly complex interconnections that seem impossible to have been produced *de novo* in the short interval between grafting and death. Evidence was sought for fusion, and the progressive accumulation of heterokaryons with bone marrow-derived nuclei in Purkinje cells has recently been described *in vivo*.[14]

Further support for cell fusion in the generation of bone marrow-derived Purkinje cells and also hepatocytes and cardiomyocytes was presented recently by Alvarez-Dolado and colleagues who carried out elegant studies *in vivo* and *in vitro* in which a reporter gene was activated only when cells fused.[15] Importantly, they considered that after some time either the two nuclei within heterokaryons fused or supernumerary nuclei were eliminated.

□ POTENTIAL CLINICAL APPLICATIONS

Pluripotent marrow cells could be used to treat tissue injury and multiple diseases of non-haematopoietic tissue in four ways:[4]

- □ transplantation of normal autologous cells
- □ enhancement or mobilisation of endogenous marrow-derived stem cells
- □ transplantation of gene-modified autologous marrow cells, and
- □ transplantation of allogeneic bone marrow cells.

The use of cell transfer strategies using these autologous or allogeneic cellular sources has biological plausibility but there are also obstacles.

Autologous transfer

Autologous (donor and recipient the same individual) sources would require the harvesting of a resident stem cell population (ie HSCs from the bone marrow or myogenic stem cells from skeletal muscle), followed by *in vitro* expansion and the use of exogenous agents to direct the differentiation to a specific lineage prior to delivery.

An autologous source of somatic stem cells would eliminate the use of immunosuppressive agents as well as any issues pertaining to donor availability as the donor and recipient are the same individual. Several issues require optimisation or definition before this technique could be applied in the clinical setting:

- □ the timing of delivery of the cellular source
- □ the limited proliferative capacity of somatic stem cells
- □ the ability efficiently to direct differentiation to a particular lineage, and
- □ the efficiency of cell transfer strategies.

Allogeneic transfer

The proven efficacy of allogeneic cell therapy (donor and recipient different individuals) using somatic stem cells underscores the potential of adult stem cells and provides the rationale for application of cell transfer strategies in the treatment of diseases. This cell transfer strategy has been successful for haematopoietic disorders, but other organs such as the heart, kidney or brain which require a functional anatomical organisation (such as synchronised cardiac contractility and correct neuronal synapses) may be less amenable to such therapy. Furthermore, there is extensive cell loss immediately following delivery due to inflammation and immune rejection. The delivery of cells into ischaemic, injured tissue with compromised vascularisation further limits this therapy.

Perhaps the most successful long-term approach would be to coerce resident stem cells within the patient's diseased organ to participate in the repair process. This strategy would conceivably require the administration of mobilising or activating agents (ie growth factors such as insulin-like growth factor and hepatocyte growth factor) that would prime the resident stem cells to re-enter the cell cycle, proliferate and differentiate to repair the damaged tissue (ie neural, cardiac, renal tissues). Such a strategy would require an enhanced understanding of the regulatory mechanisms of the resident stem cells and side effects associated with the administration of the priming agents.

Acknowledgement

This work is funded by Cancer Research UK.

REFERENCES

1 Cohnheim J. Über Entzündung und Eiterung. *Virchows Arch* 1867;**40**:1–79.
2 Anderson DJ, Gage FH, Weissman IL. Can stem cells cross lineage boundaries? Review. *Nat Med* 2001;**7**:393–5.
3 Wulf GG, Jackson KA, Goodell MA. Somatic stem cell plasticity: current evidence and emerging concepts. Review. *Exp Hematol* 2001;**29**:1361–70.
4 Herzog EL, Chai L, Krause DS. Plasticity of marrow-derived stem cells. Review. *Blood* 2003;**102**:3483–93.

5 Ferrari G, Cusella-De Angelis G, Coletta M, Paolucci E *et al.* Muscle regeneration by bone marrow-derived myogenic progenitors. *Science* 1998;**279**:1528–30.

6 Eglitis MA, Mezey E. Hematopoietic cells differentiate into both microglia and macroglia in the brains of adult mice. *Proc Natl Acad Sci USA* 1997;**94**:4080–5.

7 Alison MR, Poulsom R, Jeffery R, Dhillon AP *et al.* Hepatocytes from non-hepatic adult stem cells. *Nature* 2000;**406**:257.

8 Poulsom R, Forbes SJ, Hodivala-Dilke K, Ryan E *et al.* Bone marrow contributes to renal parenchymal turnover and regeneration. *J Pathol* 2001;**195**:229–35.

9 Brittan M, Hunt T, Jeffery R, Poulsom R *et al.* Bone marrow derivation of pericryptal myofibroblasts in the mouse and human small intestine and colon. *Gut* 2002;**50**:752–7.

10 Direkze NC, Forbes SJ, Brittan M, Hunt T *et al.* Multiple organ engraftment by bone-marrow-derived myofibroblasts and fibroblasts in bone-marrow-transplanted mice. *Stem Cells* 2003;**21**:514–20.

11 Poulsom R, Alison MR, Forbes SJ, Wright NA. Adult stem cell plasticity. Review. *J Pathol* 2002;**197**:441–56.

12 Fang TC, Alison MR, Wright NA, Poulsom R. Adult stem cell plasticity: will engineered tissues be rejected? *Int J Exp Pathol* 2004;**85**:115–24.

13 Korbling M, Estrov Z. Adult stem cells for tissue repair – a new therapeutic concept? Review. *N Engl J Med* 2003;**349**:570–82.

14 Weimann JM, Johansson CB, Trejo A, Blau HM. Stable reprogrammed heterokaryons form spontaneously in Purkinje neurons after bone marrow transplant. *Nat Cell Biol* 2003;**5**:959–66.

15 Alvarez-Dolado M, Pardal R, Garcia-Verdugo JM, Fike JR *et al.* Fusion of bone-marrow-derived cells with Purkinje neurons, cardiomyocytes and hepatocytes. *Nature* 2003;**425**:968–73.

☐ TRANSPLANTATION SELF ASSESSMENT QUESTIONS

Bone marrow cells: from development to therapy

1 The following features are found in autologous adult stem cell therapy (compared with embryonic stem cell therapy):
(a) Less infection
(b) Less hepatic failure
(c) Fewer cardiovascular problems
(d) More immunological tolerance
(e) More risk of secondary malignancy

2 The following methods are commonly used to trace bone marrow progeny cells:
(a) Y chromosome
(b) Genetic polymorphism
(c) β-galactosidase
(d) Green fluorescence protein
(e) Isotope

3 The following phrases are associated with stem cell plasticity:
(a) Turning blood into liver
(b) Turning blood into brain
(c) Cloning of Dolly, the sheep
(d) Fusion brings down barriers
(e) Graft failure due to chronic allograft nephropathy

Medicine in pregnancy

How to manage renal disease in pregnancy

Liz Lightstone

□ INTRODUCTION

Chronic kidney disease (CKD) is not uncommon, either in the form of structural kidney damage such as found in reflux nephropathy or presenting with impaired renal function with or without proteinuria. Many women with systemic diseases are predisposed to the development of kidney disease, especially during pregnancy. The presence of CKD or the development of acute kidney disease during pregnancy can significantly impact on the health of both mother and baby, occasionally with long-term consequences for both. The thesis of this chapter is that many of the problems associated with CKD in pregnancy can be addressed preconception and that good preconception care and antenatal vigilance can often offset significant problems. The key issue is to recognise those patients at risk so that pregnancies can be planned in a timely and safe manner.

□ PRECONCEPTION PLANNING

Physicians need to be aware that all women of childbearing age with chronic conditions may consider getting pregnant and may not consider that their disease will impact on such a venture. Hence, it is crucial for the issues to be raised with such patients – it is much worse if they have to face the possible adverse consequences of their decision for the first time once they are already pregnant.

Several issues need to be discussed with any woman of childbearing age who has kidney disease or a disease predisposing her to hypertension or kidney disease (notably systemic lupus erythematosus (SLE)), including the impact of:

- □ pregnancy on the disease
- □ the disease and its treatment on the chances of becoming pregnant and the pregnancy itself, and
- □ the disease and its treatment on the fetus.[1]

□ IMPACT OF PREGNANCY ON KIDNEY DISEASE

During normal pregnancy both glomerular filtration rate (GFR) and renal plasma flow increase early and dramatically. Hence, the normal range for serum creatinine is much lower in pregnant than non-pregnant women (mean creatinine 51 μmol/l vs 73 μmol/l), and the presence of a 'normal' serum creatinine in a pregnant woman may raise the suspicion of impaired renal function. However, women with impaired renal function may demonstrate a fall in creatinine in early pregnancy, suggesting significant renal reserve. Conversely, some patients with apparently normal or only mildly impaired function do not have a fall in their creatinine, raising anxiety about their underlying renal reserve. The renal hyperfiltration in a normal pregnancy is not associated with intraglomerular hypertension. In women with pre-existing kidney damage, the hyperfiltration may be associated with intraglomerular changes which can lead to accelerated loss of renal function.

This effect is clearly illustrated in Fig 1 which shows the reciprocal creatinine plot of a young woman with focal segmental glomerulosclerosis whose serum creatinine increased from 100 µmol/l to 180 µmol/l between the start and finish of her first pregnancy, consistent with more than 50% loss of function. Importantly, between pregnancies her renal function declined only slowly, but the impact of her second pregnancy was dramatic and left her at end-stage renal failure (ESRF).

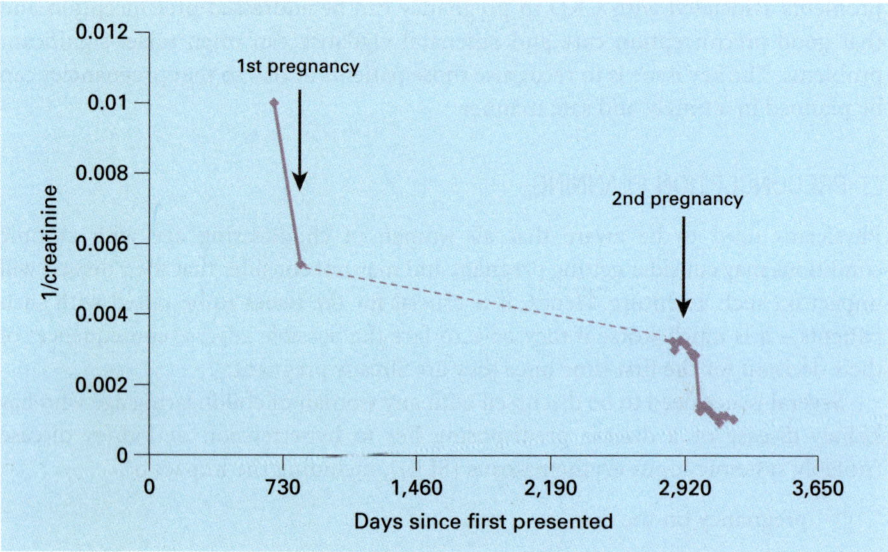

Fig 1 Reciprocal creatinine plot of a woman with focal segmental glomerulosclerosis who lost significant function in her first pregnancy and developed end-stage renal failure within four weeks of her second pregnancy, despite having had stable function for years.

Influence of renal function and hypertension

In general, however, the key predictors of outcome of pregnancy in women with kidney disease are the preconception levels of renal function and hypertension. Review of thousands of pregnancies in women with CKD (barring connective tissue diseases) suggested that a baseline creatinine below 120 µmol/l and normal blood pressure were associated with little or no impact on the underlying kidney disease, relatively low rates of obstetric complications and excellent fetal outcomes (Table 1(a) and (b)). Davison *et al* originally suggested that mild to moderate renal

Table 1(a) Influence of pre-conception serum creatinine on maternal, obstetric and long-term renal complications. Based on data from 1973–96 on 2,130 women with 3,425 pregnancies (courtesy of Professor J Davison, University of Newcastle).

Creatinine (μmol/l)	Problems during pregnancy (%)	Successful obstetric outcome (%)	Long-term renal problems (%)
<125	26	96	<3
125–250	47	89	25
>250	86	46	53

Table 1(b) Influence of preconception serum creatinine on rates of hypertension, pre-eclampsia toxaemia (PET), intrauterine growth retardation (IUGR) and preterm delivery. Based on data from 1973–96 on 2,130 women with 3,425 pregnancies (courtesy of Professor J Davison, University of Newcastle).

Creatinine (μmol/l)	Hypertension	PET (%)	IUGR and/or prematurity (%)
<125	Variable	10–20	Increased
125–250	30–50%	40	30–50
>250	Most	80	57–73

impairment (serum creatinine >120 μmol/l and <240 μmol/l) was associated with increased risk to the mother both for obstetric complications and worse long-term renal complications, whilst severe renal impairment (serum creatinine >240 μmol/l) was associated with bad maternal and fetal outcomes.[2] More recently, it has been suggested that a cut-off of above and below 180 μmol/l defines poor and better outcomes (Table 2), respectively.[3,4]

In the future, risk is more likely to be assessed on the basis of estimated GFR (using the Modification of Diet in Renal Disease (MDRD) or Cockcroft-Gault formula) rather than serum creatinine alone as the latter is an imperfect marker of renal function. The GFR can be significantly reduced whilst the creatinine remains in the 'normal' range, especially in small, vegetarian women. The worse the renal

Table 2 Influence of moderate/severe renal impairment (serum creatinine >180 μmol/l) on pregnancy, fetal and maternal outcomes. Data from 107 women with 125 pregnancies (adapted from Refs 3 and 4).

Problems in pregnancy		Successful obstetric outcome		Long-term renal problems		End-stage renal failure	
%	Range	%	Range	%	Range	%	Range
90	81–97	84	65–93	50	39-57	15	10–23

function preconception, the greater the risk of significant loss of renal function during or soon after a pregnancy. This is not a minor consideration: not only is it emotionally and physically difficult to cope with starting dialysis when pregnant or with a new baby, but the younger the starting age on dialysis the higher the risk of mortality compared with an age-matched population.

□ IMPACT OF KIDNEY DISEASE ON PREGNANCY AND THE FETUS

Many types of kidney disease can present problems in pregnancy. Women with structurally abnormal kidneys may be more predisposed to urinary tract infections (UTIs), hypertension and the development of pre-eclampsia toxaemia (PET). Women with recurrent UTIs are advised to take prophylactic antibiotics (usually cephradine nocte), certainly from the second trimester, to reduce both their frequency and the risk of pyelonephritis. Those who start pregnancy with proteinuria (whatever the underlying renal lesion) will develop increasing proteinuria throughout their pregnancy and may also be predisposed to hypertension and PET.

Heritability

An important consideration is the heritability of the condition:

- *Adult polycystic kidney disease* (APKD) is inherited in an autosomal dominant fashion. Most women who come from families with APKD are aware of the one in two risk of the child inheriting the condition but abortion is almost never considered by such patients. Patients may benefit from genetic counselling, particularly if the diagnosis of APKD is recent or made during the pregnancy.
- Several forms of *glomerulonephritis* can be inherited, the most common being the X-linked Alport's syndrome. Female carriers may be unaware they are carriers unless they have an affected male sibling. If the diagnosis of Alport's has been made in the family, genetic counselling is advised prior to conception.
- *Reflux nephropathy* has a strong genetic component and women need to be made aware that their child may be affected and should be screened in the first year of life in order to institute renal protective prophylaxis prior to the development of any scarring.

Fertility

Some diseases or their treatment impair fertility. Women with certain structural abnormalities involving the renal tract may have abnormal reproductive organs. Clearly this needs to be addressed prior to attempted conception as they may require *in vitro* fertilisation and consideration of mode of delivery. More common in renal practice are patients with SLE. The disease itself can be associated with premature menopause, but more commonly therapy with cyclophosphamide can lead to infertility in a dose- and age- dependent fashion. It is imperative to advise women of the risks of treatment, though clearly these need to be offset against the risk of lupus nephritis. Recent data suggest that inducing a temporary menopause with gonadotropin-releasing hormone agonists may protect ovaries from cytotoxic agents. Women who have had cyclophosphamide but continue to have periods need to be aware that they may still be susceptible to an early menopause and therefore, if their lupus is stable, should not postpone getting pregnant. For women with lupus who have irregular periods, it is worth referring them for a fertility assessment sooner rather than later.

Renal disease activity and timing of pregnancy

Women with conditions leading to chronic progressive renal dysfunction (eg APKD, progressive glomerulonephritis) must be advised that, if the possibility arises, they should try to get pregnant earlier in the course of their disease rather than later. The received wisdom used to be to advise women to wait to conceive until they had reached renal failure and had a stable renal transplant. This is now untenable as a strategy. With better blood pressure control and reduction of proteinuria with angiotensin-converting enzyme inhibitors (ACEI) or angiotensin-2 receptor blockers (AT2RB), renal failure is often delayed by years. Furthermore, waiting times for transplants have significantly increased and many of the newer antirejection regimens include drugs contraindicated in pregnancy. All this means that a woman with predicted ESRF may reach the menopause before she is safely transplanted and off contraindicated medications.

In contrast, women with relapsing/remitting conditions (eg lupus nephritis) should be advised not to get pregnant until their renal disease is in stable remission for about six months and they are not on immunosuppressive agents which are teratogenic or otherwise contraindicated in pregnancy (see below). Women need to be specifically advised to use contraception whilst their disease is being actively treated.

Medication

A crucial area where CKD impacts on pregnancy concerns the drugs used to treat the kidney disease.

Cytotoxic agents

The first category to consider is cytotoxic agents such as cyclophosphamide which are contraindicated and teratogenic. Women must be advised to use reliable contraception when taking such medication and to continue contraception for some months after the treatment has stopped.

A recent problem has been the introduction of mycophenolate mofetil (MMF), a potent and effective immunosuppressant in lupus nephritis, vasculitis and transplantation. MMF does not cause infertility but is strictly contraindicated in pregnancy. Since many women with lupus nephritis need to be treated for at least two years with MMF, which is now a standard lifelong drug in transplantation, this poses a major dilemma for women considering pregnancy. They have to be advised to switch to a 'safer' drug such as azathioprine before embarking on a pregnancy. The switch needs to be monitored carefully as it may be associated with relapse in lupus nephritis or rejection in transplantation.

Contraception

Contraception needs to be discussed in general: for instance, fertility returns rapidly in women with successful transplants,[5] but the likelihood of renal impairment and problematic pregnancies is much higher if conception occurs within six months of transplantation.

Angiotensin-converting enzyme inhibitors and angiotensin-2 receptor blockers

In recent years, it has become clear that strict blood pressure control and reduction of proteinuria with ACEI/AT2RB can markedly delay the progression of CKD, regardless of underlying cause. There is also a growing tendency to use statins to control hypercholesterolaemia (more common in those with nephrotic range proteinuria). Women planning a pregnancy need to be aware that many antihypertensives are contraindicated. Importantly, ACEI (and probably AT2RB), can cause a serious fetopathy particularly in the second and third trimesters. The purist approach is to recommend stopping these drugs prior to conception. However, pregnancy may not be achieved for years during which CKD may progress more rapidly in the absence of the drugs. It is therefore reasonable to counsel women that ACEI and AT2RB are contraindicated in pregnancy but are probably very low risk until about seven weeks post-conception.[6] Women need to be advised to have a low threshold for undertaking a pregnancy test and to stop the medication as soon as they know they are pregnant. They can then go on to antihypertensives known to be safe such as methyldopa and/or labetolol. Similarly patients need to know to stop their statin, non-steroidal anti-inflammatory drugs and any other inappropriate medications in early pregnancy.[7]

Other medication issues

It is also important to ensure that women are aware that many drugs are critically important to the well-being of the mother, are safe in pregnancy and should absolutely not be stopped without prior discussion. The classic error is for women to stop their steroids abruptly – this can precipitate not only an Addisonian crisis but also a relapse of their renal disease (eg lupus nephritis or steroid-dependent minimal change nephropathy). An acute relapse of any renal disease during pregnancy is associated with a worse maternal and fetal outcome.

For women who have decided to get pregnant, it is worth recommending standard measures of care such as:

- encouraging cessation of smoking (now also recognised to be an independent risk factor for progression of renal disease)

- commencement of folic acid, and
- starting low dose aspirin for those at risk of PET (eg lupus nephritis, anticardiolipin antibody (ACA) positive).

IMPACT OF KIDNEY DISEASE ON THE FETUS

The key risks to the fetus are:

- inheriting the renal condition
- being damaged by drugs used to treat the kidney disease, and
- an adverse uterine environment due to maternal hypertension, PET, uraemia (eg in pregnant dialysis patients) and/or severe proteinuria.

Whilst drugs may cause miscarriages and fetal abnormalities, the adverse uterine environment is most likely to be manifest by intrauterine growth retardation (IUGR) and preterm delivery. Women with renal disease, even when considered 'low risk', have at least a twofold increased rate of PET; they need to be advised that IUGR and preterm delivery may lead to handicap, which can be severe and permanent, and even death of the infant. The earlier the onset of PET (especially if before 28 weeks), the greater the risk to the fetus. Preterm delivery is common in women with severe renal impairment and more common in women with transplants.

MANAGEMENT OF PREGNANCY IN WOMEN WITH RENAL DISEASE

Women with significant renal disease should be carefully monitored during pregnancy and ideally jointly managed by an obstetrician and physician. They should be advised that they may not be suitable for shared care, may well have preterm deliveries – which often mean an increased rate of Caesarean section. Women need to be aware that diagnosing superimposed PET is difficult in patients with underlying hypertension and proteinuria. We recommend that women considered at risk of developing PET, worsening renal function, heavy proteinuria or with severe lupus should have regular fetal growth scans from 24 weeks. We also look for notching on the uterine artery wave forms from doppler examination – this has a strong predictive value for PET.

Women are advised to book early, especially if they are on drugs which need to be stopped. Those at risk are prescribed low-dose aspirin, while for those with nephrotic range proteinuria, low molecular weight heparin (LMWH) is advised to reduce the risk of thrombosis. LMWH is also used in those women with a history of severe prior PET, especially in the context of lupus or ACA.

Hypertension still needs to be controlled during pregnancy. The standard first-line agents are methyldopa and/or labetolol. Unopposed beta-blockade should not be used as it is associated with IUGR. Diuretics are generally to be avoided as they risk causing intravascular depletion and impaired placental flow. If a third agent is required, we usually use nifedipine which, although not licensed for use in pregnancy, has been widely used for this indication. Hydralazine can also be used but causes marked tachycardia which patients often find intolerable.

Renal function should be monitored regularly through pregnancy by measuring:

- serum creatinine
- serum albumin (recognising that this is significantly lower in normal pregnancy), and
- urine albumin or protein:creatinine ratio (24-hour urines are not necessary).

Women with moderate renal dysfunction often develop severe anaemia during pregnancy due to erythropoietin (EPO) deficiency. Once they are iron replete, EPO can be safely administered in pregnancy to avoid the need for transfusions.

At our institution, patients are seen at least monthly in a joint renal/antenatal clinic.

PROBLEMS ASSOCIATED WITH SPECIFIC DISEASES

The problems likely to be associated with specific diseases need also to be considered during pregnancy. Women with lupus nephritis should be in remission for six months prior to conceiving. Starting pregnancy with active nephritis is associated with a much worse maternal and fetal outcome. In general, women with lupus who have ACA do less well than those without. ACA positivity is associated with higher rates of spontaneous abortions and IUGR. A particular consideration in lupus is the risk of antibodies crossing the placenta and causing fetal problems. Anti-Ro or anti-La antibodies are associated with the development of fetal cardiac abnormalities, in particular congenital heart block. Women with lupus should be screened for these antibodies and, if present, offered detailed cardiac scanning at 24 weeks and thereafter as required.

As women in general now delay their pregnancies until about their 30s, it is becoming more common to see women with established diabetic nephropathy who are pregnant. In general, the outcome is defined not only by the diabetic control but also by the level of renal impairment, the severity of proteinuria and the mean arterial pressure. Very high rates of PET are seen (30% vs 15% in all pregnancies of those with type 1 diabetes vs 5% in non-diabetic pregnancies).

ASSESSING RENAL DISEASE IN PREGNANCY

The presence of proteinuria, with or without haematuria, at booking strongly suggests the presence of underlying renal disease. This may often not have been previously diagnosed. The cause can be searched for largely as if not pregnant. Blood work should include full biochemical profile, full blood count, lupus anticoagulant and an autoimmune screen (complement, antineutrophilic cytoplasmic, antinuclear and anti-dsDNA antibodies, serum immunoglobulins), as well as viral screen (hepatitis B, C and HIV). Urine should be sent for albumin:creatinine ratio and microscopy. Kidneys should be imaged with renal ultrasound and with dopplers, if necessary, for example to exclude renal vein thrombosis in women with nephrotic syndrome.

The decision that needs to be made with an early unexpected presentation is whether a renal biopsy is indicated. The more remote from term, the safer this is; especially for problems in the first trimester, it is probably better to biopsy and diagnose rather than treat blindly. However, in later pregnancy, it is usually more advisable to consider delivery if renal function is compromised (eg heavy proteinuria, worsening function) rather than contemplate renal biopsy.[8] It is occasionally impossible to distinguish active lupus nephritis from PET, but beyond 30 weeks in either situation it is probably safer to deliver and deal with the baby and mother separately.

Late renal problems

If late renal problems occur in pregnancy they may signify new renal disease or true pregnancy induced problems such as PET or related syndromes. Acute renal failure in pregnancy is now rare in the developed world. Women at risk include those who develop acute volume depletion (eg with hyperemesis, sepsis and haemorrhage). Judicious fluid and blood pressure support can often prevent the onset of established acute tubular necrosis (ATN). The pregnancy related syndromes such as abruption, PET and HELLP (haemolysis, elevated liver enzymes and low platelets) can cause ATN but can also cause specific renal lesions, classically glomerular endotheliosis.[9]

An important practical point to remember is that, although these conditions may be associated with severe oedema, the women are often intravascularly deplete and will develop worse renal function with diuretics. Fluid administration needs to be carefully monitored (ideally with central venous monitoring) as both intravascular depletion and pulmonary oedema are major risks. Post-partum, haemolytic uraemic syndrome (HUS) (non-diarrhoea associated) can cause severe and often irreversible renal failure. Cortical necrosis is a rare but devastating sequel to renal failure in pregnancy – the pregnant or recently pregnant kidney is thought to be more susceptible due to the superimposition of microthrombi on baseline glomerular endothelial dysfunction, all of which leads to irreversible renal cortical ischaemia. The classic settings for the development of cortical necrosis are massive haemorrhage (ante- or post-partum), septic abortion, HUS and severe PET.

☐ CONCLUSIONS (Table 3, overleaf)

Ideally, all patients with renal disease should have preconception counselling about the risks to them and their fetus should they become pregnant and how these may be minimised. Women with good function and minimal hypertension can be reassured that, although considered high risk, they should have a successful obstetric outcome with minimal damage to their kidneys. Women with poor renal function, problematic hypertension and/or severe proteinuria are at increased risk of declining renal function and a worse obstetric outcome. All women with kidney disease should be carefully monitored and assessed during pregnancy.

Table 3 Summary of key components of care of women with renal disease contemplating pregnancy.

Preconception	Counselling re: • risks to mother and fetus • fertility/heritability/medications
Pregnancy	Consider all high risk; centre-based care; BOOK EARLY Drugs: • stop ACEIs and NSAIDS • consider specific medications to add/stop Control hypertension and anaemia Monitor: • proteinuria • renal function • fetal growth

ACEI = angiotensin-converting enzyme inhibitor; NSAID = non-steroidal anti-inflammatory drug.

REFERENCES

1 Nelson-Piercy C. *Handbook of Obstetric Medicine*, 2nd edn. London: Taylor and Francis, 2001: ch.10.

2 Davison JM. Renal disorders in pregnancy. Review. *Curr Opin Obstet Gynecol* 2001;**13**:109–14.

3 Jones DC, Hayslett JP. Outcome of pregnancy in women with moderate or severe renal insufficiency. *N Engl J Med* 1996;**335**:226–32.

4 Jungers P, Chauveau D, Choukroun G, Moynot A *et al.* Pregnancy in women with impaired renal function. *Clin Nephrol* 1997;**47**:281–8.

5 Davison JM, Bailey DJ. Pregnancy following renal transplantation. *J Obstet Gynaecol Res* 2003;**29**:227–33.

6 How HY, Sibai BM. Use of angiotensin-converting enzyme inhibitors in patients with diabetic nephropathy. Review. *J Matern Fetal Neonatal Med* 2002;**12**:402–7.

7 Livingston JC, Maxwell BD, Sibai BM. Chronic hypertension in pregnancy. Review. *Minerva Ginecol* 2003; **55**:1–13.

8 de Swiet M, Lightstone L. Glomerular endotheliosis in normal pregnancy and pre-eclampsia. *Br J Obstet Gynaecol* 2004;**111**:191–2.

9 Smyth L, Lightstone L. The obstetric unit. In: Glynne P, Allen A, Pusey C (eds). *Acute renal failure.* London: Imperial College Press, 2002:497–509.

Congenital heart disease in pregnancy

Sara Thorne

□ INTRODUCTION

There are now more adults than children living with congenital heart disease (CHD) in the UK, reflecting the successes of congenital cardiac surgery and intervention over the last two decades. As a result, the adult CHD population is growing not only in number but also in complexity because of surgically modified disease.

It was estimated that there were 150,000 adults with CHD in the UK in 2000, 10,000 of them with complex disease. This is predicted to rise to 180,000 by 2010, with 15,000 having complex disease (a 50% increase). Most of the latter will develop late complications and require further intervention.

Half the adult CHD population are women, most of whom are well enough to consider becoming pregnant. The majority can achieve a successful pregnancy, albeit sometimes with a significant maternal and fetal risk, but in a minority pregnancy carries an unacceptable risk. Those who become pregnant require well co-ordinated multispecialty care which is both time and resource consuming. The challenges presented by these patients can be viewed as a problem, or the ability to have children can be viewed as a good measure of successful outcome.

The cardiologist needs to understand the pathophysiology of each congenital cardiac condition and its surgical modifications in order to give appropriate preconception and antenatal advice. Pregnancy causes marked circulatory changes from the first trimester. The ability to tolerate a pregnancy depends on the ability of the cardiovascular system to adapt to these changes. In a normal pregnancy, stroke volume and heart rate increase by about 17%; as a result, cardiac output increases by about 45%, peaking at 16 weeks' gestation. Plasma volume increases by 40–50%, reaching a peak at about 28 weeks' gestation, producing a dilutional anaemia. Systemic and pulmonary vascular resistance both fall, with a greater fall in the latter. Blood pressure may fall or remain unchanged.

Given these dramatic changes in cardiac physiology, how can the clinician distinguish the cardiovascular signs and symptoms of a normal pregnancy from those indicating cardiac decompensation? Any pregnant woman may have physical signs which would suggest heart failure in the non-pregnant state: she may be tired, breathless and have palpitation, a collapsing pulse, sinus tachycardia, raised jugular venous pressure, a third heart sound, a systolic flow murmur and peripheral oedema. However, extreme dyspnoea or orthopnoea, chest pain, a fourth heart sound, sinus tachycardia greater than 100 bpm at rest, atrial flutter, ventricular tachycardia, pulmonary oedema and pleural effusion are all signs of cardiac pathology requiring action.

☐ MORTALITY AND MORBIDITY

The Confidential Enquiry into Maternal Deaths (CEMD) publishes triennial figures for the UK.[1] Cardiac disease is the joint most common cause of death, being implicated in 7% (n = 42) of early maternal deaths between 1997 and 1999. A breakdown of these figures shows that the most dangerous conditions are ventricular dysfunction and pulmonary hypertension of any cause, accounting for 40% and 19% of cardiac deaths, respectively. The high number of deaths from poor ventricular function reflects the fact that the disease is often undiagnosed until revealed by a pregnancy or, in the case of the peripartum, cardiomyopathy is caused by the pregnancy itself. Most deaths due to pulmonary hypertension are also the result of previously undiagnosed disease, pulmonary hypertension is widely recognised as carrying an extremely high maternal mortality and pregnancy is strongly discouraged. Aortic dissection and acute myocardial infarction each accounted for 12% of cardiac deaths, and endocarditis for 7% in the same period. CHD does not figure highly in the CEMD figures which do not measure morbidity or the workload of units caring for women with CHD.

Maternal risk is assessed from published data and, where data are lacking, on an individualised basis (as discussed in the rest of this chapter). Fetal risk factors include any condition which puts the mother at risk, as well as maternal cyanosis (see below) and maternal drugs. The risk of recurrence of CHD is about 5% in the absence of a strong family history or specific genetic defect.

☐ CONDITIONS IN WHICH PREGNANCY IS LOW RISK

Many congenital lesions are well tolerated in pregnancy. Mild unoperated pulmonary stenosis, successfully repaired secundum atrial septal defects and anomalous pulmonary venous drainage probably confer no additional risk to the mother. Endocarditis prophylaxis is not needed in labour.

Unoperated small secundum atrial septal defects also need no antibiotic prophylaxis. However, it is easy to reverse the interatrial shunt, especially in the pregnant state with a large intra-abdominal mass, so there is a risk of paradoxical embolism and stroke if the patient develops venous thrombosis. These patients should receive low-dose aspirin throughout pregnancy and be given heparin prophylaxis and venous compression stockings for any period of immobility.

Small ventricular septal defects and persistent patent arterial ducts should be given endocarditis prophylaxis in labour, but they carry no other significant maternal risk.

Most regurgitant valvar lesions, including mitral and aortic regurgitation, are well tolerated in pregnancy provided that ventricular function is normal. The vasodilatory effects of pregnancy may be beneficial and help to counteract the additional volume loading effects of the pregnancy on the already volume loaded left ventricle.

There are many adults with successfully repaired tetralogy of Fallot. It is the commonest cyanotic condition (1 in 3,600 live births); after successful repair, survival into the fourth decade is close to that of the normal population.[2] Many patients with tetralogy of Fallot initially have a small pulmonary valve annulus, so require the placement of a patch across the annulus as part of their radical repair. As a result, the pulmonary valve is incompetent and the majority will have free pulmonary regurgitation by the time they reach the adult clinic. None the less, pregnancy is well tolerated provided that there are no other adverse sequelae. Antibiotic prophylaxis is required in labour.

☐ CONDITIONS IN WHICH PREGNANCY CARRIES A SIGNIFICANT RISK

Pregnancy may be undertaken in the following situations, but it carries a significant risk and should be managed in a specialist unit:

- Mechanical valves
- Systemic right ventricle
- Cyanotic heart disease *without* pulmonary hypertension
- Fontan circulation.

Mechanical valves

All mechanical valves require anticoagulation with warfarin to maintain valve function and prevent thromboembolism. However, warfarin crosses the placenta and causes embryopathy in the first trimester.[3] It anticoagulates the fetus, so throughout pregnancy there is a risk of fetal haemorrhage and fetal loss. If the mother is adequately anticoagulated on a daily dose of 5 mg warfarin or less, the risk to the fetus is significantly reduced.[4] Warfarin is also associated with maternal haemorrhage during labour.

Warfarin versus heparin

The alternative to warfarin is heparin which does not cross the placenta; it can be stopped shortly before delivery to reduce the risk of maternal haemorrhage. However, even if meticulously monitored, heparin is a less effective anticoagulant for mechanical valves than warfarin, and its use during pregnancy is associated with a significant risk of maternal valve thrombosis and death.[5] Warfarin is thus the safest maternal option and heparin safest for the fetus – bearing in mind that valve thrombosis may result in both maternal and fetal death.

Not all valves are equally thrombogenic: an adult sized bileaflet tilting disc valve (eg St Jude or Carbomedics valve) in the aortic position is less thrombogenic than a small single leaflet tilting disc valve (eg Bjork-Shiley valve) in the mitral position (placed before the patient was fully grown). The former may be managed with heparin and aspirin throughout pregnancy with relatively low risk, whereas the latter may face a major complication risk of up to 10% if warfarin is discontinued.

No anticoagulation regimen for a mechanical valve is safe for both the mother and the fetus, so the patient needs help to make an informed decision. The choice lies between:

1 Warfarin throughout pregnancy, converting to unfractionated heparin to allow an elective Caesarean section, thus minimising the time off heparin.

2 Heparin plus aspirin for the first and last trimesters, taking warfarin in the middle trimester.

3 Heparin plus aspirin throughout the pregnancy.

Further controversy surrounds the choice of heparin. Low molecular weight (LMW) heparin has theoretical advantages over unfractionated heparin:

- LMW heparin has a longer half-life
- a twice daily subcutaneous regimen provides 'smoother' anticoagulant cover, and
- levels are more reliably monitored, with antiXa levels dictating dose.

However, a recent study using LMW heparin in mechanical valves was stopped before adequate data were available because of maternal deaths, so it is now unlikely that data will be available on choice of heparin from a controlled study.[6]

Whichever regimen is chosen, anticoagulation and valve function need to be monitored meticulously.

Systemic right ventricle

The systemic ventricle is a morphological right ventricle in patients with either congenitally corrected transposition of the great arteries (atrioventricular and ventriculoarterial discordance) or atrial repair (eg Mustard operation) for transposition of the great arteries (atrioventricular concordance, ventriculoarterial discordance). Terminology is confusing to health professionals who do not specialise in CHD; it may be helpful to attach a diagram to the front of the patient's maternity notes (Figs 1 and 2).

In both conditions there may be pre-existing dysfunction of the right ventricle and systemic (tricuspid) atrioventricular valve, neither of which is well suited to support the systemic circulation. Additional complications for women with congenitally corrected transposition of the great arteries include complete heart block.[7,8] Sinus node dysfunction, atrial arrhythmia and pulmonary venous pathway narrowing may complicate pregnancy for those who have had a Mustard operation for transposition of the great arteries.[9]

Cyanotic heart disease *without* pulmonary hypertension

For patients with cyanosis and low or normal pulmonary vascular resistance and pulmonary arterial pressure, maternal and fetal risk is largely determined by ventricular function and the degree of cyanosis.

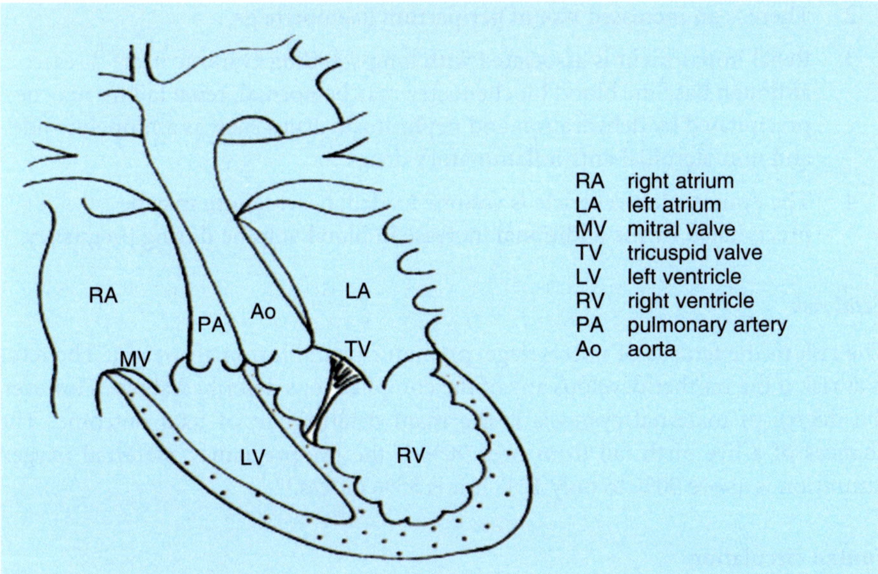

Fig 1 Congenitally corrected transposition of the great arteries.

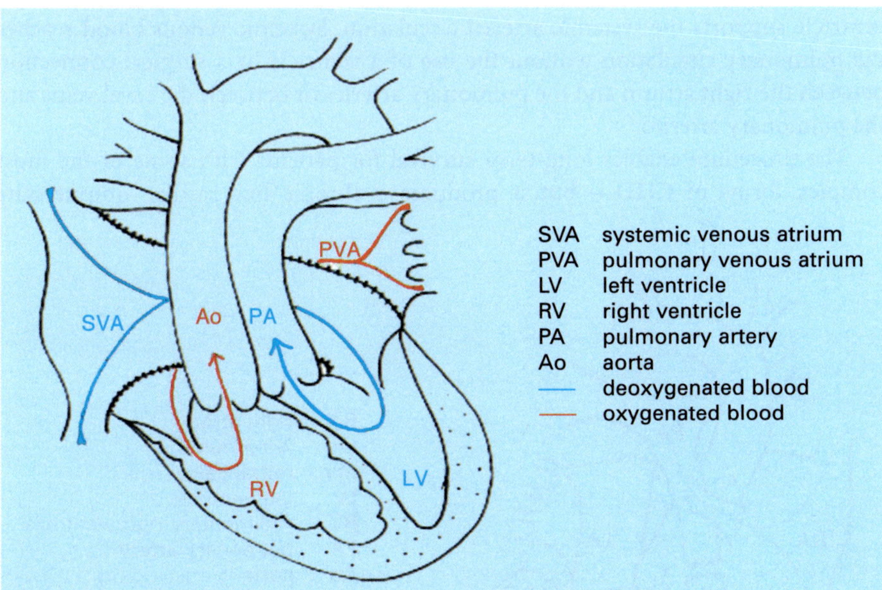

Fig 2 Mustard operation for transposition of the great arteries.

Maternal risk

1 All cyanotic patients have a right to left shunt and are therefore at risk of paradoxical embolism. Thrombosis prophylaxis is required for any period of immobility; venous lines should be fitted with air filters to avoid iatrogenic air embolism.

2 There is an increased risk of peripartum haemorrhage.

3 Renal impairment is associated with long-standing cyanotic heart disease; although baseline blood biochemistry may be normal, renal failure may be precipitated by dehydration and nephrotoxic drugs such as aminoglycosides and non-steroidal anti-inflammatory drugs.

4 The cyanotic left ventricle is volume loaded; heart failure may be precipitated by the additional increase in blood volume during pregnancy.

Fetal risk

The risk to the fetus is of miscarriage, prematurity and low birth weight. The fetus is at risk if the mother develops any of the complications described above. However, the degree of maternal cyanosis is the main determinant of fetal outcome. The chances of a live birth fall from over 90% if the pre-pregnancy maternal oxygen saturation is above 90% to only 12% if it is 85% or less.[10]

Fontan circulation

The aim of Fontan-type procedures is to abolish cyanosis and reduce ventricular volume loading in patients with a functionally single ventricle (Fig 3). The single ventricle supports the systemic arterial circulation. Systemic venous blood reaches the pulmonary circulation without the use of a ventricle by a surgical connection between the right atrium and the pulmonary arteries or between the caval veins and the pulmonary arteries.

The procedure enables long-term survival for patients with some of the most complex forms of CHD – but it produces a chronic low cardiac output state

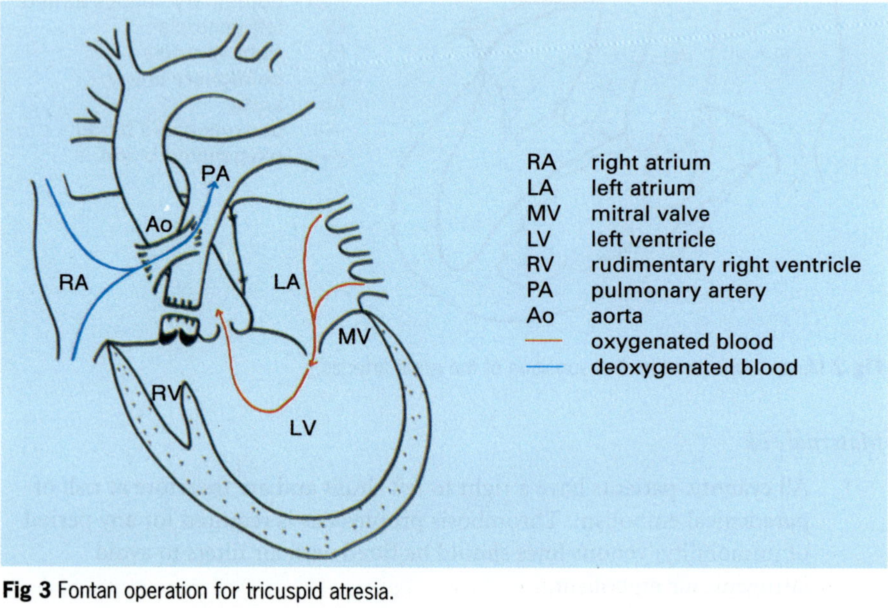

Fig 3 Fontan operation for tricuspid atresia.

dependent on a high systemic venous filling pressure and low pulmonary vascular resistance. As a result, many patients are advised against pregnancy. None the less, maternal mortality is low provided ventricular function is good, although there may be significant maternal morbidity in the form of ventricular failure and atrial arrhythmia. In addition, the risk of fetal loss is high (30%).[11]

□ CONDITIONS IN WHICH PREGNANCY IS CONTRAINDICATED

Pregnancy is high risk and should be avoided in the following conditions:

1 Severe systemic ventricular dysfunction.

2 Pulmonary hypertension of any cause.

3 Severe left-sided obstructive lesions (eg mitral and aortic stenosis, coarctation).

4 Marfan syndrome with aortic aneurysm.

Severe systemic ventricular dysfunction

Patients with severe systemic ventricular dysfunction should be counselled against pregnancy. A left ventricular ejection fraction of less than 20% or New York Heart Association class III or IV symptoms carry a risk of 7% maternal mortality. For those who wish to continue with a pregnancy there is a risk of overt heart failure, irreversible deterioration in ventricular function and fetal loss. Admission for bedrest is helpful; pharmacological treatment for heart failure is as for the non-pregnant patient except that angiotensin-converting enzyme inhibitors should be avoided because of the risk of fetal renal agenesis.

Pulmonary hypertension of any cause

Pregnancy in pulmonary hypertension, whether primary or secondary to CHD (Eisenmenger syndrome), carries a 40–50% risk of maternal death.[12,13] It is noteworthy that even modest pulmonary hypertension carries a significant risk of maternal death. There is no evidence that intervention with heparin, oxygen, nitric oxide or prostacyclin reduces mortality. Avoidance of pregnancy is the most important message (see discussion on contraception) and therapeutic termination should be offered for those who do conceive. If the patient opts to continue her pregnancy, admission for rest and treatment of right heart failure is likely to be necessary. Since even minor exertion causes a drop in arterial oxygen saturation in a pregnant patient with Eisenmenger syndrome, strict bedrest to optimise oxygen saturation may improve fetal outcome. The high risk of maternal death continues for at least two weeks after delivery and may be sudden or due to progressive hypoxia.

Severe left-sided obstructive lesions

Ideally, these lesions should be relieved before pregnancy is embarked upon.

Mitral stenosis

Mitral stenosis is usually rheumatic in origin and may not present until the patient is pregnant and becomes symptomatic for the first time. Treatment with bedrest, oxygen, diuretics and beta-blockade to decrease heart rate and allow time for left ventricular filling may allow the pregnancy to continue until the baby can be delivered safely. If, however, the patient remains breathless at rest or develops pulmonary oedema, balloon mitral valvuloplasty may be performed after the first trimester with minimal fetal risk.

Aortic stenosis

An asymptomatic woman with aortic stenosis is likely to tolerate pregnancy if she has a normal resting and exercise ECG, a normal heart rate and blood pressure response to exercise, normal left ventricular function and a pre-pregnancy mean Doppler gradient of 50 mmHg or below (peak gradient 80 mmHg or below).The Doppler-derived aortic valve gradient should rise during pregnancy as cardiac output increases. A falling gradient indicates left ventricular impairment and the patient is likely to become symptomatic, with dyspnoea, angina or syncope. Management includes bedrest, oxygen and beta-blockade to reduce heart rate and allow coronary filling time. If the patient does not respond and the fetus cannot be safely delivered, balloon aortic valvotomy or surgical replacement may need to be considered. The latter carries a high risk of fetal loss.[14,15]

Coarctation

Pregnancy in unrepaired coarctation carries a risk of uncontrolled hypertension and aortic dissection, although maternal mortality appears to be low.[16] Hypertension should be treated with high-dose beta-blockade and the fetus delivered before term (at about 35 weeks) by elective Caesarean section. Catheter balloon intervention is best avoided during pregnancy because of the increased risk of aortic dissection and rupture.

Marfan syndrome with aortic aneurysm

Aortic dissection can occur in pregnancy even in a woman with a previously normal aorta. The risk of aortic dissection during pregnancy in Marfan syndrome without aortic dilatation is about 1%. The risk is significantly higher in those with aortic root above 4 cm, cardiac involvement and a family history of dissection and sudden death; patients should be advised accordingly.[17] Repair of aortic dissection during pregnancy carries a 22% maternal mortality.[18] The main fetal risk is of recurrence (50%). Pregnant patients should be given beta-blockade and strong consideration be given to elective Caesarean section.

□ CONTRACEPTION IN CONGENITAL HEART DISEASE

Women with CHD need safe, effective contraceptive advice to allow them to plan or avoid pregnancy.

Combined oral contraceptive pill

The combined oral contraceptive (OC) pill is suitable for many women with CHD including those with repaired tetralogy of Fallot. Its cardiovascular risks relate to the prothrombotic effects of the oestrogen component, so combined OCs should be avoided in those with an intrinsic risk of thrombosis (Table 1). Warfarin anticoagulation may mitigate some of these risks, but anticoagulation control must be carefully monitored since oestrogen may reduce the anticoagulation effect of warfarin. Patients with unoperated atrial septal defect are at risk of paradoxical embolism if they develop venous thrombosis, so an alternative contraceptive method may be preferred.

Table 1 Contraindications for combined oral contraceptive use.

- Atrial arrhythmia
- Fontan circulation
- Pulmonary hypertension of any cause
- Cyanotic heart disease
- Mechanical valves
- Ischaemic heart disease
- Previous thromboembolism
- Dilated cardiomyopathy

Progesterone-only methods

There is no cardiac contraindication to progesterone-only contraception, but different methods and devices carry specific risks. The progesterone-only pill is safe for all women with cardiac disease, but its significant failure rate makes it unsuitable for those in whom pregnancy is absolutely contraindicated. The newer desogestrel-containing pill (Cerazette®) has additional anovulant effects and a higher contraceptive efficacy.

Depot progesterone injections are safe and reliable but there may be haematoma at the injection site in women who are anticoagulated. The Mirena coil is discussed below.

The subdermal progesterone implant (Implanon®) has a lower failure rate than sterilisation and there are no cardiac contraindications to its use. In common with some of the other progesterone-only preparations, it reduces or even abolishes menstrual blood loss.

Intrauterine contraceptive devices

Traditional intrauterine contraceptive devices (IUDs) carry a risk of menorrhagia, infection and vasovagal syncope at insertion – the last may be fatal in Eisenmenger syndrome. They are suitable for women with minor disease who have had a previous pregnancy. The progesterone eluting IUD (Mirena® coil) has the advantages of improved contraceptive efficacy, reduced menstrual blood loss and a lower associated risk of endocarditis.

Sterilisation

Laparoscopic sterilisation carries a risk in those patients in whom pregnancy is most dangerous (eg Eisenmenger syndrome). Now that safe and secure methods of contraception are available, sterilisation should not be routinely recommended in these patients. It is rarely appropriate to consider male sterilisation, since the male partner is likely to outlive the female with significant heart disease and may wish to have children in the future.

Providing the service

Pre-pregnancy and contraceptive counselling should begin in adolescence to allow women to plan the timing of their pregnancies and to come to terms with their childbearing potential.

Patients with complex disease benefit from a multidisciplinary approach and close collaboration between the specialist adult CHD cardiologist, the obstetric team and the obstetric anaesthetist. Joint pre-pregnancy and antenatal clinics allow the patient to be fully informed and to benefit from combined expertise throughout their pregnancy and delivery.

REFERENCES

1. Why mothers die 1997–1999. The Confidential Enquiry into Maternal Deaths in the United Kingdom. London: Royal College of Obstetricians and Gynaecologists, 2001.
2. Murphy JG, Gersh BJ, Mair DD, Fuster V *et al.* Long-term outcome in patients undergoing surgical repair of tetralogy of Fallot. *N Engl J Med* 1993;**329**:593–9.
3. Bonow RO, Carabello B, de Leon AC, Edmunds LH Jr *et al.* ACC/AHA Guidelines for the Management of Patients With Valvular Heart Disease. Executive Summary. A report of the American College of Cardiology/American Heart Association Task Force on Practice Guidelines (Committee on Management of Patients With Valvular Heart Disease). *J Heart Valve Dis* 1998;**7**:672–707.
4. Cotrufo M, De Feo M, De Santo LS, Romano G *et al.* Risk of warfarin during pregnancy with mechanical valve prostheses. *Obstet Gynecol* 2002;**99**:35–40.
5. Sbarouni E, Oakley CM. Outcome of pregnancy in women with valve prostheses. *Br Heart J* 1994;**71**:196–201.
6. Ginsberg JS, Chan WS, Bates SM, Kaatz S. Anticoagulation of pregnant women with mechanical heart valves. *Arch Intern Med* 2003;**163**:694–8.
7. Connolly H, Grogan M, Warnes CA. Pregnancy among women with congenitally corrected transposition of great arteries. *J Am Coll Cardiol* 1999;**33**:1692–5.
8. Therrien J, Barnes I, Somerville J. Outcome of pregnancy in patients with congenitally corrected transposition of the great arteries. *Am J Cardiol* 1999;**84**:820–4.
9. Clarkson PM, Wilson NJ, Neutze JM, North RA *et al.* Outcome of pregnancy after the Mustard operation for transposition of the great arteries with intact ventricular septum. *J Am Coll Cardiol* 1994;**24**:190–3.
10. Presbitero P, Somerville J, Stone S, Aruta E *et al.* Pregnancy in cyanotic congenital heart disease. Outcome of mother and fetus. *Circulation* 1994;**89**:2673–6.
11. Canobbio MM, Mair DD, van der Velde M, Koos BJ. Pregnancy outcomes after the Fontan repair. *J Am Coll Cardiol* 1996;**28**:763–7.
12. Weiss BM, Zemp L, Seifert B, Hess OM. Outcome of pulmonary vascular disease in pregnancy: a systematic overview from 1978 through 1996. Review. *J Am Coll Cardiol* 1998;**31**:1650–7.

13 Yentis SM, Steer PJ, Plaat F. Eisenmenger's syndrome in pregnancy: maternal and fetal mortality in the 1990s. *Br J Obstet Gynaecol* 1998;**105**:921–2.

14 Gopal K, Hudson IM, Ludmir J, Braffman MN *et al.* Homograft aortic root replacement during pregnancy. *Ann Thorac Surg* 2002;**74**:243–5.

15 Weiss BM, von Segesser LK, Alon E, Seifert B, Turina MI. Outcome of cardiovascular surgery and pregnancy: a systematic review of the period 1984–1996. Review. *Am J Obstet Gynecol* 1998;**179**(6Pt 1):1643–53.

16 Beauchesne LM, Connolly HM, Ammash NM, Warnes CA. Coarctation of the aorta: outcome of pregnancy. *J Am Coll Cardiol* 2001;**38**:1728–3.

17 Elkayam U, Ostrzega E, Shotan A, Mehra A. Cardiovascular problems in pregnant women with the Marfan syndrome. Review. *Ann Intern Med* 1995;**123**:117–22.

18 Lind J, Wallenburg HC. The Marfan syndrome and pregnancy: a retrospective study in a Dutch population. *Eur J Obstet Gynecol Reprod Biol* 2001;**98**:28–35.

☐ MEDICINE IN PREGNANCY SELF ASSESSMENT QUESTIONS

How to manage renal disease in pregnancy

1 The risks associated with pregnancy need to be considered in women of childbearing age with:
(a) Systemic lupus erythematosus
(b) Mitral valve disease
(c) Hypertension
(d) Reflux nephropathy
(e) End-stage renal failure (ESRF)

2 Appropriate advice to give a woman with known kidney disease considering pregnancy includes:
(a) A normal creatinine is associated with no increased risk of complications
(b) To protect her renal function she should continue her angiotensin-converting enzyme inhibitors throughout pregnancy
(c) She should stop taking hydroxychloroquine used to treat her lupus arthralgia
(d) Stopping steroids when she is pregnant is unwise and unnecessary
(e) If she has reflux nephropathy, her baby may also be at risk of the same condition

3 In women with kidney disease, a creatinine greater than 180 μmol/l increases her risk of:
(a) Preterm delivery
(b) Delivery by Caesarean section
(c) Transmitting neonatal lupus
(d) Having an macrosomic baby
(e) Developing ESRF

4 Management of pregnancies in women with known kidney disease should include:
(a) The use of low molecular weight heparin
(b) Atenolol to control blood pressure
(c) Regular growth scans
(d) Regular estimation of serum urea to assess renal function
(e) Planned elective Caesarean section no later than 38 weeks

Congenital heart disease in pregnancy

1 Aortic stenosis and pregnancy:
(a) Pregnancy is likely to be well tolerated in the asymptomatic patient with a mean pre-pregnancy aortic valve echo Doppler gradient below 50 mmHg
(b) A fall in echo Doppler-derived aortic valve gradient during pregnancy is to be expected and is not cause for concern
(c) Initial management of dyspnoea and new onset angina during pregnancy should include bedrest and beta-blockade

(d) The exercise tolerance test is a useful pre-pregnancy investigation in assessing maternal risk
(e) Aortic valve replacement during pregnancy carries a high risk of fetal loss

2 Regarding drugs and procedures in pregnancy:
(a) Heparin crosses the placenta and is teratogenic
(b) Angiotensin-converting enzyme inhibitors cause renal agenesis
(c) Beta-blockers may be used in pregnancy
(d) Balloon mitral valvuloplasty after the first trimester carries a high risk of fetal loss
(e) The maternal risk of balloon dilatation of native aortic coarctation is no higher in the pregnant than in the non-pregnant state

3 Pregnancy is usually well tolerated in:
(a) Repaired tetralogy of Fallot
(b) Eisenmenger syndrome
(c) Unoperated small ventricular septal defect
(d) Left ventricular systolic dysfunction
(e) Mitral regurgitation

4 The combined oral contraceptive pill may be used safely in the following conditions:
(a) Repaired tetralogy of Fallot
(b) Pulmonary hypertension
(c) Mild pulmonary stenosis
(d) Dilated cardiomyopathy
(e) Cyanotic heart disease

5 The following may be normal in pregnancy:
(a) Elevated jugular venous pressure
(b) Fourth heart sound
(c) Palpitation
(d) Systolic murmur
(e) Pleural effusion

Managing risk factors

The epidemic of obesity: genes versus environment

I Sadaf Farooqi

□ INTRODUCTION

Obesity is defined as a disorder in which excess body fat has accumulated such that health may be adversely affected. It is associated with substantially increased mortality from type 2 diabetes mellitus, cardiovascular and cerebrovascular diseases and certain cancers. Obesity also results in severe morbidity from musculoskeletal, gastrointestinal, psychiatric and reproductive diseases, and is associated with lowered quality of life, self-esteem and socio-economic performance.[1] The World Health Organization classification of obesity is a body mass index (BMI) exceeding 30 kg/m^2. Using this definition, it is clear that the prevalence of obesity has risen dramatically over the last 20 years. Currently, at least 20% of the population of the US and most Western countries is clinically obese and at least 50% either overweight or obese.[1] There is little doubt that the pandemic of obesity represents a significant public health problem.

The rising prevalence of obesity over a short genetic interval supports the role of environmental factors, in particular the availability of energy-dense foods and reduced requirement for physical exertion. However, there is considerable evidence from twin and family studies suggesting that the heritability of fat mass is between 40–70%.[2] It is likely that the ability to store fat in times of nutritional abundance is a positive trait selected over many thousands of years of human evolution as a means of dealing with periodic famine. This inherent propensity to store energy in an environment where there is excess energy intake and a reduction in energy expenditure during physical activity results in a tendency to excess body weight and the emergence of the current epidemic of obesity.

□ GENETIC BASIS OF COMMON OBESITY

Genetic influences are not confined to the extremes of obesity, but exert their effect across the whole range of body weight and at a population level are consistent with the polygenic inheritance of fat mass. The genetic determinants of interindividual variation in fat mass are likely to be multiple and interacting, each single variant producing only a moderate effect. The search for genetic determinants of human obesity has accelerated rapidly in recent years using various methodologies, including family-based linkage studies incorporating genome-wide scans and studies of candidate genes in population or family-based association studies (methodologies and results are reviewed in Ref 3).

□ STUDY OF EXTREME PHENOTYPES

Historical evidence, including artefacts dating from the Palaeolithic Stone Age depicting subjects with an excess of body fat, suggests that some individuals harbour the propensity to store excess energy as fat independent of diet and geographical region. The existence of such individuals provides evidence for major gene effects. Our attention to date has primarily been focused on the extreme phenotype of severe, early-onset obesity, having hypothesised that major and more highly penetrant genetic mutations were likely to be found in this condition. Over 1,000 subjects have been recruited as part of the Genetics Of Obesity Study (GOOS), a cohort of subjects with severe obesity (mean BMI >4 standard deviations above the population mean) of early onset (<10 years old). A candidate gene approach has been undertaken in subsets of this cohort, screening genes known to be involved in energy homeostasis in rodents.

□ RODENT MODELS OF OBESITY

The identification and characterisation of single gene defects in rodent obesities inherited in either a dominant (yellow, *Ay/a*) or recessive (*ob/ob, db/db, fa/fa, tb/tb)* manner has given substantial insights into:

- □ physiological disturbances that can lead to obesity
- □ metabolic and endocrine abnormalities associated with the obese phenotype, and
- □ more detailed anatomical and neurochemical pathways that regulate energy intake and energy expenditure.[4]

These studies provide the basic framework upon which the understanding of the more complex mechanisms in humans can be built.

□ LEPTIN-MELANOCORTIN PATHWAY

The initial observations in this field were made as a result of positional cloning strategies in two strains of severely obese mice (*ob/ob* and *db/db*). Severely obese *ob/ob* mice were found to harbour mutations in the *ob* gene resulting in a complete lack of its protein product leptin.[5] Administration of recombinant leptin reduced the food intake and body weight of leptin-deficient *ob/ob* mice and corrected all their neuroendocrine and metabolic abnormalities. The signalling form of the leptin receptor is deleted in *db/db* mice, which are consequently unresponsive to endogenous or exogenous leptin. The identification of these two proteins established the first components of a nutritional feedback loop from adipose tissue to the brain. However, it is thought that the physiological role of leptin in humans and rodents might be to act as a signal for starvation because, as fat mass increases, further rises in leptin have a limited ability to suppress food intake and prevent obesity.

Considerable attention has focused on deciphering the hypothalamic pathways that co-ordinate the behavioural and metabolic effects downstream of leptin. The first-order neuronal targets of leptin action in the brain are anorectic (reducing food intake) pro-opiomelanocortin (POMC) and orexigenic (increasing food intake) neuropeptide-Y/Agouti-related protein (NPY/AgRP) neurones in the hypothalamic arcuate nucleus, where the signalling isoform of the leptin receptor is highly expressed.[6] mRNA for the long form of the leptin receptor is expressed by 40% of POMC neurones in the arcuate nucleus and POMC expression is regulated positively by leptin. POMC is sequentially cleaved by prohormone convertases (PC) to yield peptides, including α-melanocyte stimulating hormone (α-MSH), that play a role in feeding behaviour. There is clear evidence in rodents that α-MSH acts as a suppressor of feeding behaviour, probably through the melanocortin 4 receptor (MC4R). In fact, targeted disruption of MC4R in rodents leads to increased food intake, obesity, severe early hyperinsulinaemia and increased linear growth. Heterozygotes have a phenotype intermediate between homozygotes and wild-type mice.[7]

□ HUMAN MONOGENIC OBESITY SYNDROMES

Congenital leptin deficiency

The first monogenic human obesity syndrome to be reported was congenital leptin deficiency. Two severely obese cousins in a highly consanguineous family of Pakistani origin were found to have undetectable levels of serum leptin. They were homozygous for a frameshift mutation in the *ob* gene (ΔG133) resulting in a truncated protein that was not secreted.[8] These children were severely hyperphagic, constantly demanding food, with an intense drive to eat that was never satisfied. They developed severe disabling obesity (the 8-year-old girl weighed 86 kg and the 2-year-old boy weighed 29 kg) characterised by an excess deposition of fat.

Mild hyperinsulinaemia, advanced skeletal maturation, impaired T cell mediated immunity and hypogonadotropic hypogonadism are other features seen in three leptin deficient subjects from a Turkish family homozygous for a missense mutation in the *ob* gene.[9]

Studies of the heterozygote members of the ΔG133 families indicate that their leptin levels are lower than ethnically matched control subjects; this partial leptin deficiency results in increased fat mass (mean 23% more than predicted).[10] Thus, the phenotype of human leptin deficiency due to mutations in the *ob* gene is remarkably similar to that seen in leptin-deficient rodents.

Three leptin-deficient children have been treated with daily subcutaneous injections of recombinant human leptin for up to four years, with sustained beneficial effects on appetite, fat mass, hyperinsulinaemia and hyperlipidaemia (Fig 1). The major impact of leptin on human energy balance was mediated via its suppressive effects on food intake, with a marked reduction in caloric consumption during a test meal, associated with parental reports of a near-normalisation of eating behaviour in the domestic setting.[9] Leptin administration permits the full

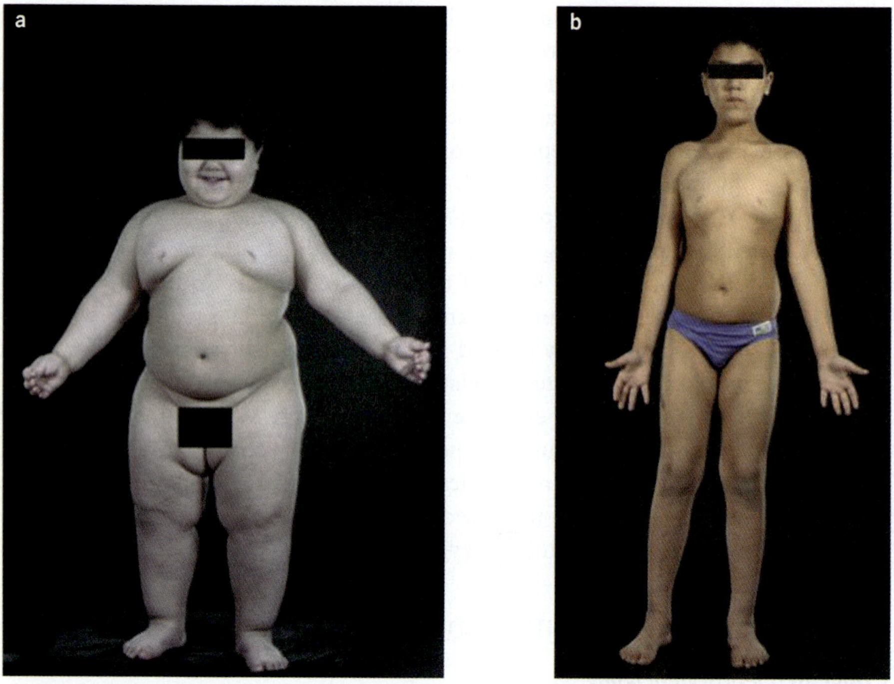

Fig 1 Clinical response to leptin therapy in a child with congenital leptin deficiency: **(a)** before treatment, weighing 42 kg at three years old; **(b)** after treatment, weighing 32 kg at seven years old.

progression of appropriately timed puberty, but does not appear to cause precocious activation of the pubertal process in younger children (Fig 2).

Although this syndrome is rare, these studies have established that leptin has profound effects on appetite in humans and may act as a metabolic gate for the onset of puberty at an appropriate developmental age.[9]

Leptin receptor deficiency

A mutation in the leptin receptor has been reported in one consanguineous family. Affected individuals were homozygous for a mutation that truncates the receptor before the transmembrane domain, and the mutated receptor circulates bound to leptin.[10] There are a number of phenotypic similarities with the leptin-deficient subjects. Leptin receptor-deficient subjects in this family were also born of normal birth weight, exhibiting rapid weight gain in the first few months of life, with severe hyperphagia and aggressive behaviour when denied food. In contrast, some neuroendocrine features were unique to leptin receptor deficiency. The presence of mild growth retardation in early childhood in these subjects, together with impaired basal and stimulated growth hormone secretion, decreased insulin-like growth factor-1 (IGF-1) and IGF-BP3 levels and evidence of hypothalamic hypothyroidism, suggest that loss of the leptin receptor results in a more diverse phenotype than loss of its ligand, leptin.[11]

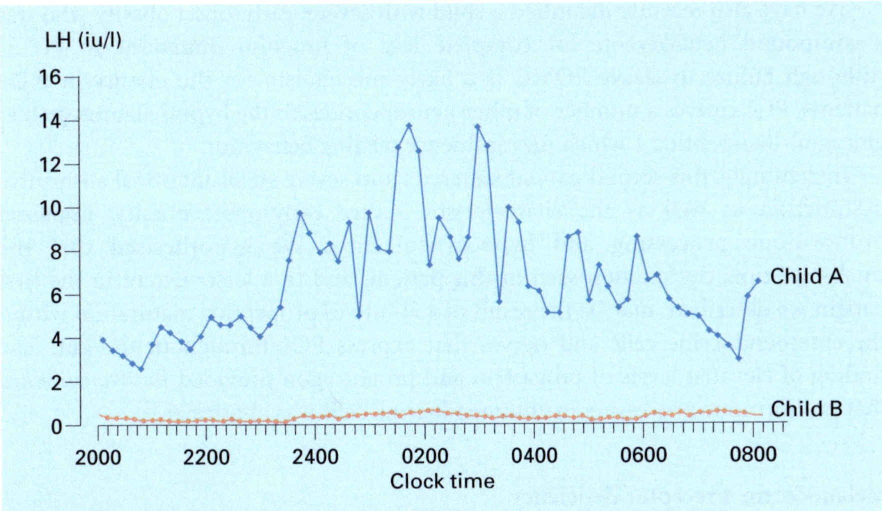

Fig 2 Leptin therapy is associated with pulsatile gonadotrophin secretion at an appropriate developmental age in child A (age 11 years) compared with child B (age 5 years) (LH = luteinising hormone).

Pro-opiomelanocortin deficiency

Two unrelated obese German children with homozygous or compound heterozygous mutations in POMC have been reported.[12] These children were hyperphagic, developing early-onset obesity as a result of impaired melanocortin signalling in the hypothalamus. They presented in neonatal life with adrenal crisis due to isolated ACTH deficiency (POMC is a precursor of ACTH in the pituitary) and had pale skin and red hair due to the lack of MSH function at melanocortin 1 receptors in the skin. We and others have identified a heterozygous missense mutation (Arg236Gly) in POMC that disrupts the dibasic amino acid processing site between β-MSH and β-endorphin. This mutation results in an aberrant β-MSH/β-endorphin fusion peptide which binds to MC4R with an affinity identical to that of α- and β-MSH but with a markedly reduced ability to activate the receptor.[13] Thus, this cleavage site mutation in POMC may confer susceptibility to obesity through a novel molecular mechanism.

Prohormone convertase 1 deficiency

Further evidence for the role of the melanocortin system in the regulation of body weight in humans comes from the description of a 47-year-old woman with severe childhood obesity, abnormal glucose homeostasis, very low plasma insulin but elevated levels of proinsulin, hypogonadotropic hypogonadism and hypocortisolaemia associated with elevated levels of POMC. She was a compound heterozygote for mutations in PC1, which cleaves prohormones at pairs of basic amino acids, leaving C-terminal basic residues which are then excised by carboxypeptidase E (CPE).[14]

We have also recently identified a child with severe, early-onset obesity who was a compound heterozygote for complete loss of function mutations in PC1.[15] Although failure to cleave POMC is a likely mechanism for the obesity in these patients, PC1 cleaves a number of other neuropeptides in the hypothalamus such as glucagon-like-peptide 1 which may influence feeding behaviour.

Intriguingly, this second patient suffered from severe small-intestinal absorptive dysfunction as well as the characteristic severe early-onset obesity, impaired prohormone processing and hypocortisolaemia. We hypothesised that the small-intestinal dysfunction seen in this patient, and to a lesser extent in the first patient we described, may be the result of a failure of propeptide maturation within the enteroendocrine cells and nerves that express PC1 throughout the gut. The finding of elevated levels of progastrin and proglucagon provided *in vivo* evidence that prohormone processing in enteroendocrine cells was abnormal.[15]

Melanocortin 4 receptor deficiency

Heterozygous mutations in MC4R have been reported to cause a dominantly inherited obesity syndrome in different ethnic groups. In a study of 500 severely obese probands, approximately 5% were found to harbour pathogenic mutations in the *MC4R* gene, making this the commonest monogenic cause of obesity thus far described in humans.[16] A small number of homozygotes for MC4R mutations have been described, but the heterozygotes in these families have an intermediate phenotype consistent with a co-dominant mode of inheritance.[16]

Detailed phenotypic studies of patients with MC4R mutations reveal that this syndrome is characterised by an increase in lean body mass and bone mineral density, increased linear growth throughout childhood, hyperphagia and severe hyperinsulinaemia.[16] These features are similar to those seen in MC4R knock-out mice, suggesting the preservation of the relevant melanocortin pathways between rodents and humans. Of particular note is the finding that the severity of receptor dysfunction seen in *in vitro* assays can predict the amount of food ingested at a test meal by the subject harbouring that particular mutation.[16]

We have studied in detail the signalling properties of many of these mutant receptors. The information obtained should help to advance the understanding of structure/function relationships and potentially provide *in vitro* support for the use of MC4R agonists in this group of patients.[17] Importantly, it has not been possible to demonstrate evidence for dominant negativity associated with these mutants, suggesting that *MC4R* mutations are more likely to result in a phenotype through haplo-insufficiency.

☐ DISCUSSION

Although these monogenic syndromes are rare, an improved understanding of the precise nature of the inherited component of severe obesity has undoubted medical benefits and helps to dispel the notion that obesity represents an individual defect in behaviour with no biological basis. For individuals at highest risk of the complications of severe obesity, such findings provide a starting point for providing more rational mechanism-based therapies, as successfully achieved for congenital leptin deficiency.

The concept that environmental factors operate on an underlying pool of genes that contributes to obesity susceptibility in the general population has important implications for our approach to the prevention and treatment of obesity. First, it would help identify pathways in humans responsible for energy homeostasis, thereby clarifying the relevance of such pathways as targets for pharmacological intervention. Secondly, different subsets of genetic variants may determine responses to environmental manipulations such as calorie restriction, altered macronutrient balance or exercise regimens. A number of recent advances are likely to make significant contributions to the search for obesity genes, including the completion of a draft of the human genome sequence and the discovery and cataloguing of single nucleotide polymorphisms, the most prevalent source of sequence variation throughout the human genome. These efforts promise to enhance our ability to identify risk-conferring genes for complex traits such as obesity.

REFERENCES

1 Kopelman PG. Obesity as a medical problem. Review. *Nature* 2000;**404**:635–43.

2 Barsh GS, Farooqi IS, O'Rahilly S. Genetics of body-weight regulation. Review. *Nature* 2000;**404**:644–51.

3 Comuzzie AG. The emerging pattern of the genetic contribution to human obesity. Review. *Best Pract Res Clin Endocrinol Metab* 2002;**16**:611–21.

4 Leibel RL, Chung WK, Chua SC Jr. The molecular genetics of rodent single gene obesities. Review. *J Biol Chem* 1997;**272**:31937–40.

5 Zhang Y, Proenca R, Maffei M, Barone M *et al.* Positional cloning of the mouse obese gene and its human homologue. *Nature* 1994;**372**:425–32.

6 Schwartz MW, Woods SC, Porte D Jr, Seeley RJ, Baskin DG. Central nervous system control of food intake. Review. *Nature* 2000;**404**:661–71.

7 Huszar D, Lynch CA, Fairchild-Huntress V, Dunmore JH *et al.* Targeted disruption of the melanocortin-4 receptor results in obesity in mice. *Cell* 1997;**88**:131–41.

8 Montague CT, Farooqi IS, Whitehead JP, Soos MA *et al.* Congenital leptin deficiency is associated with severe early-onset obesity in humans. *Nature* 1997;**387**:903–8.

9 Farooqi IS, Matarese G, Lord GM, Keogh JM *et al.* Beneficial effects of leptin on obesity, T cell hyporesponsiveness, and neuroendocrine/metabolic dysfunction of human congenital leptin deficiency. *J Clin Invest* 2002;**110**:1093–103.

10 Farooqi IS, Keogh JM, Kamath S, Jones S *et al.* Partial leptin deficiency and human adiposity. *Nature* 2001;**414**:34–5.

11 Clement K, Vaisse C, Lahlou N, Cabrol S *et al.* A mutation in the human leptin receptor gene causes obesity and pituitary dysfunction. *Nature* 1998;**392**:398–401.

12 Krude H, Biebermann H, Luck W, Horn R *et al.* Severe early-onset obesity, adrenal insufficiency and red hair pigmentation caused by POMC mutations in humans. *Nat Genet* 1998;**19**:155–7.

13 Challis BG, Pritchard LE, Creemers JW, Delplanque J *et al.* A missense mutation disrupting a dibasic prohormone processing site in pro-opiomelanocortin (POMC) increases susceptibility to early-onset obesity through a novel molecular mechanism. *Hum Mol Genet* 2002;**11**:1997–2004.

14 Jackson RS, Creemers JW, Ohagi S, Raffin-Sanson ML *et al.* Obesity and impaired prohormone processing associated with mutations in the human prohormone convertase 1 gene. *Nat Genet* 1997;**16**:303–6.

15 Jackson RS, Creemers JW, Farooqi IS, Raffin-Sanson ML *et al.* Small-intestinal dysfunction accompanies the complex endocrinopathy of human proprotein convertase 1 deficiency. *J Clin Invest* 2003;**112**:1550–60.

16 Farooqi IS, Keogh JM, Yeo GS, Lank EJ *et al.* Clinical spectrum of obesity and mutations in the melanocortin 4 receptor gene. *N Engl J Med* 2003;**348**:1085–95.

17 Yeo GS, Lank EJ, Farooqi IS, Keogh J *et al.* Mutations in the human melanocortin-4 receptor gene associated with severe familial obesity disrupts receptor function through multiple molecular mechanisms. *Hum Mol Genet* 2003;**12**:561–74.

The management of hypertension: what the trials have taught us

Anthony Heagerty

□ INTRODUCTION

It is estimated that 20% of the adult UK population have a degree of raised blood pressure sufficient to increase the risk of stroke or heart disease. Hypertension management has evolved against the background of rapidly accumulating evidence, now overwhelmingly persuasive, that lowering blood pressure is associated with reduction in mortality and morbidity. Increasingly refined clinical trial design has led to answers to most questions about optimal therapy and target levels to achieve. This review addresses several issues key to hypertension management.

□ ARE NEWER CLASSES OF DRUGS SUPERIOR TO OLDER AGENTS?

New classes of drugs include calcium-channel blockers (CCB), angiotensin-converting enzyme inhibitors (ACEI), angiotensin II receptor blockers (ARB) and α-adrenoreceptor antagonists. Strong evidence for the efficacy of CCBs and ACEIs in placebo-controlled trials was provided by an overview involving more than 17,000 patients, but the evidence for differences between drug classes was weaker in larger studies involving 37,000 patients.[1]

A number of important conclusions have now emerged from other investigations:

1. An increased awareness that the level of systolic blood pressure is as prognostically important as diastolic blood pressure, and that isolated systolic hypertension is the predominant form of raised blood pressure as we grow older. Far from being an irreversible part of the ageing process, blood pressure can also be lowered with drugs in the older age group and favourable outcomes on stroke and heart disease observed.
2. New classes of drugs are being used in outcome trials to test further the claim that they could be superior to beta-blockers and diuretics.
3. A landmark study which addressed the concerns about lowering blood pressure too far demonstrated that lowering diastolic pressure below 90 mmHg did not cause increased mortality or morbidity.[2]

There has recently been a further attempt to examine the evidence for the superiority of new drugs. A search was made for outcome trials that tested drugs to lower blood pressure in normotensive and hypertensive patients without overt heart failure at enrolment. Other criteria were:

- □ a randomised controlled design
- □ publication in a peer reviewed journal
- □ a sample size of 100 patients or more
- □ inclusion of patients with hypertension, with follow-up assessment of blood pressure and cardiovascular events of at least two years.[3]

Nine studies were found involving more than 62,000 hypertensive patients who had been randomised to conventional therapy with diuretics or beta-blockers or initial treatment with newer agents such as CCBs, ACEIs or α-adrenoreceptor antagonists. CCBs and ACEIs offered similar overall cardiovascular protection to conventional therapy. There was some evidence that CCBs provided more reduction in the risk of stroke and less reduction in the risk of myocardial infarction (MI). Overall, the findings confirmed the previous meta-analysis. The emerging message is clear: older and newer antihypertensive drugs confer similar protection.

There have now been three more major outcome studies, two of which demand close scrutiny because they appear at first glance to offer evidence that ACEIs or ARBs could provide extra added value.

HOPE (for explanation of studies see end of text)

HOPE was not strictly a study in hypertensive patients. It included more than 9,000 high risk patients with declared circulatory problems, in particular impaired cardiac function, with vascular disease or diabetes plus one other cardiovascular risk factor, and known to have a low ejection fraction or symptomatic heart failure. The patients were randomised to ramipril (up to a maximum dose of 10 mg) or placebo as additional therapy to their pre-existing treatment regimen for five years.[4] The primary outcome was a composite of MI, stroke and cardiovascular death. The outcome was dramatic: on ramipril there was a 22% reduction in the composite end-point, with 20% reduction in MI, 32% reduction in stroke and 26% reduction in cardiovascular death.

In their original report the trial co-ordinators stated that the small impact on blood pressure could not account for these particular large benefits. However, a subsequent examination of a small subset of patients from the HOPE trial using ambulatory blood pressure monitoring suggested that the falls in pressure were far larger than first appreciated, and that adopting the meta-analysis approach of Staessen *et al*[3] indicated that even the initially reported small falls in blood pressure were sufficient to explain the beneficial outcome observed.

LIFE

The second trial suggesting a favourable effect on cardiovascular outcomes independent of pressure used losartan, an ARB. In LIFE, more than 9,000 patients were randomised to receive losartan or atenolol in a double-blind, parallel group design. Primary outcomes included non-fatal stroke and mortality due to MI such as sudden death, heart failure or other cardiovascular causes. Losartan significantly reduced relative risk in all patients and to a greater extent in a subgroup of diabetics.[5] There is clear evidence for a small superior effect of losartan on systolic blood pressure. Incorporating the patient data into the Staessen meta-analysis, it is clear that the superior impact on blood pressure influenced the outcome.

ALLHAT

The most recent trial, ALLHAT, addressed prospectively whether the outcome of fatal coronary heart disease (CHD) or non-fatal MI is reduced in high risk patients with hypertension treated with a CCB (amlodipine), an ACEI (lisinopril) or an α-adrenoreceptor antagonist (doxazosin). Each class of drugs was compared with diuretic treatment (chlorthalidone).[6] Secondary outcomes included all-cause mortality, stroke and other cardiovascular events.

In order to evaluate possible heterogeneity in the cardiovascular disease effects of the various agents previously suggested by the meta-analysis approach, ALLHAT was designed with a large sample size (9,000–15,000 patients per intervention arm) and a long follow-up (4–8 years). Such a large-scale investigation also allowed the relative benefit of various agents to be examined in high risk hypertensive subgroups such as older patients, black patients and diabetics. Hypertensive men and women aged 55 years or older with at least one additional risk factor for CHD were included.

The results of ALLHAT are impressive. Chlorthalidone was found to be superior to doxazosin and the α-adrenoreceptor arm was terminated controversially early. This was because there were more cases of non-fatal heart failure on doxazosin, which is not surprising given that patients already on treatment could be recruited into this study. Therefore, it was inevitable that some patients with left ventricular dysfunction would be randomised to receive no diuretic and would deteriorate. All-cause mortality was the same in all groups. However, it is important to point out that systolic pressures were significantly higher with amlodipine (0.8 mmHg) and lisinopril (2 mmHg) than with chlorthalidone. Diastolic pressure was lower on amlodipine (0.8 mmHg). Lisinopril, amlodipine and chlorthalidone achieved control of hypertension (less than 140/90 mmHg) in 61%, 66% and 68% patients, respectively. In terms of secondary outcomes, chlorthalidone was superior (perhaps predictably) in preventing heart failure and better than lisinopril in preventing stroke.

As an important side issue, the safety concerns about long-acting CCBs were allayed by this trial. Once again, the overall impression was that the level of systolic blood pressure lowering achieved is the sole determinant of cardiovascular and cerebrovascular outcomes.

Conclusion

At present, there is no evidence that the newer classes of drugs are superior to older agents; the level of blood pressure achieved is the most important factor.

☐ DO ANY ANTIHYPERTENSIVE DRUG CLASSES AFFORD PARTICULAR PROTECTION?

This question of whether any class of blood pressure lowering drugs is especially protective is worth addressing since meta-analyses have suggested that CCBs are superior to other agents in terms of protecting against stroke. In addition, some evidence in ALLHAT suggests that chlorthalidone is better than lisinopril in preventing stroke, combined cardiovascular disease and heart failure. The ALLHAT trial clearly demonstrates that any class differences can be ascribed to the target blood pressure achieved. Subsequent detailed meta-analyses confirm that it is the differences in blood pressure between drug classes that explain any differences in impact on end-points measured.[7] In terms of established cerebrovascular disease, the study of most interest is PROGRESS in which the combination of an ACEI and a diuretic showed a dramatic reduction in stroke recurrence even in normotensive patients.[8] Staessen has incorporated this study into his meta-analysis and demonstrated clearly that the impact is a result of a lowering of blood pressure even in those who present with levels within the normal range.

Conclusion

The unequivocal conclusion is that an assiduous control of blood pressure will lead to dramatic falls in cerebrovascular accidents.

Diabetic nephropathy

Perhaps the area to receive the most attention is the use of antihypertensive drugs to retard the development of diabetic nephropathy where inhibition of the renin angiotensin system by either ACEI or ARB appears to confer class-specific benefit. However, once again the claims require close scrutiny. The number of cases of renal failure in even the largest outcome trials is small. Investigators have looked at a variety of surrogate end-points including:

- ☐ changes in renal function, such as serum creatinine, creatinine clearance or glomerular filtration rate
- ☐ incidence of renal dysfunction or failure
- ☐ changes in urine albumin excretion
- ☐ development of new microalbuminuria
- ☐ progression to overt proteinuria.

The area has been comprehensively reviewed by Zanchetti and Ruilope.[9] They identified 13 studies which have investigated renal dysfunction in diabetic patients. Class-specific benefits were difficult to establish over and above what would be expected as a result of lowering blood pressure. For example, seven of 10 trials reported blunting of proteinuria proportional to the blood pressure lowering achieved. Three trials investigating microalbuminuria and six progression to proteinuria also showed benefit with antihypertensive drugs proportional to the blood pressure control achieved. The authors concluded that it is not a class-specific effect but, once again, depends on the degree of blood pressure control brought about by good drug therapy programmes.

Non-diabetic renal disease

Protection against non-diabetic renal disease has been reviewed by Jafar *et al.*[10] To date, there have been 11 randomised controlled trials each involving over 100 patients. The authors compared ACEI with non-ACEI treatment of blood pressure in non-diabetic renal disease in 1,860 patients who had been followed for 2.2 years. The blood pressure fall on ACEIs was 4.5/2.3 mmHg greater and most benefit was observed in patients on this class of drug. The authors again concluded that the superior effect on blood pressure with ACEIs was responsible for the beneficial outcomes.

Type 2 diabetes

Perhaps the most important observation with the newer classes of antihypertensive drugs is in the area of 'prevention' of the development of type 2 diabetes. Outcome studies using CCBs (INSIGHT and ALLHAT), ACEIs (HOPE, CAPP, ALLHAT and CHARM) and ARBs (LIFE) have all demonstrated that the newer agents appear over the short term to reduce the number of new cases of type 2 diabetes. The explanation may be vasodilatation induced by these drugs as a result of a favourable effect on skeletal blood flow because of their pharmacological mode of action. Improving blood flow to skeletal muscle could in theory reduce insulin resistance and diminish the risk of the development of the overt diabetic syndrome. Studies are currently ongoing to establish whether this is a genuine finding. If it is, it represents a major step forward in our attack against diabetes – a disease reaching epidemic proportions in a number of westernised societies.

□ WHAT LEVEL OF BLOOD PRESSURE SHOULD BE ACHIEVED?

Most of the data that have framed policy statements on target levels of blood pressure to be achieved come from the HOT trial.[2] In principle, HOT established that diastolic blood pressure could be reduced below 90 mmHg without producing increased mortality or morbidity. This was also reported in SHEP. The consensus from the Joint National Committee on Prevention, Detection, Evaluation and the Treatment of High Blood Pressure, the European Society of Hypertension and the British Hypertension Society (BHS) guidelines is to aim for a blood pressure below 140/85 mmHg. Diabetics are at increased risk of blood pressure-associated complications and should have their target level reduced to below 130/80 mmHg.

The new UK general practitioner (GP) contract will initially allow a level of less than 150/90 mmHg for hypertensive patients, but inevitably this will be reduced as time goes by and more patients are diagnosed and treated. The implications are that a substantial number of patients will receive more than one antihypertensive drug in order to achieve target pressures. The BHS advocates the ABCD approach (Fig 1).[11] This algorithm is based on the fact that patients with hypertension can often be broadly divided into those who have a high renin or a low renin state. They are therefore best treated initially by antihypertensive agents which inhibit renin (ACEI, ARB and beta-blockers) or those which do not (CCBs or diuretics), respectively. Long established data indicate that younger people have higher renin levels than those above 55 years or Afro-Caribbeans. In consequence, the A or B drugs which reduce blood pressure by suppressing the activity of the renin angiotensin cascade are generally more effective in younger people, while CCBs and diuretics should perhaps be used as first-line therapy in older Caucasians or Afro-Caribbeans of any age.

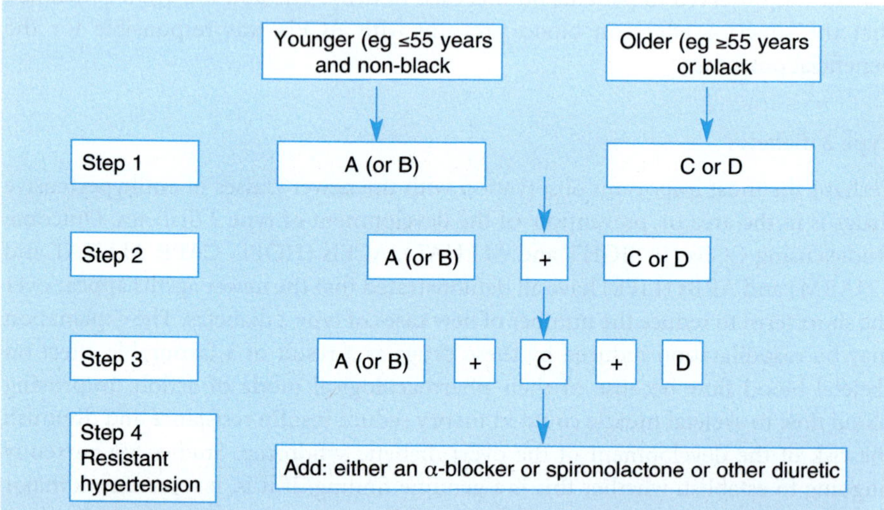

Fig 1 The British Hypertension Society recommendations for combining blood pressure lowering drugs: the ABCD Rule (A = angiotensin-converting enzyme inhibitor; B = beta-blocker; C = calcium-channel blocker; D = diuretic (thiazide)).[11]

□ WHAT DRUGS GIVE ADDED VALUE TO HYPERTENSION MANAGEMENT?

The two principal classes of drugs that must be considered in the management of essential hypertension in the 21st century are antiplatelet agents (salicylates) and lipid-lowering drugs, in particular statins. The indications for these are as follows

- □ *Antiplatelet therapy*, in particular low-dose aspirin (75 mg), should be prescribed to hypertensive patients who have previously had cardiovascular events, provided that there is no evidence of a risk of a bleeding diathesis. Blood pressure should be controlled to 150/90 mmHg or less. The evidence in hypertension suggests that therapy should be instituted in patients over 50 years of age[2] with a calculated 10-year total cardiovascular risk in excess of 20%.

- *Lipid-lowering therapy* should be offered to all patients up to the age of 80 with active CHD, peripheral arterial disease, history of ischaemia, stroke and long-standing type 2 diabetes whose total cholesterol is above 3.5 mmol/l, with the goal of reducing it by about 30%. Patients without overt cardiovascular disease or with recent onset type 2 diabetes should also receive lipid-lowering therapy if their estimated 10-year cardiovascular risk is over 20% and their total cholesterol over 3.5 mmol/l.

This is the gold standard for therapy. The new GP contract will suggest a threshold for treatment as a total cholesterol of 5 mmol/l or greater. With time, these recommendations are expected to become more strict.

CONCLUSIONS

The management of hypertension has become clearer with the emergence of an increased evidence base. Alongside the evidence, the clinician will be able to select from an increasingly large number of drugs, irrespective of price as generic representatives of each class are now increasingly available. Targeting therapy to the high risk patient has been demonstrated to be associated with an enormous impact in terms of reduction in mortality and morbidity.

Trial acronyms

ALLHAT	Antihypertensive and Lipid-Lowering Treatment to Prevent Heart Attack Trial
CAPP	Captopril Prevention Project
CHARM	Candesartan in Heart Failure Assessment in Reduction of Mortality
HOPE	Heart Outcomes Prevention Evaluation
HOT	Hypertension Optimum Treatment
INSIGHT	International Nifedipine Study Intervention as a Goal in Hypertension Treatment
LIFE	Losartan Intervention for Endpoint Reduction in Hypertension
PROGRESS	Perindopril Protection Against Recurrent Stroke Study
SHEP	Systolic Hypertension in the Elderly Programme

REFERENCES

1 Neal B, MacMahon S, Chapman N. Effects of ACE inhibitors, calcium antagonists, and other blood-pressure-lowering drugs: results of prospectively designed overviews of randomised trials. Blood Pressure Lowering Treatment Trialists' Collaboration. *Lancet* 2000;**356**: 1955–64.

2 Hansson L, Zanchetti A, Carruthers SG, Dahlöf B *et al.* Effects of intensive blood-pressure lowering and low-dose aspirin in patients with hypertension: principal results of the Hypertension Optimal Treatment (HOT) randomised trial. HOT Study Group. *Lancet* 1998;**351**:1755–62.

3 Staessen JA, Wang JG, Thijs L. Cardiovascular protection and blood pressure reduction: a meta-analysis. *Lancet* 2001;**358**:1305–15.

4 Yusuf S, Sleight P, Pogue J, Bosch J *et al.* Effects of an angiotensin-converting-enzyme inhibitor, ramipril, on cardiovascular events in high-risk patients. The Heart Outcomes Prevention Evaluation Study Investigators. *N Engl J Med* 2000;**342**:145–53.

5 Lindholm LH, Ibsen H, Dahlöf B, Devereux RB *et al.* Cardiovascular morbidity and mortality in patients with diabetes in the Losartan Intervention For Endpoint reduction in hypertension study (LIFE): a randomised trial against atenolol. *Lancet* 2002;**359**:1004–10.

6 ALLHAT Officers and Coordinators for the ALLHAT Collaborative Research Group. Major outcomes in high-risk hypertensive patients randomized to angiotensin-converting enzyme inhibitor or calcium channel blocker vs diuretic. The Antihypertensive and Lipid-Lowering Treatment to Prevent Heart Attack Trial (ALLHAT). *JAMA* 2002;**288**:2981–97.

7 Wang JG, Staessen JA, Heagerty AM. Ongoing trials: what should we expect after ALLHAT? *Curr Hypertens Rep* 2003;**5**:340–5.

8 PROGRESS Collaborative Group. Randomised trial of a perindopril-based blood-pressure-lowering regimen among 6,105 individuals with previous stroke or transient ischaemic attack. *Lancet* 2001;**358**:1033–41.

9 Zanchetti A, Ruilope LM. Antihypertensive treatment in patients with Type-2 diabetes mellitus: what guidance from recent controlled randomized trials? Review. *J Hypertens* 2002;**20**:2099–110.

10 Jafar TH, Schmid CH, Landa M, Giatras I *et al.* Angiotensin-converting enzyme inhibitors and progression of nondiabetic renal disease. A meta-analysis of patient-level data. *Ann Intern Med* 2001;**135**:73–87.

11 Williams B, Poulter NR, Brown MJ, Davis M *et al.* Guidelines for management of hypertension: report of the fourth working party of the British Hypertension Society, 2004-BHS IV. *J Hum Hypertens* 2004;**18**:139–85.

What to do about hormone replacement therapy

Howard Jacobs

□ INTRODUCTION

Medical advice to postmenopausal woman has undergone an extraordinary change in the last few years. As recently as a decade ago doctors who did not recommend long-term hormone treatment (HT) were considered irresponsible, patients who did not accept their advice, feckless. Now, for reasons that will be examined in this review, long-term HT is under a cloud. Most women seem to have quickly appreciated the need for a radical change in practice and the reasons for it. Doctors, however, are only slowly conceding that postmenopausal HT has not realised the promises made to their patients on its behalf.

Faced with the several new sets of data, the Committee on Safety of Medicines recently issued guidance on HT to patients and doctors,[1] consistent with advice provided by other agencies such as the US Food and Drug Administration, the European Committee for Proprietary Medicinal Products and a consensus statement from a conference on HT by the Royal College of Physicians of Edinburgh (RCPE) in 2003.[2] However, important voices disagree with the position adopted by these bodies, for instance the British Menopause Society, whose consensus statement would have us believe that nothing of clinical relevance has happened.[3] Women have been ill served by the way some of the medical profession have responded to the new information concerning the long-term outcome of HT. Their sincerity is not to be doubted but their wisdom may be questioned.

Another aspect of the context in which long-term HT is presently administered is worth noting. In the US, 46 million prescriptions for Premarin were written in 2000, a figure hardly more staggering than that describing their value – more than $1 billion in that one year alone. In the UK, more than 100 products are now licensed for treatment of postmenopausal women. Poised to fill the gap when doctors finally abandon long-term prescription of HT are complementary and alternative medicines (CAM). The federal budget for CAM in the USA grew from $2 million in 1998 to $68.7 million in 2000. It seems that quite a number of women risk leaving the frying pan of ineffective and risky allopathic medicine for the fire of evidence-free CAM. Given that the few controlled trials of CAM products that have been conducted have shown little or no benefit,[4] it is not a heartening prospect. The biology of some CAM products may yet hold surprises – certainly their safety, particularly long term, has not been examined with the same intensity as expected for medicinal products.[5]

☐ THE HISTORICAL POSITION

The Nurses' Health Study

The field of menopausal medicine was for many years dominated by results from the Nurses' Health Study, an observational account of the outcome of long-term postmenopausal HT in more than 70,000 female nurses. Data were first reported in 1985, the most recent report being published 15 years later.[6] The main finding was that current users of HT had a 40% lower risk of coronary heart disease (CHD) than never users. There were problems of interpretation with this study because outcome was not related to dose or duration of treatment and the risk of stroke was increased. None the less, its optimistic conclusion dominated thinking and, backed by a meta-analysis that included additional observational studies,[7] it led to a widely accepted notion that long-term postmenopausal HT prevented heart attacks and prolonged life. A plausible context of beneficially affected surrogates and mechanisms was assembled.

There had always been concern over bias as an explanation for the findings of these observational studies, but its extent was fully realised only with the publication of randomised controlled trials (RCTs) of HT (Table 1).

Table 1 Sources of bias in observational studies.

Selection	HT as part of a healthy lifestyle
Adherence	A marker for characteristics that confer protection, independent of medication prescribed
Surveillance	Requirement for prescriptions increases contacts with doctors
Survivors	People who become ill often stop HT, so persistent users are less likely to have been ill and so more likely to survive
Publications	Positive studies are more likely to be published than negative ones

HT = hormone therapy.

☐ THE NEW INFORMATION

Heart disease

The change in attitude to long-term HT for postmenopausal women is a direct outcome of the publication of results from two large RCTs. The first, the Heart and Estrogen Progestin Replacement Study (HERS),[8] which tested whether HT prevented further heart attacks in postmenopausal women, was a trial of HT as a method of secondary prevention. In this study, 1,300 postmenopausal women (average age at entry 67 years) were randomly assigned to HT (details given below) and 1,383 to placebo. The first report was published after 4.1 years, the second, an open label extension (HERS II), after 6.8 years. There was no reduction in the risk of further heart attack.

The second study, the Women's Health Initiative (WHI),[9] a trial of HT as a method of primary prevention, tested whether long-term HT prevented heart attacks in healthy postmenopausal women. In this study, 8,506 women (average age at entry

63 years) were randomly assigned to HT and 8,102 to placebo. The study was planned to last eight and half years, but was terminated after 5.2 years because of evidence that treatment caused more harm than benefit, to a degree predetermined by the Data Monitoring Committee as requiring the trial's termination.

The most important outcomes are shown in Table 2. Treatment with HT was associated with more heart attacks than treatment with placebo, also with an increase in the number of women suffering strokes (mainly thrombotic) and pulmonary emboli. There was a statistically significant increase in the number of cases of invasive breast cancer in the women assigned to HT. Serious adverse events offset benefit attributable to HT (fewer osteoporotic fractures and colon carcinomas).

Table 2 Major outcomes of the Women's Health Initiative (WHI) trial.[9]

Outcome	HR	95% CI	Cases per 10,000 women-years
Coronary heart disease	1.29	1.02–1.63	+7
Breast cancer	1.26	1.00–1.59	+8
Stroke	1.41	1.07–1.85	+8
Pulmonary embolus	2.13	1.39–3.25	+8
Colorectal cancer	0.63	0.43–0.92	–6
Endometrial cancer	0.83	0.47–1.47	
Hip fracture	0.66	0.45–0.98	–5
Total mortality	*0.98*	*0.82–1.18*	
*Global index**	*1.15*	*1.03–1.28*	*+19*

*A statistic devised by the WHI to represent the overall balance between beneficial and adverse outcomes.
CI = confidence interval; HR = hazard ratio.

These alarming results immediately triggered several important questions:

1 *Internal validity*: did the trial answer the questions it asked? For example, was the sample size appropriate, was there true randomisation, blinding, a control group, were losses to follow-up minimised and was the analysis by intention-to-treat? Perhaps the only question to which the answer was unsatisfactory concerned blinding. A larger number of women in the treatment group experienced bleeding than in the placebo group. Because bleeding required investigation, this effect of HT differentially unblinded patients and doctors. None the less it is unlikely that unblinding explains the alarming excess of adverse over beneficial effects.

2 *External validity*: were the results of the RCTs generalisable? The subjects in the WHI were asymptomatic and of an average age a decade or so older than women usually given HT (only 30% were in their 50s). The age of menopause was not described.

3 *Should the results be considered specific to the regimen used?* The medication in both HERS and WHI was PremPro (Table 3), at the time the most widely prescribed combined (oestrogen with progestogen) continuous HT preparation in the USA. It has never been available in the UK although similar ones are available (Table 3). Much has been made of a putative cardiotoxic effect of medroxyprogesterone acetate (MPA),[10] the progestogen contained in PremPro. It seems unlikely that MPA should shoulder the blame alone for the adverse outcome, not least because more comprehensive and subtle analyses of these and earlier studies have failed to substantiate a beneficial cardiovascular effect of HT.[11] When the results of RCTs and the re-analyses of the observational studies are considered together with the vital statistics of CHD – that is, that there is no increase in the rate of increase in heart attacks in women at the age of the menopause (Figs 1(a) and (b))[12] – it is hard to escape the conclusion that HT does not provide postmenopausal women with protection from heart attacks. Indeed, the evidence from WHI and HERS is that HT *impairs* cardiovascular status (namely, the increased risks of CHD, stroke and pulmonary embolus shown in Table 2).

Table 3 Constituents of PremPro, the preparation used in the Heart and Estrogen Progestin Replacement Study and Women's Health Initiative trial, and of similar products available in the UK.

Preparation	Constituents
PremPro	Premarin 0.625 mg + MPA 2.5 mg
Similar preparations available in the UK	
Premique	Premarin 0.625 mg + MPA 5 mg
Premique cycle	Premarin 0.625 mg + MPA 10 mg
Prempak C	Premarin 0.625 mg + NG 0.15 mg
Indivina	EV 1–2 mg + MPA 2.5–5 mg
Tridestra	EV 2 mg + MPA 20 mg

EV = oestradiol valerate; MPA = medroxyprogesterone acetate; NG = norgestrol.

Breast cancer

The duration dependent increase in the risk of invasive breast cancer reported in the WHI RCT (Table 2) mirrors the observational results reported in 1995 by the worldwide Collaborative Group[13] and more recently by the UK Million Women Study (MWS).[14] The figures from these different types of study (Table 4) show that combined treatment with oestrogen and progestogen is associated with 3–4 times more invasive breast cancers than treatment with oestrogen alone.

Addition of progestogen to oestrogen is routinely advised to protect the uterus from overstimulation with its potential for causing endometrial cancer. Differences in the impact of the two steroids on breast and uterine tissue provide a plausible mechanism

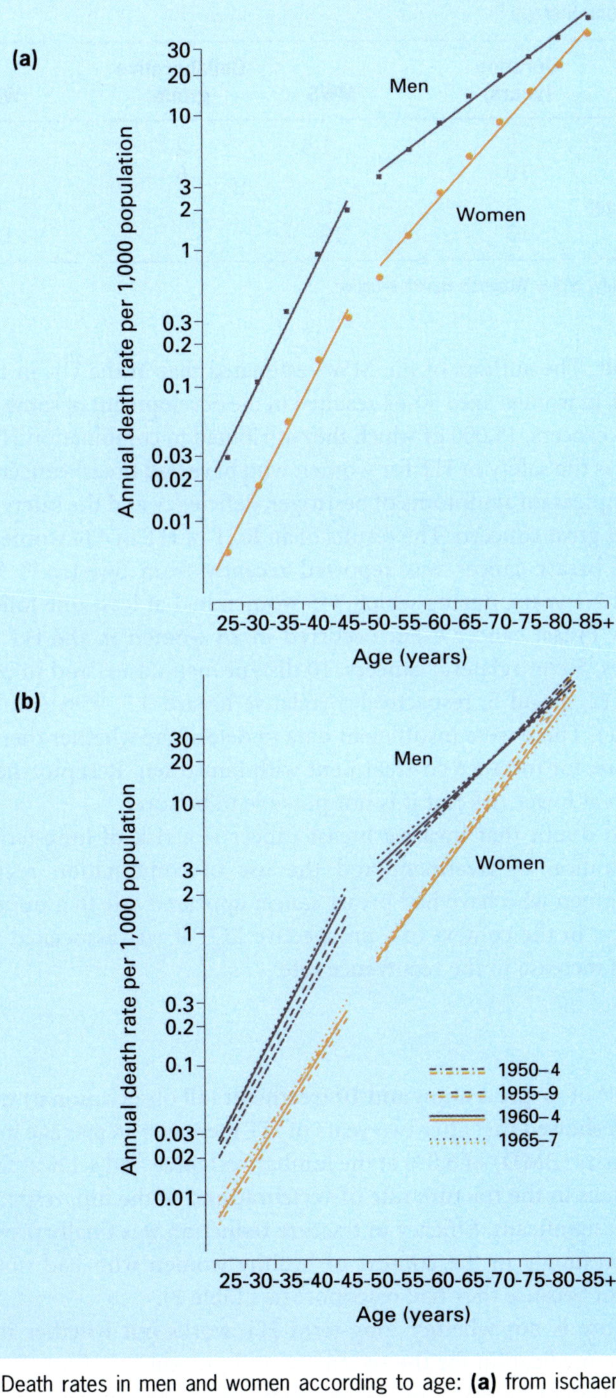

Fig 1 Death rates in men and women according to age: **(a)** from ischaemic heart disease (IHD) (England and Wales 1970–1974); **(b)** from arteriosclerotic and degenerative heart disease (England and Wales 1950–1967).[12] (Coronary heart disease or IHD was classified as arteriosclerotic and degenerative heart disease up to 1967.)

Table 4 Number of additional cases of breast cancer per 1,000 women aged 50-64 attributable to postmenopausal hormone therapy.[14]

Treatment regimen	Duration (years)	MWS	Collaborative group	WHI
Oestrogen alone	5	1.5	2	
	10	5	6	
Oestrogen + Progestogen	5	6		6
	10	19		18

MWS = Million Women Study; WHI = Women's Health Initiative.

for this clinical result. The authors of the MWS estimated that in the UK in the last decade the use of HT in women aged 50-64 resulted in the development of some 20,000 extra invasive breast cancers, 15,000 of which they attributed to combination HT.

A separate issue is the safety of HT for women who have had breast cancer in the past. Many suffer unpleasant symptoms of oestrogen deficiency and the safety of HT has been a subject of great concern. The results of an RCT of HT in 434 women with successfully treated breast cancer was reported recently from Sweden.[15] After a median duration of 2.1 years, during which 345 women had at least one follow-up examination, a new breast cancer event occurred in 26 women in the HT group (11 local recurrences, 5 contralateral cancers, 10 distant metastases) and in eight in the non-HT group (2, 1 and 5, respectively) (relative hazard 3.5, 95% confidence interval (CI) 1.5–8.1). There were insufficient data to determine whether there were any protective factors, for instance co-treatment with tamoxifen. Receptor-negative cases may have been at lower risk but it is not possible to be sure.

There can be no doubt that invasive breast cancer is a risk of long-term HT, increasing with duration of treatment and the use of combination regimens. Although HT for women who have had breast cancer appeared safe in a number of observational studies, in the context of a prospective RCT it was associated with a more than threefold increase in the recurrence rate.

Osteoporosis

A systematic review[16] of 47 prevention and 10 treatment (all observational) trials in osteoporotic women showed that after two years of HT there was an average increase of bone mineral density (BMD) of 6.8% at the lumbar vertebrae and 4.1% at the hip. The 34% and 13% falls in the fracture rate of vertebrae and of the hip, respectively, were not statistically significant. Efficacy in fracture reduction was finally proven by the WHI RCT, interestingly in the context of healthy women who had not been selected for treatment because they had osteoporosis (Table 2).

The issue therefore is not whether long-term HT works but whether it is an appropriate first-line medication for the treatment and prevention of osteoporosis. An important limitation of the effect of HT on the postmenopausal skeleton is that benefit is lost soon after HT is withdrawn; to maintain protection, treatment must necessarily be long term. The data shown in Tables 2 and 4, together with the knowledge that bisphosphonates are equally, if not more, efficacious[16] explains why the regulatory agencies concluded that HT is not an appropriate medication for first-line prevention of osteoporosis.

Clearly, reassurance is needed about the safety of the alternatives to HT taken long term, but at present it seems unlikely that they will be associated with more severe or a greater number of adverse outcomes than HT.

Depression and dementia

In HERS, only the women with flushing attacks who were assigned to HT had improved mental health and fewer depressive symptoms; those without vasomotor symptoms showed no improvement.[17] HT had no effect on cognitive function. In the much larger WHI study, a four-year follow-up of 4,532 women aged 65 years or older at enrolment showed an alarming doubling of the risk of dementia (hazard ratio 2.05, CI 1.21–3.48), representing an additional 23 cases per 10,000 women-years.[18] This increase was possibly caused by cerebrovascular disease because there was also a 31% increase in the risk of ischaemic stroke in the women on HT.

Whatever the mechanism, these results lend no support to the idea that HT prevents dementia.

□ CONCLUSIONS

This review has emphasised changes in our thinking about the value of long-term HT that have resulted predominantly – but not exclusively – from the impact of two large prospective RCTs. Another important feature of the present approach to assessing data in this field is to move away from measurements of surrogate markers of risk (eg lipid subfractions, BMD) in favour of observable clinical end-points, such as the number of heart attacks and fractures that occur during treatment.

I think that the combination of lack of efficacy with the reported rate of serious adverse events makes prescription of long-term HT ill advised, to say the least. Is there any place at all for HT in postmenopausal women? Currently, an important role remains for HT in the control of vasomotor instability and the consequences of genital atrophy – no other agent has yet been found to be as effective. As with all medications, the correct dose of HT is the lowest that works, prescribed while the patient is symptomatic and discontinued when symptoms no longer occur when treatment is withdrawn. At present, for the woman whose uterus is intact, addition of progestogen to treatment with oestrogen remains necessary to avoid overstimulation. It may be that many of the undesirable systemic effects of the combination may be avoided by applying the gestogen directly to the endometrium, for example by means of a progestogen medicated intrauterine device. Progestogen is not required in hysterectomised women. Prevention of osteoporosis may be a fortunate, if temporary, benefit of short-term HT treatment, but long-term management to preserve skeletal strength requires a series of measures in which HT plays little part. Heart disease in women needs to be assessed in the same spirit as it is in men, with the same attention paid to issues of lifestyle, diet, blood pressure and lipid profile because HT does not prevent heart attacks in postmenopausal women.

REFERENCES

1 CMO issues urgent safety message advising HRT should not be used first-line in the prevention of osteoporosis in women aged 50 and over. http://www.druginfozone.nhs.uk/Record%20Viewing/viewRecord.aspx?id=524952

2 Consensus statement on hormone replacement therapy (HRT), Royal College of Physicians of Edinburgh, October 2003. http://www.rcpe.ac.uk/esd/consensus/hrt_03.html

3 Managing the menopause. British Menopause Society Council Consensus statement on Hormone Replacement Therapy. http://www.the-bms.org/conses_stat.htm

4 Kronenberg F, Fugh-Berman A. Complementary and alternative medicine for menopausal symptoms: a review of randomized, controlled trials. Review. *Ann Intern Med* 2002;**137**: 805–13.

5 Amato P, Marcus DM. Review of alternative therapies for treatment of menopausal symptoms. *Climacteric* 2003;**6**:278–84.

6 Grodstein F, Manson JE, Colditz GA, Willett WC *et al.* A prospective, observational study of postmenopausal hormone therapy and primary prevention of cardiovascular disease. *Ann Intern Med* 2000;**133**:933–41.

7 Grady D, Rubin SM, Petitti DB, Fox CS *et al.* Hormone therapy to prevent disease and prolong life in post menopausal women. Review. *Ann Intern Med* 1992;**117**:1016–37.

8 Hulley S, Grady D, Bush T, Furberg C *et al.* Randomized trial of estrogen plus progestin for secondary prevention of coronary heart disease in postmenopausal women. Heart and Estrogen/progestin Replacement Study (HERS) Research Group. *JAMA* 1998;**280**:605–13.

9 Rossoux JE, Anderson GL, Prentice RL, LaCroix AZ *et al*; Writing Group for the Women's Health Initiative Investigators. Risks and benefits of estrogen plus progestin in healthy postmenopausal women: principal results from the Women's Health Initiative randomized controlled trial. *JAMA* 2002;**288**:321–3.

10 Sitruk-Ware R. Alternatives for optimal hormone replacement therapy. *Climacteric* 2003;**6**(Suppl 2):11–6.

11 Barrett-Connor E. Clinical Review 162: cardiovascular endocrinology 3: an epidemiologist looks at hormones and heart disease in women. Review. *J Clin Endocrinol Metab* 2003;**88**: 4031–42.

12 Heller RF, Jacobs HS. Coronary heart disease in relation to age, sex, and the menopause. *BMJ* 1978;**1**;472–4.

13 Breast cancer and hormone replacement therapy: collaborative reanalysis of data from 51 epidemiological studies of 52,705 women with breast cancer and 108,411 without breast cancer. Collaborative Group on Hormonal Factors in Breast Cancer. *Lancet* 1997;**350**:1047–59; erratum *Lancet* 1997;**350**:1484.

14 Beral V; Million Women Study Collaborators. Breast cancer and hormone-replacement therapy in the Million Women study. *Lancet* 2003;**362**:419–27; erratum *Lancet* 2003;**352**:1160.

15 Holmberg L, Anderson H; HABITS steering and data monitoring committees. HABITS (hormonal replacement therapy after breast cancer – is it safe?), a randomised comparison: trial stopped. *Lancet* 2004;**363**:453–5.

16 Cranney A, Guyatt G, Griffith L, Wells G *et al*; Osteoporosis Methodology Group and The Osteoporosis Research Advisory Group. Meta-analyses of therapies for postmenopausal osteoporosis. IX: Summary of meta-analyses of therapies for postmenopausal osteoporosis. *Endocrine Rev* 2002;**23**:570–8.

17 Hlatky MA, Boothroyd D, Vittinghoff E, Sharp P, Whooley MA; Heart and Estrogen/Progestin Replacement Study (HERS) Research Group. Quality-of-life and depressive symptoms in postmenopausal women after receiving hormone therapy: results from the Heart and Estrogen/Progestin Replacement Study (HERS) trial. *JAMA* 2002;**287**:591–7.

18 Shumaker SA, Legault C, Rapp SR, Thal L *et al*; WHIMS Investigators. Estrogen plus progestin and the incidence of dementia and mild cognitive impairment in postmenopausal women: the Women's Health Initiative Memory Study: a randomized controlled trial. *JAMA* 2003;**289**: 2651–62.

☐ MANAGING RISK FACTORS SELF ASSESSMENT QUESTIONS

The epidemic of obesity: genes versus environment

1 Congenital leptin deficiency:
(a) Is an autosomal or recessive disorder
(b) Is associated with premature obesity
(c) Is associated with immune deficiency
(d) Is associated with primary hypothyroidism
(e) Is associated with developmental delay

2 Pro-opiomelanocortin deficiency:
(a) Is associated with Addison's disease
(b) Causes hyperphagia
(c) Causes red hair
(d) Has been identified in several ethnic groups
(e) Is associated with loss of skin pigmentation

3 Melanocortin 4 receptor deficiency:
(a) Is dominantly inherited
(b) Is associated with growth failure
(c) Causes hyperphagia
(d) Causes reproduction failure
(e) Is the commonest cause of obesity

The management of hypertension: what the trials have taught us

1 Bendrofluazide:
(a) Improves glycaemia control
(b) Is effective in lowering systolic blood pressure
(c) Is superior to calcium-channel blockade in reducing stroke
(d) Has a dose-dependent blood pressure lowering profile
(e) Can cause hypokalaemia

2 In type 2 diabetes:
(a) When microalbuminuria is present, 90% of patients have hypertension
(b) All patients should receive lipid-lowering therapy
(c) Angiotensin-converting enzyme inhibitors (ACEIs) are contraindicated
(d) Beta-blockers should not be prescribed
(e) Hypertension management has no influence on diabetic complications

3 The ALLHAT trial:
(a) Suggested that ACEIs were superior to diuretics in protecting against stroke and heart disease
(b) Reported that calcium antagonists should be used as first-line antihypertensive therapy

(c) Reported that diuretic therapy was effective in most groups of patients
(d) Stated that ACEIs were best used in Afro-Caribbean patients
(e) Suggested that the level of achieved blood pressure during treatment determined outcome in terms of stroke and coronary heart disease development

What to do about hormone replacement therapy

1 The rate of increase with age of coronary heart disease:
(a) Decelerates after the menopause
(b) In women is not influenced by smoking
(c) Falls after five years of postmenopausal hormone treatment (PHT)
(d) In women is influenced by attention to lifestyle (eg weight reduction, aerobic exercise)
(e) In women is not related to lipid levels

2 Concerning breast cancer in women:
(a) The rate of increase decelerates after the menopause
(b) The incidence increases with duration of PHT
(c) Risk is increased by combined PHT
(d) The risk of a recurrence is increased by oestrogen treatment in women who have completed a course of treatment for breast cancer
(e) Is an insignificant risk of short-term PHT

3 Osteoporosis in postmenopausal women:
(a) Is usually caused by postmenopausal oestrogen deficiency
(b) Has been shown by randomised controlled trial to be preventable by PHT
(c) Is correctable by PHT
(d) Should be treated by PHT as first-line treatment
(e) Does not respond to bisphosphonates in postmenopausal women

Institute of Physics and Engineering in Medicine

The clinical use of functional electrical stimulation in neurological rehabilitation

Ian Swain and Paul Taylor

□ INTRODUCTION

Electrical stimulation is not a new technique; it dates back to the Ancient Greeks who used rubbed amber and torpedo fish to produce a number of physiological responses, primarily to cause muscular contractions. Its development followed that of advances in physics by Volta and Faraday during the 18th and 19th centuries which led to more reliable, controllable sources of electricity, and in neurophysiology as a result of the work of Galvani and Duchenne. Various researchers then showed that denervated muscles respond to stimulation only by connecting and disconnecting a direct current source and do not respond to alternating or Faradic current. However, there was a contraction when a muscle was stimulated by a Faradic current via an intact motor neurone. All the work described in this chapter refers to the use of functional electrical stimulation (FES) in upper motor neurone conditions in which the muscle is contracted via nerve stimulation. If there is damage to the peripheral nervous system, for example by a prolapsed lumbar disc, the resulting denervated muscles can still be directly stimulated, although the length of the pulses required means that work to date is limited to the research laboratory.

Over the last twenty years electrical stimulation has been used to treat a wide range of clinical conditions. It is not possible to cover all these in detail in this chapter; for more information, readers should consult the web sites of the International Functional Electrical Stimulation Society[1] and the International Neuromodulation Society.[2]

The uses of FES are shown in Table 1. Some of these (eg pain relief, cochlear implants, pacemakers) are widely used in the clinical environment, whereas others (eg visual prostheses) are still in the research stage. This review will concentrate on the middle ground, discussing techniques that have been developed to a level where they are now clinically applicable without the need for bioengineering support but where they are not widely used in the NHS. These are primarily devices to improve gait or restore limited hand function following neurological conditions such as stroke, multiple sclerosis, spinal cord injury, head injury and cerebral palsy.

□ HISTORY OF FUNCTIONAL ELECTRICAL STIMULATION

The first functional use of electrical stimulation to improve gait was performed by Liberson in 1961[3] who used electrical stimulation successfully to correct foot drop

Table 1 Conditions in which functional electrical stimulation is used.

- Pacemakers and cardiac assistance
- Limb movement
- Bladder and bowel control
- Cochlear implants
- Visual prostheses
- Deep brain stimulation for tremor
- Scoliosis correction
- Pain relief
- Tissue regeneration
- Phrenic pacing for high level tetraplegics
- Treatment of facial palsy

as a result of a stroke. Despite the passage of 40 years, routine treatment using FES is still not available in the UK – or indeed in any other country as far as the authors are aware – even though in this country alone there may be up to 100,000 people who would benefit from such devices.

It was not until 1997 that Burridge *et al* published the first randomised controlled trial (RCT) to show clinical benefit of an FES based orthosis, the Odstock Dropped Foot Stimulator (ODFS).[4] Prior to that, the few RCTs that did exist concentrated on the physiological changes rather than on increase in function.[5]

Today, developments in microelectronics and computing can provide increased function for a large number of people with neurological disabilities. Some of these are implanted devices in which electrodes are directly attached to the nerves or sutured to the surface of the muscle. An example of such an implanted system is the FreeHand system, developed at Case Western Reserve University in Cleveland, Ohio,[6] designed to enable gripping function in people with tetraplegia. An alternative approach is to use electrodes on the skin to stimulate the muscles transcutaneously, as in devices like the ODFS[4] and the Handmaster.[7]

In Salisbury, a number of different FES treatments are provided for patients with neurological and musculoskeletal impairments, the most common being one- and two-channel transcutaneous systems to improve walking, and exercise regimens to strengthen muscles and reduce spasticity in both the upper and lower limbs. There are also implanted devices like the FreeHand system combined with surgical techniques such as tendon transfer, and FES combined with medical treatments such as botulinum toxin injections. These treatments necessitate medical, therapy and engineering staff working closely together in the clinical environment to provide the most appropriate treatment.

☐ RESEARCH BACKGROUND

Work in Salisbury has concentrated on the development of simple practical devices which are affordable for the NHS and of sufficient flexibility to be applicable in a variety of clinical conditions. There are considerable advantages in having the engineering and clinical services working closely together; this has ensured that the present generation of stimulators has been developed to meet a clinical need that was determined as a result of treating patients.

The MkIII Odstock dropped foot stimulator

The MkI ODFS was designed as part of a Department of Health (DH) trial. A number of modifications were made as clinical experience increased, culminating in the MkIII ODFS which is in use today (Fig 1).

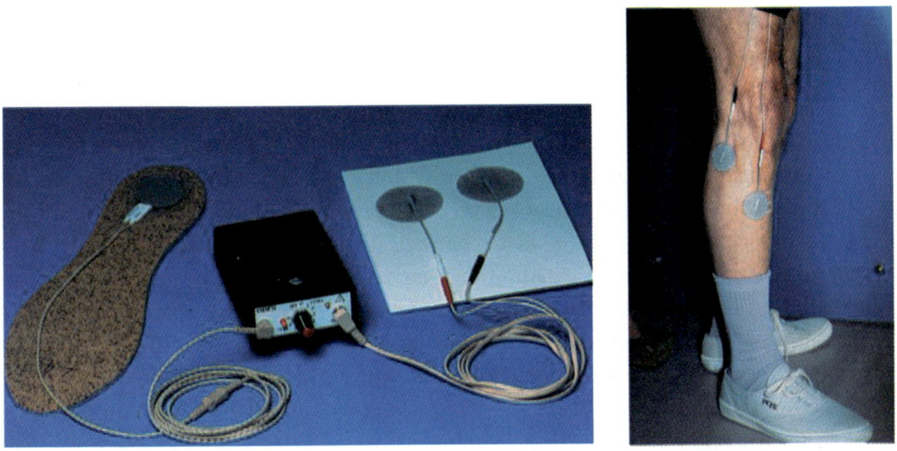

Fig 1 The Odstock Foot Dropped Stimulator showing standard electrode positions.

The MkIII ODFS is a single-channel, foot-switch triggered stimulator designed to elicit dorsiflexion of the foot by stimulation of the common peroneal nerve (maximum amplitude 100 mÅ, 350 μs pulse, 40 pps). Skin-surface electrodes are typically placed over the common peroneal nerve as it passes over the head of the fibula and the motor point of tibialis anterior. The rise and fall of the stimulation envelope and the extension after heel strike can be adjusted to prevent both a stretch reflex in the calf muscles and 'foot flap' due to the premature ending of dorsiflexion. The provision of dorsiflexion and eversion enables the foot to clear the ground more easily during swing phase. This reduces the compensatory mechanisms such as circumduction and hip hitching, hence reducing effort, which in turn can lead to a reduction in associated reactions. Repeated use of the stimulator can lead to a more 'normal' gait pattern being learnt. Heel strike with evasion is achieved at initial contact, so weight bearing is made along the centre line of the foot; stability at the ankle is therefore increased, making gait safer and increasing confidence.

The ODFS was the subject of an RCT in which 32 stroke patients who had had a stroke more than six months previously were randomly allocated to a treatment group who used the device and received 12 sessions of physiotherapy or to a control group who received only physiotherapy.[4] Compared with the controls, the treatment group showed a significant increase in:

- walking speed
- reduction in effort, as measured by the Physiological Cost Index (PCI) (defined as the change in heart rate divided by walking speed)
- Hospital Anxiety and Depression score, and
- reduction in quadriceps spasticity.

The ODFS has been widely used since then for a variety of neurological conditions.[8] It has been recognised by the Development and Evaluation Committee of the South-West Regional Health Authority and the Royal College of Physicians of England in their guidelines on stroke.[9]

Other stimulators

The design of the other stimulators used in the department at Salisbury is also achieved through the same iterative design process. In addition to exercise stimulators, there is a two-channel version which can be used for stimulation either of the bilateral common peroneal nerve or of one common peroneal nerve and a separate muscle group.[10] In the two-channel stimulator, only one foot switch is required to control both channels, the relative timing being adjusted when the system is first fitted. Therefore, the system can be used in swing phase to stimulate hamstrings to achieve greater knee flexion, in stance phase to stimulate gluteae to improve hip extension or with quadriceps to improve knee stability.

CLINICAL SERVICE

Referrals are taken from general practitioners and hospital consultants. Patients have an initial assessment and, if appropriate, they start on a treatment programme. Careful referral criteria have meant that over 82.5% of people referred are suitable for treatment. When the equipment is provided, the patient is seen on consecutive days:

- *1st day*: the technique is explained and the patient taught how to find the optimum electrode positions.
- *2nd day*: the patient attends wearing the equipment so that any possible problems can be readily corrected.

The patient is seen again after six weeks and three months, then every six months throughout the time the device is used. If there are few problems, the monitoring interval might be extended to one year. For people using the walking systems, walking speed and the effort involved, measured by the PCI, are recorded both with and without the stimulator at each appointment in order to monitor progress. The patient selection criteria ensure that 86% of people starting treatment are still using the ODFS one year after first issue.

A telephone helpline is available so that any problems can be solved rapidly. Patients are also given spares of certain items such as foot switches to prevent any inconvenience. A user survey showed a high level of patient satisfaction; patients also said that they were more confident and that walking was less effort.[11]

☐ RESULTS

To date, 1,683 patients have been seen in the Salisbury FES clinic with a range of disabilities arising from many different pathologies, although difficulty in walking due to a cerebrovascular accident (CVA) forms the largest group. The breakdown of patients by their primary pathology and function is shown in Table 2.

To consider the long-term effect of the clinical service, this review will concentrate on the two largest patient groups seen at Salisbury: those using an ODFS following a stroke and those with MS.

Table 2 Patients seen in the Salisbury functional electrical stimulation clinic, by pathology and function (n = 44).

Breakdown			
By pathology		**By function**	
Cerebrovascular accident	786	Walking	1,233
Multiple sclerosis	391	Hand function	350
Spinal cord injury	108	Paraplegic standing/ lower limb exercise	282
Cerebral palsy	53		
Other (TBI, PD, FSP etc)	345	Facial	25
		Assisted cough	1

N.B: some patients have treatment to enhance more than one function.
FSP = familial spastic paraplegia; PD = Parkinson's disease; TBI = traumatic brain injury.

Stroke

Despite having seen 786 patients with a stroke, complete data over 3½ years are available only on 44 patients (Table 3), for a variety of reasons including missed appointments. It is also because over the past few years the number of patients has increased dramatically, most of whom have not used the system for sufficient time for analysis. The longest any stroke patient has used a stimulator is over 10 years. All data were analysed by the Wilcoxon signed ranks test. There is no significant difference between any of the results at 4½ months and 3½ years.

Multiple sclerosis

The results presented in Table 4 were calculated from subjects for whom there are complete data, including those who have a two-channel system for bilateral foot drop. Thus, people were not included if they could walk the set 10 m course only when using the stimulator. Comparisons were made using the Wilcoxon signed ranks test.

Unlike the results for people after CVA, there is no carry over in the MS patients. There is, however, a continued orthotic gain at each of the assessments. After 72 weeks they are still walking slightly faster and with less effort when using the stimulator than without stimulation at the initial appointment, although the difference is not statistically significant.

Table 3 Effects of functional electrical stimulation following cerebrovascular accident at initial assessment, 18 weeks and 3½ years (n = 44).

	Median PCI (heartbeat m^{-1})		**Mean speed (ms^{-1})**	
	No stimulation	**Stimulation**	**No stimulation**	**Stimulation**
Initial assessment:	0.73	0.61	0.49	0.56
OG		$p < 0.01$		$p < 0.01$
After 18 weeks:	0.64	0.51	0.63	0.71
OG		$p < 0.01$		$p < 0.01$
CO	NS		$p < 0.01$	
TOE		$p < 0.01$		$p < 0.01$
After 3½ years:	0.68	0.57	0.58	0.66
OG		$p < 0.01$		$p < 0.01$
CO	NS		$p < 0.01$	
TOE		$p < 0.01$		$p < 0.01$

Orthotic gain (OG): the difference between Physiological Cost Index (PCI) or walking speed, with and without stimulation at any given appointment.
Carry over (CO): the difference between walking speed or PCI at a set time period compared with the initial assessment.
Total orthotic effect (TOE): the difference between PCI or walking speed with stimulation at a set time period compared with values without stimulation at the initial assessment.

Table 4 Effects of functional electrical stimulation in people with multiple sclerosis at initial assessment, 18 weeks and 72 weeks (n = 61).

	Median PCI (heartbeat m^{-1})		**Mean speed (ms^{-1})**	
	No stimulation	**Stimulation**	**No stimulation**	**Stimulation**
Initial assessment:	0.57	0.49	0.64	0.75
OG		$p < 0.01$		$p < 0.01$
After 18 weeks:	0.55	0.46	0.67	0.78
OG		$p < 0.01$		$p < 0.01$
CO	NS		NS	
TOE		$p < 0.01$		$p < 0.01$
After 72 weeks:	0.65	0.52	0.60	0.69
OG		$p < 0.01$		$p < 0.01$
CO	$p < 0.01$*		$p < 0.01$*	
TOE		NS		NS

* Without stimulation the walking ability of subjects had significantly deteriorated over the 72 weeks.
See Table 3 for key.

The difference between the response of people following CVA and with MS is illustrated in Fig 2 which compares the single-channel ODFS users. The CVA group showed a significant improvement in walking speed and PCI both with and without the ODFS over 72 weeks. In contrast, the walking ability of the people with MS improved when they used the stimulator, but deteriorated over time without the stimulator.

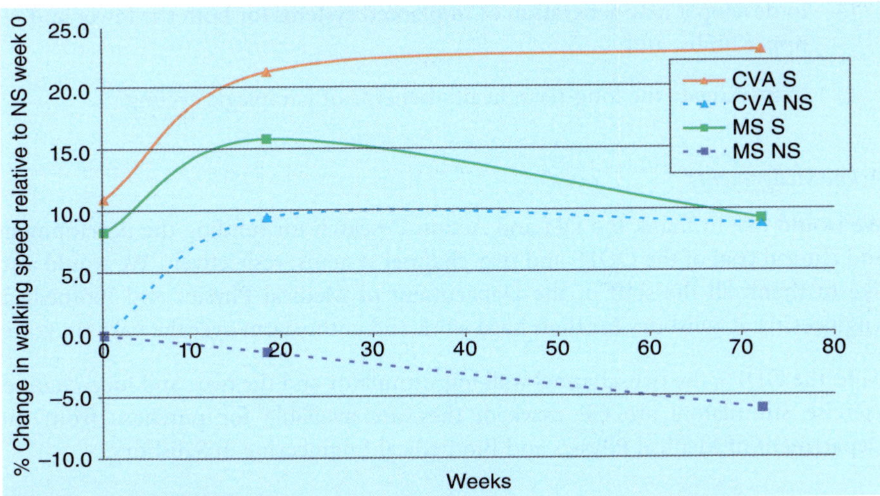

Fig 2 Median percentage change in walking speed for cerebrovascular accident (CVA) (n = 116) and multiple sclerosis (MS) (n = 42) using the single-channel Odstock Foot Dropped Stimulator. Initial walking speeds: CVA 0.57 ms^{-1}, MS 0.68 ms^{-1} (NS = no stimulation; S = stimulation).

☐ STAFF TRAINING

Part of the initial funding from the DH was to establish a training course to facilitate dissemination of FES throughout the NHS. We consider training of staff to be vitally important and see FES as a mode of treatment, not simply an electronic device. Therefore, equipment is never sold directly to patients, only to clinicians who have completed one of our training courses. To date, over 60 such courses have been held, most in the UK but recently some also in other countries (South Africa, Qatar, Turkey). Over 600 clinicians have been trained. A list of future training courses is available on our web site.[12]

☐ DISCUSSION

The results obtained with the 3½-year follow-up period are similar to those reported previously,[4,8] although it is encouraging that the effect seen at 4½ months does not diminish with time despite ageing of the patients. Although not unexpected, it is interesting to note the difference between users following CVA and those with MS. It appears that in the latter group the ODFS works primarily as an orthosis, whereas CVA use of the ODFS has a significant therapeutic effect. Nevertheless, those with MS still obtain significant benefit: 93% of 125 MS patients who started using the ODFS between 1999 and 2001 were still using it after one year.

☐ FUTURE WORK

At present, an RCT on the use of FES in MS and a pilot study into its effects in Parkinson's disease are being undertaken. The Salisbury FES clinic is also part of two multicentre projects:

- to develop a new generation of implanted systems for both the lower and upper limbs, and
- to investigate the long-term health benefits of paraplegic cycling.

Acknowledgements

We would like to thank the DH and Action Research for funding the development and clinical trial of the ODFS and two-channel systems, respectively. We would also like to thank all the staff of the Department of Medical Physics and Biomedical Engineering at Salisbury for their hard work and enthusiasm over the past ten years.

Note: the ODFS, the two-channel walking stimulator and the two- and four-channel exercise stimulators are CE marked; they are available for purchase from the Department of Medical Physics and Biomedical Engineering in Salisbury.

REFERENCES

1 www.ifess.org

2 www.neuromodulation.com

3 Liberson WT, Holmquest HJ, Scot D, Dow M. Functional electrotherapy: stimulation of the peroneal nerve synchronized with the swing phase of the gait of hemiplegic patients *Arch Phys Med Rehabil* 196l;**42**:101–5.

4 Burridge JH, Taylor PN, Hagan SA, Wood DE, Swain ID. The effects of common peroneal stimulation on the effort and speed of walking: a randomized controlled trial with chronic hemiplegic patients. *Clin Rehabil* 1997;**11**:201–10.

5 Glanz M, Klawannsky S, Stason W, Berkey C, Chalmers TC. Functional electrostimulation in poststroke rehabilitation: a meta-analysis of randomized controlled trials. *Arch Phys Med Rehabil* 1996;**77**:549–53.

6 Bhadra H, Kilgore KL, Peckham PH. Implanted stimulators for restoration of function in spinal cord injury. *Med Eng Phys* 2001;**23**:19–28.

7 Hendricks HT, Ijzerman MJ, de Kroon JR, in't Groen FA, Zilvold G. Functional electrical stimulation by means of thc 'Ness Handmaster Orthosis' in chronic stroke patients: an exploratory study. *Clin Rehabil* 2001;**15**:217–20.

8 Taylor PN, Burridge JH, Dunkerley AL, Wood DE *et al.* Clinical use of the Odstock dropped foot stimulator: its effect on the speed and effort of walking. *Arch Phys Med Rehabil* 1999;**80**:1577–83.

9 National Clinical Guidelines for Stroke 2000. London: Royal College of Physicians of London, 2000.

10 Taylor PN, Wright PA, Burridge JH, Mann GE, Swain ID. Correction of bilateral dropped foot using the Odstock 2 Channel Stimulator (O2CHS). 4th Annual Conference of the International FES Society, Sendai, Japan, August 1999:257–60. ISBN 4-9980783-0-5.

11 Taylor PN, Burridge JH, Dunkerley AL, Lamb A *et al.* Patients' perceptions of the Odstock Dropped Foot Stimulator (ODFS). *Clin Rehabil* 1999;**13**:439–46.

12 www.salisburyfes.com

Advances in renal dialysis technology: recent developments and future prospects

Nicholas Hoenich

□ INTRODUCTION

Patients with progressive renal disease undergo a loss in renal function that eventually necessitates treatment to sustain life, either by dialysis or transplantation. Dialysis is a diffusive process that replaces the excretory function of the kidneys. The concept of replacing the human kidney by artificial means has been known since the 19th century, but the first dialytic systems were not developed until the 1940s when dialysis was used for the treatment of acute renal failure (ARF). This early approach used a semipermeable, cellulose-based tubular membrane, through which the blood flowed. The membrane was wound around a wooden drum which rotated and was immersed in a bath containing a solution of electrolytes. Access to the patient was via a glass cannula and the system was anticoagulated with hirudin (Fig 1(a) and 1(b)).

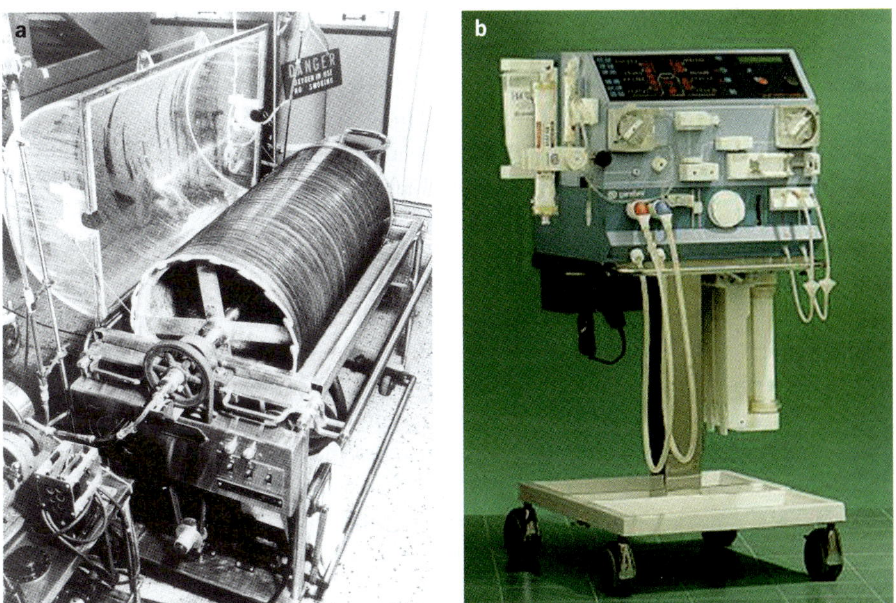

Fig 1 (a) A Kolff rotating drum dialysis machine used for the treatment of acute renal failure circa 1950; **(b)** a current haemodialysis machine capable of permitting the production of ultrapure dialysis fluid.

With the advent of more durable methods of vascular access, the technique evolved to the treatment of chronic renal failure, first in hospital and, from the mid-1960s, in the patient's own home. It has been estimated that in mid-2001, some 1.1 million patients worldwide, 17,500 of whom are in the UK, received treatment by dialysis for irreversible renal failure. The therapy also continues to be used for the treatment of ARF.

The process of dialysis may be considered as the clearing of toxic substances from the blood and the removal of excess water by a membrane exchange process. Several technological elements are involved:

- access to the patient's circulation
- an extracorporeal circuit containing the artificial kidney or dialyser
- equipment to manufacture the electrolyte solution (dialysis fluid) and to monitor the safety of the process.

This review will discuss the latest technical developments and future advances in these areas.

ACCESS TO THE CIRCULATION

Blood flow rates of 200–400 ml/min through the extracorporeal circuit are necessary to facilitate efficient dialysis. Such blood flow rates are generated by the use of a peristaltic pump within the extracorporeal circuit. The ability to achieve adequate dialysis depends critically on the blood flow rate and the ability of the patient's vascular access to deliver the required flow. This clinical need has led to developments designed to monitor the patient's vascular access and its ability to supply such flow rates at the bedside. A number of techniques are available, but there is no universal agreement as to which is the best.[1]

A surgically created arteriovenous fistula is the preferred method of vascular access for the provision of blood flow. However, many patients receiving treatment are elderly and have vascular disease; in such patients, the formation of an arteriovenous fistula presents considerable challenges. Alternative methods of vascular access such as semipermanent central venous catheters and grafts are used, but central venous lines are associated with a high incidence of infection.[2] Current understanding is incomplete regarding the roles played by the material and the technique as established infection is frequently difficult to eradicate even if the catheter is changed. Curtailment of the incidence of infection in newly inserted catheters is facilitated by the use of antibiotic coatings and novel catheter locking solutions such as Neutrolin (Biolink Corporation, Norwell, MA).[3]

The use of grafts as well as the formation of arteriovenous fistulae alters flow dynamics within the vasculature; this contributes to the development of intimal hyperplasia and the formation of thrombus at the anastomosis site. To gain a deeper insight into the evolution of this process, and to permit the development of improved vascular constructions, computational fluid dynamic techniques are being used to provide a better understanding of the flow fluid dynamics in the region of the anastomosis.[4] Technology to destroy the thrombus using a small diameter wire inserted into the access and delivering low-power acoustic energy has also been developed and is currently undergoing clinical trials.

The inability to use the patient's existing vasculature for access has resulted in new methods for accessing the circulatory system. Emergent techniques undergoing clinical trials are subcutaneously implanted devices with valves.[5,6] As vascular access remains the 'Achilles heel' of dialysis, considerable endeavour is likely to be placed on the resolution of current problems. Such work is likely to focus on:

- minimisation of trauma by improved needle design
- development of new strategies to minimise turbulence at surgical anastomoses
- elucidation of the molecular and cellular biology of neointimal hyperplasia
- the development of local therapies to block the process of intimal hyperplasia, and
- understanding how bacteria grow and proliferate on material surfaces to facilitate the development of materials with endothelial characteristics.

EXTRACORPOREAL CIRCUIT

The extracorporeal circuit facilitates flow through the dialyser. The flow is generated by a peristaltic pump whose design has remained unchanged over the past three decades. The tubing is generally manufactured from polyvinyl chloride (PVC), a material that incorporates plasticisers to provide flexibility. The most commonly used plasticiser is di(2-ethylhexyl)phthalate, a compound known to have toxicological potential, and elevated levels of which have been found in the blood of patients undergoing regular dialysis therapy.[7]

Minimising exposure to plasticisers may be achieved by coating lumen of the blood tubing to prevent its leeching. New materials are now in production based on hydrocarbons in which flexibility is achieved by the dimensional configuration of the carbon atoms and which do not contain plasticisers. They are gradually replacing the widely used PVC, whose disposal by incineration remains a controversial issue.

The dialyser

The extracorporeal circuit also contains the dialyser or artificial kidney. Early dialysers were bulky, non-disposable and required manual rebuilding and sterilisation after use. Today, most treatments use hollow-fibre designs based on the classical shell and tube heat exchange (Fig 2). Such designs are cost-effective for the production of large volumes and can be manufactured in different sizes to meet clinical requirements relatively easily. However, they are subject to flow maldistribution both within and outside the fibres which leads to loss of efficiency.

As treatment times have shortened, the ability to maintain and deliver a highly efficient therapy has become an important requirement. The application of fluid

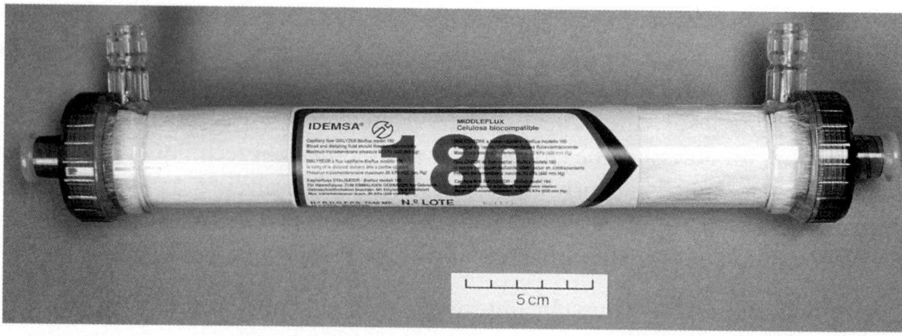

Fig 2 A currently used hollow-fibre haemodialyser. Dialysers such as this are able to provide up to 2.4 m^2 surface area. Blood flows through the lumen of the fibres, and dialysis fluid produced by the haemodialysis machine flows on the outside of the fibres.

dynamic analysis of flow aberrations has led to the development of production techniques designed to eliminate such issues.[8]

The dialyser membrane

The membrane within the dialyser represents a large (1–2 m^2) non-physiological surface to which blood is exposed during treatment. This results in the activation of both the cellular and immune systems. It is now recognised that the induction of the immune response is associated with the synthesis and release of pro-inflammatory cytokines (tumour necrosis factor α, interleukin-1 (IL-1) and IL-6). They contribute to an increased risk of infections and infectious mortality of dialysis patients and also to a pro-inflammatory state engendered by atheromatous disease. Increased emphasis has been placed on the improvement of the biocompatibility of the material, and a large proportion of treatments are now undertaken using membrane materials with improved biocompatibility compared with the classically used membranes based on cellulose in the 1970s. A variety of materials based on polymer blends and incorporating microdomain structures are available.[9]

Conventional dialysis

Conventional dialysis is principally a diffusive process favouring the selective removal of low molecular weight toxins. The attribution of complications of dialysis to inadequate removal of large molecular weight toxins has resulted in a shift from conventional dialysis to methods such as haemodiafiltration or haemofiltration that involve convective solute transport and favour the removal of larger weight solutes. Such techniques have been facilitated by new technology as well as membranes with more open pore structures.[10]

New developments

The increased permeability in the absence of selectivity leads to the loss of low molecular weight proteins and amino acids. Treatments therefore need to be selective in their solute removal. Such selectivity may be achieved by the use of sorbents, and future approaches will focus on the use of bonded antibodies to sorbent materials to confer the desired specificity.[11]

The blood and dialysis fluid flows within the dialyser are laminar. Microfluidic devices utilising the unique diffusion characteristics of such flows are already in use in laboratories; they have the potential to reduce the size of the device and provide a vehicle for the wearable artificial kidney.[12] In parallel, the rapid understanding of the cellular and molecular basis of organ function and disease processes is being translated into new therapeutic approaches using devices containing cells. Such devices offer a radical departure from current treatments in that they are additionally able to replace metabolic and endocrine functions of the kidney. Clinical studies of such devices are currently in progress.[13]

□ HAEMODIALYSIS MACHINES AND MONITORING

Dialysis is a process that takes several hours. Early dialysis systems were simple and used manual mixing of the ingredients of the dialysis fluid, with no monitoring except that of the patient. The application of dialysis to the treatment of end-stage renal failure, as well as the realisation that treatment could be undertaken in the patient's own home, led to the development of more sophisticated dialysis machines. These continuously blended dialysis fluid from treated water and a concentrated salt solution, measured the quality and temperature of the fluid produced, monitored the pressures and detected air in the extracorporeal circuit. Such machines were subject to technical problems during use, so patient safety became an important focus. This led to the development and application of internationally recognised and applied safety standards that ensure the patient is not placed at risk in the event of a fault developing during treatment.

Modern haemodialysis machines

Haemodialysis machines now make extensive use of microprocessor technology and, in addition to providing the basic functions discussed above, they also:

- permit control of fluid removal during treatment
- allow individualisation of electrolyte concentrations in the dialysis fluid to meet differing clinical requirements
- automatically prepare the system pretreatment by performing safety checks, and
- can be linked to computers.

Computer linkage allows treatments to be monitored in remote locations such as satellite dialysis units or in the patient's home. Specific software enables multiple patient monitoring and prioritisation of response to alarms. Further developments in this area will capitalise on the developments in both information technology and computing to lead to surveillance systems combined with integrated clinical support applications.[14]

☐ PROBLEMS WITH DIALYSIS

Changes in patient demographics

In parallel with the technological changes associated with dialysis there has been a change in the patients undergoing dialysis. Over the past decade there has been a rapid growth in the number of patients over 65 years of age accepted for renal replacement therapy; this has adversely influenced morbidity and mortality associated with treatment. Increased emphasis is currently being placed on improving these aspects of therapy; technology is playing an important role here.

Treatment adequacy

Statistical associations between urea removal, a measure of treatment adequacy, and survival have been widely described. The assessment of adequacy is retrospective and requires blood sampling pre- and post-treatment. Real-time monitoring techniques for the quantification of dialysis adequacy are now available, using either a specific sensor for urea or for a surrogate molecule such as sodium chloride (which has a similar molecular weight to urea). They are able to provide information relating to the delivered therapy on a sessional basis, permitting timely intervention to be initiated in the event of non-delivery of the prescribed therapy.[15] Further developments in this field will extend to molecules beyond urea and utilise specific sensors or a more global assessment using ultraviolet adsorption.[16]

Blood pressure

Many patients undergoing regular dialysis treatment are hypertensive. The pathophysiology of hypertension in the dialysis population is complex, involving different factors that interact and modulate each other. These include:

- ☐ expanded extracellular volume
- ☐ sympathetic and/or vasoconstrictor system overactivity
- ☐ inappropriate production of renin
- ☐ decreased vascular compliance
- ☐ retention of toxic substances with vasoconstrictor activity, and
- ☐ therapy with erythropoietin.

The difficulty of controlling blood pressure in the dialysis patient has been recognised since the beginning of the dialysis era. However, as treatment normalises the expanded extracellular volume by removal of fluid, it was generally accepted that normal blood pressure levels could be achieved by 'adequate' ultrafiltration in most patients. This assumption was based on the use of dialytic sessions longer than practised today. Despite improvements in dialysis technology, many patients, particularly the elderly and those with diabetes, experience cardiovascular instability or hypotension during dialysis arising from the conflict between faster and more efficient treatment and the limitations imposed by human physiology.

Hypotension during dialysis is dependent on both the amount of fluid requiring removal and the fluid removal rate. An important element of the former is accurate knowledge of the patient's dry weight (the weight corresponding to euvolaemia). This weight is usually clinically established but may be subject to inaccuracy. New approaches to establishing dry weight include the use of multifrequency electrical bioimpedance to monitor patient hydration status before and during treatment and real-time measurement of plasma volume to monitor vascular refilling in response to fluid removal during treatment.[17] Other technological approaches to modulate cardiovascular instability during treatment include:

- modulation of fluid removal (ultrafiltration profiling)
- isothermic dialysis, and
- the use of pulse-wave analysis to provide a continuous non-invasive blood pressure and cardiac function monitoring throughout treatment.[18]

As many of these parameters can be monitored in real time, linkage to feedback control algorithms to provide a degree of control during treatment is possible; such an approach requires further work on algorithm refinement. Clearly, patients also need to be adequately instructed about the importance of reducing their interdialytic sodium and water intake, to limit interdialytic weight gain and obviate the need for high ultrafiltration rates during treatment.

Cardiovascular and infection complications

Cardiovascular problems are the most frequent cause of mortality in dialysis patients, with infection the second most common. The contribution to these problems arising from the dialysis membrane is recognised and has led to the development of more biocompatible membranes in which both the induction of pro-inflammatory cytokines and the activation of the immune system are reduced. The increasing recognition that microbial products present in the dialysis fluid also contribute has led to improvements in its microbiological quality by the development of techniques to minimise the presence in the fluid of such contaminants.[19]

CONCLUSIONS

Haemodialysis represents an area of medicine in which technology is applied to the delivery of treatment on a routine basis. The technology in use today enables treatment to be safely performed either in hospital or in the patient's own home. It has also played an important role in reducing treatment times as well as nursing workload. Important issues remain relating to treatment outcomes and patient quality of life, and technology is being applied to address these aspects of dialysis therapy.

The challenge ahead is in providing this life-prolonging therapy to all patients who need it in such a way that it improves their quality of life at a cost that society can afford. Technology can continue to contribute in a meaningful way in a number of different areas. However, such developments are costly; strong evidence of benefit needs to be demonstrated for their use clinically, such as a lower rate of hospitalisation or other positive outcome measures. In the current financial climate this may be a limiting factor for major technological advances.

REFERENCES

1 Lok CE, Bhola C, Croxford R, Richardson RM. Reducing vascular access morbidity: a comparative trial of two vascular access monitoring strategies. *Nephrol Dial Transplant* 2003;**18**:1174–80.

2 Anel RL, Yevzlin AS, Ivanovich P. Vascular access and patient outcomes in hemodialysis: questions answered in recent literature. Review. *Artif Organs* 2003;**27**:237–41.

3 Shah CB, Mittelman MW, Costerton JW, Parenteau S *et al.* Antimicrobial activity of a novel catheter lock solution. *Antimicrob Agents Chemother* 2002;**46**:1674–9.

4 Leuprecht A, Perktold K, Prosi M, Berk T *et al.* Numerical study of hemodynamics and wall mechanics in distal end-to-side anastomoses of bypass grafts. *J Biomech* 2002;**35**:225–36.

5 Moran JE. Subcutaneous vascular access devices. Review. *Semin Dial* 2001;**14**:452–7.

6 Rayan SS, Terramani TT, Weiss VJ, Chaikof EL. The LifeSite Hemodialysis Access System in patients with limited access. *J Vasc Surg* 2003;**38**:714–8.

7 Dine T, Luyckx M, Gressier B, Brunet C *et al.* A pharmacokinetic interpretation of increasing concentrations of DEHP in haemodialysed patients. *Med Eng Phys* 2000;**22**:157–65.

8 Gastaldon F, Brendolan A, Crepaldi C, Frisone P *et al.* Effects of novel manufacturing technology on blood and dialysate flow distribution in a new low flux 'alpha Polysulfone' hemodialyzer. *Int J Artif Organs* 2003;**26**:105–12.

9 Deppisch R, Gohl H, Smeby L. Microdomain structure of polymeric surfaces – potential for improving blood treatment procedures. Review. *Nephrol Dial Transplant* 1998;**13**:1354–9.

10 Bowry SK. Nano-controlled membrane spinning technology: regulation of pore size, distribution and morphology of a new polysulfone dialysis membrane. *Contrib Nephrol* 2002;**137**:85–94.

11 Grovender EA, Kellogg B, Singh J, Blom D *et al.* Single-chain antibody fragment-based adsorbent for the extracorporeal removal of beta2-microglobulin. *Kidney Int* 2004;**65**:310–22.

12 Weigl BH, Bardell RL, Kesler N, Morris CJ. Lab-on-a-chip sample preparation using laminar fluid diffusion interfaces – computational fluid dynamics model results and fluidic verification experiments. *Fresenius J Anal Chem* 2001;**371**:97–105.

13 Humes HD, Weitzel WF, Bartlett RH, Swaniker FC, Paganini EP. Renal cell therapy is associated with dynamic and individualized responses in patients with acute renal failure. *Blood Purif* 2003;**21**:64–71.

14 Prado M, Roa L, Reina-Tosina J, Palma A, Milan JA. Virtual center for renal support: technological approach to patient physiological image. *IEEE Trans Biomed Eng* 2002;**49**:1420–30.

15 Gotch FA. On-line clearance: advanced methodology to monitor adequacy of dialysis at no cost. *Contrib Nephrol* 2002;**137**:268–71.

16 Fridolin I, Magnusson M, Lindberg LG. On-line monitoring of solutes in dialysate using absorption of ultraviolet radiation: technique description. *Int J Artif Organs* 2002;**25**:748–61.

17 Hoenich NA, Levin NW. Can technology solve the clinical problem of 'dry weight'? *Nephrol Dial Transplant* 2003;**18**:647–50.

18 Lambie SH, McIntyre CW. Developments in online monitoring of haemodialysis patients: towards global assessment of dialysis adequacy. *Curr Opin Nephrol Hypertens* 2003;**12**:633–8.

19 Nakatani T, Tsuchida K, Sugimura K, Yoshimura R, Takemoto Y. Investigation of endotoxin adsorption with polyether polymer alloy dialysis membranes. *Int J Mol Med* 2003;**11**:195–7.

Advances in ultrasonic imaging

Peter Wells

□ INTRODUCTION

Approximately 17% of all medical imaging procedures worldwide are undertaken using ultrasound, compared with about 3% which use radionuclides, 5% magnetic resonance imaging (MRI) and 75% X-rays or computed tomography (CT). Thus, ultrasonic imaging is extremely important in diagnosis, and indeed has a vital role in developing as well as in developed countries.

Ultrasound was first used in medical diagnosis about 50 years ago and is now a mature technology. Most medical practitioners are familiar with the appearance of modern ultrasonic scans. These images, like CT and MRI scans, are two-dimensional representations of anatomical sections and usually quite easily interpreted by those familiar with them. They provide anatomical information and, in some circumstances, also functional information. Ultrasonic imaging is particularly effective in the study of soft tissue structures because the presence of gas or bone degrades the quality of the image. The main clinical applications are in obstetrics, internal medicine, cardiology, vascular studies and ophthalmology, but there is hardly a branch of medicine in which ultrasonic diagnosis is not able to make a contribution.

The performance of ultrasonic imaging has steadily improved up to the present time but numerous opportunities remain for further advances in the future. Recent improvements and potential advances are described in this chapter.

□ SCANNERS AND TRANSDUCERS

There are four main groups of ultrasonic scanners:

1 Simple systems to investigate simple clinical problems.

2 More sophisticated systems, operated by skilled users.

3 Advanced systems, a workhorse of imaging specialists.

4 Niche systems for specialist applications.

Manufacturers are continuously improving the function and utility of their systems and adding incremental features to extend the attractiveness of their products.

A new class of scanners is beginning to emerge: small devices made practicable by advances in microelectronics and transducer technology. The performance of these scanners can approach that of the highest quality traditional devices. Ultimately, there may be a scanner in every doctor's pocket.

The performance of an ultrasonic scanner depends to a large extent on the design and characteristics of the ultrasonic probe, the central component of which is the transducer which converts electrical energy into ultrasound and vice versa. The trend is to develop transducers with ever greater bandwidths, since this allows advanced signal processing techniques to be used. More complex arrays of transducers are being developed, with increasingly small transducer elements and with the electronics increasingly integrated with the probes.[1]

Finally, new transducer materials and devices are beginning to emerge. Composite ferroelectric transducers, made up of piezoelectric elements embedded in plastics, have led to a revolution in transducer bandwidth improvement. For the future, microfabrication techniques hold out the promise of producing two-dimensional ultrasonic transducer arrays which, as discussed later, should enable three-dimensional imaging to become commonplace.[2]

☐ COMPOUND IMAGING

Ultrasonic compound scanning was conceived nearly 50 years ago, but its benefits have become available in modern instruments only recently with the development of advanced transducer arrays.[3] In compound imaging, several image frames are acquired from different directions by a stationary transducer array and superimposed in real time. This reduces speckle in the image, sharpens the edges between structures and masks shadows caused by strong absorbers. The images are aesthetically pleasing and often easier to interpret than traditional images.

☐ EXTENDED-FIELD-OF-VIEW IMAGING

The field of view that can be obtained by a stationary transducer array is necessarily limited. Extended-field-of-view imaging uses image registration techniques to measure the ultrasonic probe motion. The operator moves the probe continuously along the scan line; this generates a two-dimensional panoramic view without the disadvantage of having to measure the position of the transducer with external sensors.[4]

☐ CODED EXCITATION

In traditional pulse-echo imaging, the pulse transmitted into the tissue is as brief as possible in order to maximise the spatial resolution. This requires a broad-band transducer and the receiver, also being broad-band, has a poor noise performance. With coded transmission excitation, a long pulse is transmitted into the tissue. The pulse has a characteristic shape so that its echoes can be recognised and compressed into short pulses by signal processing during reception.[5] This improves the signal-to-noise ratio and results in higher resolution at greater penetration than possible with short pulse transmission.

☐ THREE-DIMENSIONAL IMAGING

In traditional two-dimensional imaging, the ultrasonic beam is scanned through a plane of tissues within the patient. By changing the position of the probe during the scanning process, the observer is able to build up in their mind's eye a three-dimensional picture of the scanned anatomy. This requires a good deal of skill, and the results of the examination are often better described to non-imaging experts in words rather than in pictures.

Information can be acquired from a three-dimensional tissue volume either by moving a two-dimensional scan plane, mechanically or manually, or by exploring the tissue by electronically sweeping the beam direction from a two-directional transducer array.[6] The image of the three-dimensional tissue volume can be displayed as a three-dimensional segmented surface of selected anatomical structures or as a semitransparent three-dimensional tissue volume. With the development of advanced computer graphics, it is now becoming possible to display the information as a pictorial representation of what would be seen under direct vision.[7] This approach is in its infancy but when fully implemented promises to remove much of the skill needed at the moment to interpret image information.

□ INTRAVASCULAR, ENDOSCOPIC AND INTRACAVITARY SCANNING

In traditional transcutaneous ultrasonic imaging, the closeness of the probe to the structure of interest is limited by it having to make contact with the skin. In intravascular, endoscopic and intracavitary scanning, the probe is close to the imaged tissue so that penetration is minimal.[8] Tissue attenuation is therefore less of a problem, so the ultrasonic frequency can be increased. The result is that the spatial resolution is relatively high, although this may be limited by the size of the aperture of the ultrasonic transducer which is itself limited by the size of the available anatomical access.

□ CONTRAST AGENTS

The echoes that give rise to traditional ultrasonic images occur as the result of differences in the density and speed of ultrasound in the constituent parts of tissues, whether at structural or cellular level. At the ultrasonic frequencies used for abdominal scanning, blood is relatively anechoic. During the last 20 years there has been a huge growth of interest in the potential of ultrasonic contrast agents to change the echogenicity of tissues[9] and, in particular, of blood. There are three main classes of ultrasonic contrast agents:

1 Gas-filled microspheres.

2 Solid particle contrast agents.

3 Multimodal contrast agents.

Gas-filled microspheres

Gas-filled microspheres are small enough to pass through the capillaries of the lung. They can be injected intravenously where they subsequently enhance the echogenicity of blood because they are strong scatterers. The scattering can be linear, non-linear or result from ultrasonically-induced destruction of microbubbles.

Solid particle contrast agents

One of the exciting possibilities for the development of ultrasonic contrast agents is that they may turn out to be targetable, as distinct from being merely blood-borne. The most interesting results so far have been obtained with solid particle, as distinct from microbubble, contrast agents. Ultrasound is scattered more strongly by particles of materials that differ from tissues both in density and speed of ultrasound than by the tissues themselves and, because the particles are very small, they have the potential to be targeted immunologically. Indeed, contrast agent-enhanced ultrasonic imaging seems to have the potential to replace some radionuclide scanning in functional studies.

Multimodal contrast agents

The third group are multimodal contrast agents; these are able to change the contrast not only of ultrasound images but also of other images such as those produced by magnetic resonance. One example of such an agent is a gadolinium-labelled microbubble.

□ HARMONIC IMAGING

In traditional ultrasonic imaging, the receiver is tuned to receive echoes scattered from the tissue at the same frequency as that of the transmitted ultrasonic pulse. Because of the non-linear properties of microbubble contrast agents, the backscattered ultrasound has energy not only at the same frequency as that of the transmitted ultrasound but also at harmonic frequencies, in particular at the second harmonic frequency. This means that the receiver can be tuned to twice the frequency of the transmitted ultrasound and a useful signal still be received from the microbubbles. The effect is that echoes from the microbubbles in the blood are enhanced in relation to the echoes from the surrounding tissues.

Microbubbles are relatively strongly non-linear. Tissue itself is also non-linear, but not to such a marked extent. Nevertheless, following transmission, second harmonics can build up in the ultrasonic pulse as it travels through tissue. Consequently, the receiver can be tuned to the second harmonic frequency; this has a number of advantages:[10]

1. Image clutter is reduced because the distortion and reverberation of the transmitting beam in the superficial tissue, which takes place at the fundamental frequency before the second harmonics have developed, are minimal.
2. The side-lobe patterns of the transmitting and receiving beams are not identical since they correspond to different frequencies.
3. The receiving beam is narrower than the transmitting beam, so the spatial resolution is improved.

Echoes from stationary tissue can be further suppressed by pulse harmonic imaging.[11] In this process, consecutive pulses having opposite polarities produce echoes of the same shapes but opposite polarities when originating from linear scatterers; these cancel each other when the consecutive echo wavetrains are added together. The echoes from non-linear scatterers are not identical, however, and produce a harmonic signal when added together. This technique is proving a powerful way of improving the spatial resolution and noise performance of ultrasonic imaging and is now widely used.[12]

□ OTHER ADVANCES

Microscanning

Traditional ultrasonic imaging uses frequencies typically in the range 3–10 MHz, although the frequency may be as high as 30 MHz in some intravascular applications. The corresponding wavelengths of ultrasound are 0.5–0.15 mm, extending down to 0.02 mm at the highest frequency. These wavelengths roughly correspond to the highest spatial resolution that can be achieved. However, if only a short penetration is required, frequencies typically of 50 MHz and above can be used. The corresponding resolution is around 30 mm or better. The images are detailed and the resolution may even approach the subcellular level. The process, known as microscanning,[13] is relatively novel but of great relevance, for example for the imaging of small animals, particularly those being used in genetic research.

Elasticity imaging

Elasticity imaging displays changes in the mechanical elasticity of the tissues, as distinct from their ultrasonic backscattering characteristics.[14] There are various methods of elasticity imaging. In one example, the motion of the scatterers within the tissue volume can be observed whilst the tissue is vibrated or compressed. The relative movement of the scatterers within harder tissues is much less than within softer tissues; an image of the elasticity can be produced by processing the scatterer motion information. In a sense, elasticity images can be thought of as representative of what a clinician might detect by palpation, but the information can be obtained from deeper structures and more quantitatively.

Vector Doppler imaging

One of the limitations of the ultrasonic Doppler technique for the measurement of blood flow is that the shift frequency depends on the velocity, a vector the magnitude of which depends upon the angle between the directions of the ultrasonic beam and the flow. Several attempts have been made to overcome this limitation. For example, in vector Doppler imaging, two or more ultrasonic beams are directed through the region of interest and the true flow speed can be determined by trigonometrical processing of the acquired data.[15]

Continuous wave ultrasonic Doppler tomography

Traditional Doppler ultrasonic imaging depends on the shift in the backscattered frequency that occurs as the result of relative motion between the tissue or the flowing blood and the ultrasonic beam. The possibility of producing images by artificially introducing relative motion is now beginning to be explored.[16] The process is analogous to backprojection reconstruction imaging: by rotating the tissue specimen in a stationary ultrasonic beam, the Doppler frequency spectra correspond to the distances between the axis of rotation and the radial positions of the ultrasonic scatterers. Research is at an early stage and initial results have been quite promising. It seems likely that continuous wave ultrasonic Doppler tomography may produce images of, for example, the breast with a resolution perhaps five times better than that possible using pulse-echo techniques at the same frequency.

☐ VISIONS OF THE FUTURE

Ultrasonic imaging has the advantages of safety, high performance and low cost in comparison with other techniques. It should soon become technically possible to construct an ultrasonic scanner small enough to fit into a doctor's pocket. This could be used as a commonplace diagnostic tool alongside the stethoscope, blood pressure monitor and clinical thermometer.

Real-time, three-dimensional imaging is becoming a practical possibility with the development of two-dimensional ultrasonic transducer arrays. The display of the three-dimensional information using techniques already in common use in CT imaging presents few technical problems. The challenge will be to produce images representing reality, as distinct from those which need expert interpretation.

Ultrasonic contrast agents are already widely used. The possibility that they might be immunologically targeted is becoming a reality. Target-specific ultrasonic imaging techniques could expand the horizons of functional studies and perhaps replace some of those that currently depend on radionuclides.

Ultrasonic microscanning is currently limited to the examination of tissue specimens, superficial structures and small animals. Research into the development of *in vivo* microscanners is underway; it may soon be possible to use needle-mounted, very high frequency ultrasonic transducers for histological examination of tissues at short range without the need for biopsy.

Ultrasonic elasticity imaging already shows great promise, particularly because the contrast mechanism is different from and complementary to that of most other imaging methods. Remote non-invasive palpation of deep-seated structures within the body should open up new areas of opportunity for the diagnostician.

REFERENCES

1 Light ED, Davidsen RE, Fiering TA, Hruschka TA, Smith SW. Progress in two-dimensional real-time arrays for volumetric imaging. *Ultrason Imaging* 1998;**20**:1–15.

2 Foster FS. Transducer materials and probe construction. *Ultrasound Med Biol* 2000; **26**(Suppl 1):S2–5.

3 Entrekin RR, Jago JR, Kofoed SC. Real-time spatial compound imaging technical performance in vascular applications. In: Halliwell M, Wells PN (eds). *Acoustical Imaging.* New York: Plenum Press, 2000;**25**:331–42.

4 Weng L, Tirumalai AP, Lowery CM, Nock LF *et al.* US extended-field-of-view imaging technology. *Radiology* 1997;**203**:877–80.

5 Pedersen MH, Misaridis TX, Jensen JA. Clinical evaluation of chirp-coded excitation in medical ultrasound. *Ultrasound Med Biol* 2003;**29**:895–905.

6 Lees W. Ultrasound imaging in three and four dimensions. Review. *Semin Ultrasound CT MR* 2001;**22**:85–105.

7 Sarvazyan AP, Lizzi FL, Wells PN. A new philosophy of medical imaging. *Med Hypotheses* 1991;**36**:327–35.

8 Bom N, Carlier SG, van der Steen AF, Lancée CT. Intravascular scanners. *Ultrasound Med Biol* 2000;**26**(Suppl 1):S6–9.

9 Burns PN. Contrast agents for Doppler ultrasound. In: Taylor KJ, Burns PN, Wells PN (eds). *Clinical Applications of Doppler Ultrasound*, 2nd edn. New York: Raven Press, 1995:367–79.

10 Tranquart F, Grenier N, Eder V, Pourcelot L. Clinical use of ultrasound tissue harmonic imaging. *Ultrasound Med Biol* 1999;**25**:889–94.

11 Leen E. Ultrasound contrast harmonic imaging of abdominal organs. Review. *Semin Ultrasound CT MR* 2001;**22**:11–24.

12 Burns P, Wilson S, Simpson DH. Pulse inversion imaging of liver blood flow: improved method for characterizing focal masses with microbubble contrast. *Invest Radiol* 2000; **35**:58–71.

13 Wells PN. Advances in ultrasound: from microscanning to telerobotics. Review. *Br J Radiol* 2000;**73**:1138–47.

14 Ophir J, Alam SK, Garra B, Kallel F *et al.* Elastography: ultrasonic estimation and imaging of the elastic properties of tissues. *Proc Inst Mech Eng* 1999;**213**:203–33.

15 Dunmire B, Beach KW, Labs KH, Plett M, Strandness DE Jr. Cross-beam vector Doppler ultrasound for angle-independent velocity measurements. *Ultrasound Med Biol* 2000;**26**: 1213–35.

16 Liang HD, Halliwell M, Wells PN. Continuous wave ultrasonic tomography. *IEEE Trans Ultrason Ferroelectr Freq Control* 2001;**48**:285–92.

☐ INSTITUTE OF PHYSICS AND ENGINEERING IN MEDICINE SELF ASSESSMENT QUESTIONS

The clinical use of functional electrical stimulation in neurological rehabilitation

1 Functional electrical stimulation (FES) can be used for each of the following conditions:
(a) Poliomyelitis
(b) Familial spastic paraplegia
(c) Motor neurone disease
(d) Brachial plexus lesions
(e) Traumatic brain injury

2 Contraindications for FES are:
(a) Mild spasticity
(b) Pregnancy
(c) Uncontrolled oedema
(d) Diabetes
(e) Uncontrolled epilepsy

3 Special precautions (eg simultaneous physiological monitoring) should be taken on the first assessment if the patient:
(a) Has a pacemaker
(b) Is known to suffer from autonomic dysreflexia
(c) Has poor circulation in the legs
(d) Has mild hypertension

4 In order to use an FES walking system patients should:
(a) Be able to walk at least 10 m
(b) Be able to climb a flight of stairs
(c) Be able to walk at least 100 m
(d) Be able to achieve a positive heel strike without stimulation
(e) Already wear an orthosis

5 Possible complications:
(a) Skin allergy
(b) Deep vein thrombosis
(c) Walking deteriorates when no stimulation
(d) Muscle atrophy

Advances in renal dialysis technology: recent developments and future prospects

1 Dialysis therapy is able to:
(a) Remove all uraemic toxins
(b) Correct electrolyte abnormalities
(c) Replace the metabolic functions of the human kidney

2 Common complications associated with dialysis therapy are:
(a) Inadequate removal of urea
(b) Hypertension
(c) Metabolic acidosis
(d) Inflammation

3 Complications associated with vascular access include:
(a) Inflammation of the vessels
(b) Infection
(c) Clotting
(d) Intimal hyperplasia

4 The technology used in renal replacement therapy has:
(a) Improved mortality and morbidity
(b) Reduced intradialytic complications
(c) Allowed treatment to be performed in the patient's own home

Advances in ultrasonic imaging

1 The performance of an ultrasonic scanner depends on:
(a) The physical size of the scanner
(b) The bandwidth of the transducer
(c) The excitation of the transducer
(d) The use of contrast agents
(e) The signal processing in the receiver

2 Ultrasonic compound scanning:
(a) Enhances shadows in the image
(b) Can be performed in real time
(c) Reduces speckle in the image
(d) Blurs the edges between structures
(e) Cannot be performed with a transducer array

3 Intravascular scanning:
(a) Produces high-resolution images
(b) Has no penetration limitation
(c) Requires a low ultrasonic frequency
(d) Involves a compromise between resolution and aperture
(e) Is inadequate because it is not transcutaneous

4 Contrast agents:
(a) Must contain gas
(b) Can be small enough to cross the lung capillaries
(c) Can sometimes be immunologically targeted
(d) Can be multimodal
(e) Can suppress the echoes from blood

5 Elasticity imaging:
(a) Is impossible with ultrasound
(b) Requires the application of an external force
(c) Is more sensitive than manual palpation
(d) Depends on differences in scatterer displacement
(e) Always requires a Doppler signal

Lumleian Lecture

Growth hormone: from molecule to mortality

Michael Sheppard

□ INTRODUCTION

Growth hormone (GH) is a 22 kDa protein secreted from the anterior pituitary gland in an episodic pattern central to the regulation of growth. GH induces metabolic changes indirectly through the induction of insulin-like growth factor-1 (IGF-1) expression or directly on tissues such as liver, muscle, bone or fat. The GH receptor (GHR) is a transmembrane protein with an extracellular domain that binds to GH; the intracellular domain interacts with other proteins to regulate cellular functions of the target cell. GH has two binding sites and dimerisation of the GHR is required for signal transduction.

It has become increasingly clear that excess levels of GH are harmful in inducing symptoms as well as resulting in increased mortality in subjects exposed to high levels of GH. This review will discuss:

- the current approaches to managing acromegaly, with evidence that mortality rates can now be restored to normal by inhibitors of GH secretion
- the development of new agents which will antagonise GH actions
- the risks of GH deficiency (GHD), and
- the increasing evidence that GH and IGF-1 may be related to morbidity and mortality in a variety of circumstances.

□ ACROMEGALY

Acromegaly is caused by GH hypersecretion and the resulting elevated levels of circulating IGF-1. The underlying abnormality in more than 98% of cases is a pituitary GH-producing tumour. The disease is typically diagnosed 10–15 years after the presumed onset of GH hypersecretion because of the slow, insidious progression of the disease and lack of symptoms. Clinical manifestations of acromegaly can be divided into those due to:

- local tumour expansion with compression of surrounding structures (headaches, visual field loss, hypopituitarism), and
- excess GH and IGF-1 secretion.

The most common biochemical consequences of acromegaly are impaired glucose tolerance or overt diabetes, and insulin resistance. Cardiovascular disease is an important clinical consequence. The importance of sleep apnoea as a cause of morbidity has become increasingly apparent. The relationship between acromegaly and cancer risk remains controversial, with the strongest evidence for an increased risk of colorectal cancer. Acromegaly decreases life expectancy, with a two- to threefold increase in mortality, major causes of death including cardiovascular, cerebrovascular and respiratory diseases. The morbidity produced by acromegaly is much more difficult to quantify.

Management of acromegaly

The clinical management of acromegaly has changed dramatically in recent years.[1,2] The two most important advances are:

- the recognition that the increased mortality associated with acromegaly can be reversed by optimal treatment (Table 1), and
- the development of effective inhibitors of GH secretion and action as major adjuncts to the traditional approaches of surgery and radiotherapy.

Table 1 Acromegaly treatment objectives.

- Reduction or stabilisation of pituitary tumour size
- Reversal of symptoms and signs to the greatest extent possible
- Correction of abnormal biochemistry
- Prevention of disease recurrence
- Avoidance of hypopituitarism

In view of the absence of sensitive clinical parameters, cure has been defined arbitrarily as normalisation of biochemical parameters. There is logic in this approach as there is now increasing and convincing evidence that effective biochemical control can reduce mortality to that of the general population. There is general agreement that control of disease is achieved when mean GH levels are below 5 mU/l, nadir GH after an oral glucose load is less than 2 mU/l and circulating IGF-1 is reduced to an age-adjusted normal range. However, controversy remains about the relative importance of GH and IGF-1 values in determining post-treatment control status. Virtually all evidence from epidemiological studies has related GH values and not IGF-1 values to long-term morbidity and mortality; post-treatment mean GH values below 5 mU/l are associated with a mortality no different from the general population.

Surgery

Trans-sphenoidal surgery remains the most cost-effective and rapid initial treatment of choice for most patients with acromegaly. However, using the rigorous criteria given above to interpret the surgical results obtained by an experienced operator in an expert unit, approximately 80% of patients with microadenomas and fewer than 50% of patients with macroadenomas can be defined as controlled. Many patients who undergo initial surgery will therefore require additional therapy such as radiation and/or medical therapy to alleviate potentially disabling signs and symptoms and to control GH and IGF-1 levels.

Somatostatin analogues

Somatostatin analogue therapy has proved an effective adjunctive therapy in patients already treated with surgery and/or radiotherapy. In addition, several studies in which newly diagnosed acromegalics were given a short course of subcutaneous octreotide before surgery report similar reductions in GH and IGF-1 levels to those observed in patients given octreotide after surgery. Studies of depot somatostatin analogues with prolonged release – Sandostatin LAR (octreotide), Lanreotide SR and Lanreotide Autogel – have also included patients who have not received pituitary surgery or radiotherapy. Sandostatin LAR was as effective both as primary therapy and as adjunctive therapy in patients previously treated with surgery and/or radiotherapy.

There is increasing interest in the use of somatostatin analogue therapy to induce shrinkage of GH-producing tumours. The prospective UK Primary Octreotide Therapy Study Group found over 30% tumour shrinkage in 73% of 27 patients with newly diagnosed acromegaly treated with subcutaneous octreotide and Sandostatin LAR as primary medical therapy for up to 48 weeks.[3] Several other studies using these three depot somatostatin analogues also reported tumour shrinkage in excess of 30% in 20–100% of subjects, although most studies involved small numbers. Substantial tumour shrinkage thus occurs in a significant subset of acromegalic patients.

It was concluded from these observations that if the possibility of surgical cure is low and if there is no visual compromise, medical treatment with octreotide or lanreotide alone should be as effective biochemically and clinically as surgery followed by octreotide or lanreotide, and that it may be a reasonable primary therapeutic modality.[4]

Long-term outcome associated with acromegaly was determined using the West Midlands Acromegaly Database (419 patients).[5] Mortality was increased in the subgroup of patients with GH levels above 4 mU/l (measured as the mean of a GH day profile, GH values across an oral glucose tolerance test (GTT) or a random GH level). IGF-1 levels have been proposed as first-line investigation for the diagnosis and therapeutic monitoring of acromegaly, but in this large study there was no increase in mortality in the subgroup with raised serum IGF-1. On the basis of these data, serum IGF-1 does not appear to be a reliable marker of long-term risk. This study has also shown reduced life expectancy following pituitary radiotherapy. Treatment with radiotherapy was associated with increased mortality (relative risk 1.67), with cerebrovascular disease the predominant cause of death (standard mortality ratio (SMR) 4.42).

There is mounting evidence that in the subgroup of patients in whom surgery is unlikely to result in a cure, long-term treatment with depot somatostatin analogues as primary therapy is a safe and effective option. Somatostatin analogues may cause significant tumour shrinkage (Table 2).

Table 2 The treatment of acromegaly: conclusions.

- Control of GH hypersecretion, and presumably GH action, is worthwhile
- Medical inhibitors of GH hypersecretion and action are effective clinically and biochemically
- Aggressive therapy to normalise GH and/or IGF-1 levels should be instituted at diagnosis and during follow-up of all patients
- Radiotherapy may be associated with increased mortality
- Tumour shrinkage occurs in a high proportion of patients treated with somatostatin analogues
- Primary medical therapy with somatostatin analogues may be effective for patients with either micro- or macroadenomas

GH = growth hormone; IGF = insulin-like growth factor.

Growth hormone receptor antagonist

Pegvisomant, a GH receptor antagonist, represents an innovative concept in the medical management of acromegaly.[6] Of the nine amino acid substitutions in this GH analogue, one inhibits functional dimerisation of GH receptors and the other eight are within the region responsible for receptor binding; this gives the antagonist a kinetic advantage over native GH, enabling saturation of all GHs. Pegvisomant inhibits GH activity and not GH secretion, so serum GH concentrations are not a valid marker for treatment efficacy; serum IGF-1 level is the only biochemical marker of efficacy. Pegvisomant does not control pituitary tumour growth; its efficacy does not depend on the characteristics of the tumour, such as size and thus feasibility of surgical removal, radiosensitivity or dopamine and somatostatin receptor density. It is a competitive receptor antagonist and should potentially be effective in all patients, regardless of the nature of the pituitary adenoma.

In the first major study of pegvisomant in the treatment of acromegaly in which 112 patients were treated for 12 weeks, there was normalisation of IGF-1 in up to 89%. In a more extensive study of 90 patients treated for over 12 months, 97% achieved normal serum IGF-1 levels.[7] There were significant improvements in overall well-being, symptom scores for perspiration, fatigue and paraesthesiae, and improvements in soft tissue swelling. Metabolic parameters also improved, with decreased fasting insulin and glucose levels.

The risk of any treatment of acromegaly that does not attempt to control tumour growth is that there will be a gradual increase in tumour size or that the blockade of GH action could induce negative feedback mechanisms to stimulate tumour expansion – analogous to Nelson's syndrome following bilateral adrenalectomy in Cushing's disease. There is thus a need for high quality IGF-1 assays with robust age- and gender-matched reference ranges and careful follow-up of all patients with regular imaging of tumour size.

□ ADULT GROWTH HORMONE DEFICIENCY

The presence of GHD in adulthood can have had either childhood or adult onset. The most common type of deficiency with childhood onset is idiopathic, while that of acquired GHD in adults is caused by a pituitary adenoma and its treatment (surgery or radiotherapy). GHD may occur in isolation or in association with other pituitary hormone deficiencies. GH is usually the first anterior pituitary hormone to be lost in patients with large non-functioning adenomas following surgery or radiotherapy. Unlike the poor growth associated with GHD in childhood, none of the features of GHD in adults is pathognomonic for the condition. GHD in adults has therefore to be defined using biochemical criteria, now generally agreed to be a peak GH response of less than 3 μg/l during an insulin tolerance test in patients with existing hypothalamo-pituitary disease or who received GH during childhood.

In adult life, GHD is associated with significant changes in biological variables such as body composition, physical performance, insulin status, bone mineral density (BMD), lipid profile and quality of life (QoL) measures.[8] Studies have documented increased cardiovascular risk factors in patients with hypopituitarism, including visceral obesity, glucose intolerance, insulin resistance, hyperlipidaemia, vascular endothelial dysfunction and, in some studies, hypertension. These risk factors have been attributed to GHD. Decreased BMD has been reported in GHD, and hypopituitary patients have an increased risk of fracture. This situation is complicated by the presence of gonadal steroid deficiency and the appropriateness of dosing schedules of glucocorticoid therapy. Adults with GHD have a lower perceived QoL and higher levels of psychological distress than healthy controls. Characteristic features are depressed mood, increased anxiety, lack of energy, social isolation and impaired well-being. Replacement therapy with GH has shown beneficial effects on body composition (reducing fat mass and increasing muscle mass), bone quality, cardiovascular risk factors and QoL, but there are no data on the effects of GH treatment on mortality.

Hypopituitarism, growth hormone deficiency and mortality

Four retrospective studies have examined mortality in patients with hypopituitarism, all confirming increased mortality compared with age-matched controls. A prospective study by the West Midlands Hypopituitary Database investigated total and specific-cause mortality in more than 1,000 patients with hypopituitarism and attempts were made to identify factors contributing to the excess mortality.[9]

West Midlands Hypopituitary Database

The West Midlands hypopituitary database, established in 1990, includes patients with underlying pituitary disease from 16 referral centres across the West Midlands region (population ca 5.5 million, ca 10% of the UK population).

We followed up 1,014 patients from January 1992 to January 2000. The number of observed deaths was 181 compared with the 96.7 expected (SMR 1.87). Univariate analysis indicated that mortality was higher in women (SMR 2.29) than in men (SMR 1.57), in younger patients, in those with an underlying diagnosis of craniopharyngioma (SMR 9.28) and in the 353 patients treated with radiotherapy (SMR 2.32 vs 1.66). Excess mortality was attributed to cardiovascular, respiratory and cerebrovascular causes, contributed to by a marked increase in cerebrovascular deaths in patients who underwent radiotherapy (SMR 4.36 vs 1.64). There was no effect of hormonal deficiency on mortality, except for gonadotropin deficiency which, if untreated, was associated with excess mortality. Adult GHD has been implicated as having a vital role in mediating increased vascular mortality in hypopituitarism. GH replacement is known to have beneficial effects, but there are no data on the effects of GH treatment on mortality. Risks of radiotherapy must be balanced against the undoubted efficacy of treatment in reducing the recurrence rate of non-functioning pituitary tumours.

□ HEIGHT, LEG LENGTH, CANCER RISK AND INSULIN-LIKE GROWTH FACTOR-1

A large body of literature supports the existence of an association between height and cancer risk.[10]

Height

Taller individuals have a 20–60% increased risk of a range of cancers. Associations have been reported particularly for breast, prostate, colorectal, thyroid and haematopoietic cancers. The component of height most often associated with increased risk is leg length (a marker for growth before puberty). The three main environmental factors influencing childhood growth are nutrition, ill health and psychological well-being, of which nutritional status before puberty may be the most important. Height *per se* clearly does not cause cancer, but simply acts as a biological marker for some other exposure. Confounding factors such as social class, smoking and body mass index have been ruled out. A proposed link is to circulating levels of GHs and growth factors.

Insulin-like growth factors

IGFs have been implicated as having a role in the development of cancer, and height may act as a marker for their levels. Cross-sectional studies of children demonstrate that IGF-1 levels are associated with stature. Recent research showed that raised levels of IGF-1 or low levels of IGF-BP3 are associated with increased risks of prostate, premenopausal breast and colorectal cancers and, interestingly, that height-cancer associations are found for these cancers. The biological link with IGF-1 includes:

- protection of damaged cells from apoptosis, thus increasing the potential to become cancerous
- potent stimulation of cell turnover, and
- amplification of effects of DNA-damaging agents.

There is also considerable evidence for the important role of nutrition in regulating IGF-1.

Insulin-like growth factor-1 and heart failure

Several experimental investigations have emphasised the favourable effects of IGF-1 on left ventricular remodelling, partly through its anti-apoptotic effects. In a community-based study 717 elderly people without known myocardial infarction or heart failure were followed for 5–9 years.[11] Those with higher IGF-1 levels developed heart failure less often than those with lower levels. If confirmed, these data suggest that maintenance of optimal levels of IGF-1 in the elderly may reduce the risk for heart failure.

□ CONCLUSIONS

These extensive clinical observations and literature reports suggest that optimal levels of circulating GH and IGF-1 are required to maintain normal health. Excess GH levels and GHD both appear to be associated with increased mortality (Fig 1), and restoration of GH levels to normal restores the mortality risk to that of the normal population.

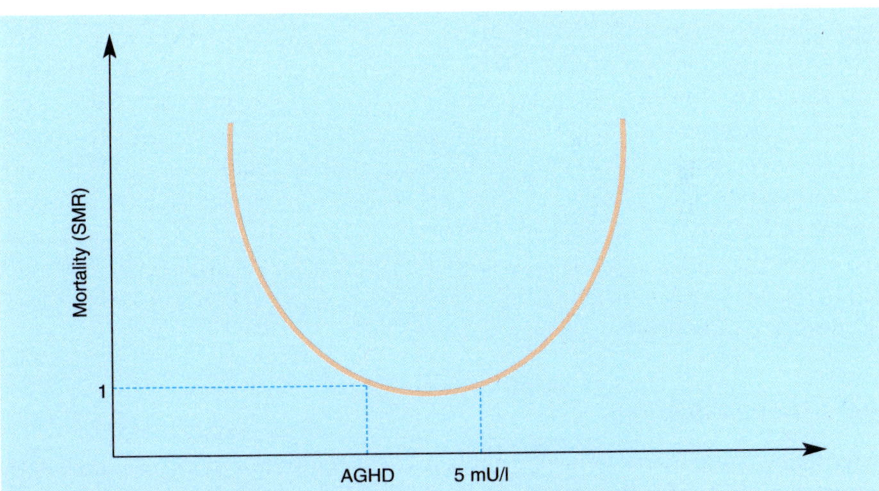

Fig 1 U-shaped curve. Clinical observations and literature reports suggest that optimal levels of circulating growth hormone (GH) and insulin-like growth factor-1 are required to maintain normal health. Excess levels of GH and GH deficiency appear to be associated with increased mortality (AGHD = adult growth hormone deficiency; SMR = standardised mortality ratio).

REFERENCES

1 Guistina A, Barkan A, Casanueva FF, Cavagnini F *et al.* Criteria for cure of acromegaly: a consensus statement. Review. *J Clin Endocrinol Metab* 2000;**85**:526–9.

2 Melmed S, Casanueva FF, Cavagnini F, Chanson P *et al.* Guidelines for acromegaly management. Review. *J Clin Endocrinol Metab* 2002;**87**:4054–8.

3 Bevan JS, Atkin SL, Atkinson AB, Bouloux PM *et al.* Primary medical therapy for acromegaly: an open, prospective, multicenter study of the effects of subcutaneous and intramuscular slow-release octreotide on growth hormone, insulin-like growth factor-I, and tumour size. *J Clin Endocrinol Metab* 2002;**87**:4554–63.

4 Sheppard MC. Primary medical therapy for acromegaly. Review. *Clin Endocrinol (Oxf)* 2003; **58**:387–99.

5 Ayuk J, Clayton RN, Holder G, Sheppard MC *et al.* Growth hormone and pituitary radiotherapy, but not serum insulin-like growth factor-I concentrations, predict excess mortality in patients with acromegaly. *J Clin Endocrinol Metab* 2004;**89**:1613–7.

6 Trainer PJ. A giant's step forward. *Clin Endocrinol (Oxf)* 2002;**56**:423–5.

7 van der Lely AJ, Hutson R, Trainer PJ, Besser GM *et al.* Long-term treatment of acromegaly with pegvisomant, a growth hormone receptor antagonist. *Lancet* 2001;**358**:1754–9.

8 Stavrou S, Kleinberg DL. Diagnosis and management of growth hormone deficiency in adults. Review. *Endocrinol Metab Clin North Am* 2001;**30**:545–63.

9 Tomlinson JW, Holden N, Hills RK, Wheatley K *et al.* Association between premature mortality and hypopituitarism. West Midlands Prospective Hypopituitary Study Group. *Lancet* 2001;**357**:425–31.

10 Gunnell D, Okasha M, Smith GD, Oliver SE *et al.* Height, leg length, and cancer risk: a systematic review. *Epidemiol Rev* 2001;**23**:313–42.

11 Vasan RS, Sullivan LM, D'Agostino RB, Roubenoff R *et al.* Serum insulin-like growth factor I and risk for heart failure in elderly individuals without a previous myocardial infarction: the Framingham Heart Study. *Ann Intern Med* 2003;**139**:642–8.

Croonian Lecture

The marvellous harmony of the nervous parts: the origins of multiple sclerosis

Alastair Compston

□ THE PATHOGENESIS OF MULTIPLE SCLEROSIS

The central concept underlying ideas on the pathogenesis of multiple sclerosis (MS) is that inflammatory events cause acute injury of axons and myelin. This has recently been challenged on the basis that tissue remote from areas of macroscopic inflammation is abnormal. Lesions sampled ultra-early in the course of the disease show loss of oligodendrocytes in the absence of inflammatory injury. There is pathological evidence for disease heterogeneity, with some cases showing oligodendrocyte apoptosis. These data suggest a primary disease process independent from immune mediated inflammation – a view favoured in the 19th century by Charcot who first made the emerging story of MS coherent. However, a preferred formulation is that the inflammatory and degenerative components are interrelated and should not be considered as competing events. Together, the phases of symptom onset, recovery, persistence and progression in MS can be summarised as:

- □ functional impairment with intact structure due to direct effects of inflammatory mediators
- □ demyelination and axonal injury with recovery through plasticity and remyelination, and
- □ chronic axonal loss due to failure of enduring remyelination from loss of trophic support for axons normally provided by cells of the oligodendrocyte lineage.

Cell death may occur in response to a state of injury from which protection would be anticipated under more favourable growth factor conditions. Conversely, optimal growth factor environment may save cells from otherwise lethal events occurring at the cell membrane. However, pieces are missing from this story. Pathologists have dissected the unitary concept of MS and proposed heterogeneity. MS is not one disease but four, each having a different aetiology – so what is known about aetiology and where should the search start?

□ THE ORIGINS OF MULTIPLE SCLEROSIS

Sutherland[1] established differential prevalence rates for MS in Scotland during the early 1950s; these mapped more closely to the distribution of Nordic people than to any geographical gradient. Later, the idea evolved that MS was disseminated throughout Europe by Norse invaders, thus accounting for its contemporary distribution (the Viking hypothesis).[2] Orcadians are considered an extreme ultra-European population but, neurologically speaking, from where did they get MS?

Until recently, the diagnosis of neuromyelitis optica was reserved for patients having a single episode of spinal cord and optic nerve or chiasmal disease, occurring in either order. It is recognised now that both the optic nerve and spinal cord features may recur, sometimes several times, but without clinical involvement elsewhere in the central nervous system. Magnetic resonance imaging (MRI) typically shows a long diffuse spinal abnormality quite unlike the discrete circumscribed lesions of MS, with high signal in the optic nerves or chiasm but a conspicuous absence of brain lesions. Although there is often an excess of white cells, the cerebrospinal fluid is conspicuous for the relative absence of oligoclonal bands.[3] Pathologically, the extensive spinal lesions are associated with necrosis and cavitation, acute axonal injury, loss of oligodendrocytes, inflammatory infiltrates and perivascular deposition of immunoglobulin and complement.[4] These are the features of a predominantly T helper 2 (Th2) immune response with prominent humoral mechanisms and they epitomise the type 2 pathology of MS.

Optico-spinal disease

Epidemiological studies of demyelinating disease have tended to separate neuromyelitis from MS – whilst noting that the latter often has a specifically different phenotype in Asian populations with disproportionate involvement of the spinal cord and optic nerves. Putting together neuromyelitis optica (monophasic or relapsing) with the Asian phenotype of MS allows the comparison of the frequencies of optico-spinal and (Western) relapsing-remitting MS. The result is rather striking. With the availability of local expertise in clinical neurology, it became clear that demyelinating disease in Africa, Asia, the Orient and in Aboriginal populations is typically optico-spinal, whereas (throughout most of the 20th century) relapsing-remitting MS matching the phenotype seen in northern Europeans has been distinctly uncommon.

Osuntokun[5] first applied sound epidemiological principles to the study of demyelinating disease in Nigeria. He found two possible cases of MS, 12 with acute disseminated encephalomyelitis, 95 with neuromyelitis optica and 33 with either acute bilateral optic neuritis or transverse myelitis. Thus, over 90% of all patients had optico-spinal disease. This has been confirmed in all studies, large and small, from the African continent.

The high frequency of optico-spinal disease is again apparent in India, Malaysia, Korea, Hong Kong, Japan, the Aboriginal populations of North and South America and those of African ancestry who reached the North American continent by sea.

The history of movements of people

Asia, the Orient, the Americas and into Europe is the route taken by man coming out of Africa. Contemporary analyses of human origins now use a combination of ephemeral, archaeological, linguistic and molecular genetic analyses of mitochondrial (mt) or Y chromosome markers to chart these movements.[6,7] The original lineage of *homo sapiens* (L) arose from *homo erectus* in Africa 150,000 years BP (before present). L1 re-emerged and expanded, but remained mainly in Africa and the Mediterranean (including Sardinia) from 100,000 BP with displacements by subsequent lineages (L2/L3) from 80,000 BP. L3 left Africa for Arabia via the Yemen in 50,000 BP. Their descendants, identified by mutations of mt DNA in the female migrants (N and M), made it to Australia, Asia and Turkey by 30,000 BP, and from Asia to North (25,000 BP) and South America (14,000 BP). Discrete subpopulations of N and M in European, Indian, African, Asian (and American) and Australian populations are identified by mt markers.

Europe was settled in the Upper Palaeolithic era (40,000 years BP). This group is marked by mt DNA haplogroups U5, H, V, I, W, T and K. Later, European man was threatened by climate change. Survivors chilled out during the last Ice Age (20,000 BP) in Iberia, the southern Mediterranean and the Ukraine, eventually giving rise to 70–80% of European descendants. With retreat of the ice (15,000 BP), repopulation occurred in the Neolithic period (10,000 BP) from Iberia (haplogroup V) and the Ukraine – but in came a new wave from Anatolia carrying mt DNA haplogroup J (originating from N) around 8,500 BP. They drifted thereafter with the movement of farming as hunter-gatherers ate their way into northern Europe, gaining a further contribution of the H, T and K mt haplogroups. Their descendants represent 20% of the present population. The language markers of these founders are Finno-Ugrian, proto-Indo-European (Neolithic arriving with the Anatolian wave and haplogroup J) and Basque (Ice Age survivors), respectively. Orkney and Shetland have no Palaeolithic history. They were populated from Meso- or early-Neolithic mainland Scotland, tweaked by the Norse interests of the 5th and 6th centuries AD imposing *élite dominance*, and again from Scotland in the 15th century.

The relevance to MS of this history is that MS in general, and the optico-spinal form in particular, is associated with haplogroup J/T[8] in northern Europeans but not in Basques in whom the frequencies of haplogroups J and T are reduced. Is it too glib to suggest that optico-spinal MS, present at low frequency in the out-of-Africa population, reached Europe with the Neolithic migration – carried not in saddlebags but tucked in the genes?

Perhaps transitional cases provide the archaeological record. Harding[9] described eight women presenting with bilateral sequential optic neuropathy, later developing symptoms consistent with demyelination outside the visual system. MRI abnormalities typical of demyelination were present in the seven who were scanned. All eight patients had matrilinear relatives affected by Leber's hereditary optic neuropathy and the 11778 mutation. There the genetic trail goes cold. Pathological mutations of mt DNA are not associated with MS in systematic screening of unselected patients nor with the neuromyelitis optica phenotype amongst Caucasians or Japanese. Thus, haplogroup J and T are population markers but do not harbour a pathological mutation. In that case, where should the search for genes that determine susceptibility to MS be focused?

Genetic search in MS

Because of linkage disequilibrium, susceptibility genes making even a small contribution to a disease process may still be identifiable by screening nearby anonymous markers, thus obviating the need directly to hit the disease locus itself. When polymorphisms that increase susceptibility to disease arise in a founder group, these will initially be located amongst a large group of linked genes. This block is subject to recombination during subsequent meioses and is gradually whittled down as the population expands. It follows that the progeny of this founder will share segments of DNA identical-by-descent over several generations, but this linkage disequilibrium degrades over time. Susceptibility genes can then no longer be identified by association mapping. The population is now in linkage equilibrium.

For younger populations, or more recently introduced alleles, the degree of linkage disequilibrium may be sufficient to use markers remote from the disease promoting polymorphism to track the genetic basis for susceptibility. Although the loss of founder mt DNA markers is significant, those that are transmitted survive longer as population markers than do nuclear genes. Therefore it may be easier to identify an mt DNA population marker than the nuclear genes putatively introduced with that founder group. It follows that the ancient susceptibility genes for MS will be hard to identify by association mapping. Conversely, susceptibility genes represented in the European population may still be trapped in large blocks of linkage disequilibrium and easier to find. Although estimates for the extent of linkage disequilibrium are changing, empirical evidence suggests that this may be relatively extensive. Recombination is not uniformly distributed, as assumed, but concentrated in hot spots separating regions of marked linkage disequilibrium averaging around 25 kb.

Starting with the founder alleles that arrived by chance with haplogroup J/T in the proto-European population, genetic drift and selection for survival from epidemic disasters of the Middle Ages may have concentrated the optico-spinal susceptibility genes and exposed the expanding population to the immunological consequences of these and additional mutations. Systematic filtration of high risk groups would have culled individuals and genotypes not well suited to surviving the waves of infectious disease and selected others for their immunological advantages.

Identification of the events that drove these changes in the genetic make-up of the emerging European population remains shrouded in the mists of history, but the answer must lie in one or more of the public health upheavals of the 15th–17th centuries resulting from infectious disease. The price paid is autoimmunity.

The major histocompatibility complex

The major suspect for having got the genetics wrong is the major histocompatibility complex (MHC). Its many polymorphisms are considered to be the 'tombstones' of long-standing battles for supremacy between the immune system and infectious pathogens. Removed from the microbial environment, these alleles saddled the progeny of their ancestral survivors with an inconvenient pro-inflammatory genetic heritage. MS is associated with and linked to alleles of the MHC, especially DR15/DQ6 (DRB1*1501, DRB5*0101, DQB1*0602) in Europeans.[10]

Although the immune repertoire was fixed long before *homo sapiens* made an appearance, it takes rather little licence to speculate that modifications of the proto-European genetic repertoire changed the nature and style of the immune response. *Neo*-MS (the Western phenotype) may have emerged because the Th2 immune response of neuromyelitis optica switched as a result of this genetic filtration and a changing microbial environment. A Th1 immune response enhancing T cell and memory responses then dominated, overriding the optico-spinal specificity, exposing new and more ubiquitous antigens and increasing the frequency of episodes – thus altering the course and phenotype. Thereafter, relapsing-remitting multifocal MS became the pattern as frequency of the disease increased during the 19th century and beyond due to population expansion, increased awareness and (perhaps) a genuine increase in incidence.

The role of Epstein-Barr virus

If there was a genetic time bomb waiting to go off, what lit the fuse? At some point, there was a specific microbial challenge which led to the appearance of MS and its subsequent increase in frequency. Lang *et al*[11] showed that a T cell receptor specificity present in MS (Hy.2E11) recognises a residue of myelin basic protein (MBP) (85–99) in the context of DRB1*1501 restriction, and an epitope of Epstein-Barr virus (EBV) (residues 627–641) in association with DRB5*0101. Four T cell receptor peptide contacts are identical for MBP and EBV. Thus, there is molecular mimicry.

EBV has probably been around for at least 10,000 years. Could cultural change have exposed a window of autoimmune opportunity through changes in age at infection and with markedly different biological consequences, as is well established for enterovirus infection and paralytic poliomyelitis? Patients with demyelinating disease report later age at infection by measles, mumps, rubella and especially EBV compared with controls selected for the same frequency of HLA-DR2 (to match for at least one marker of genetic susceptibility).[12] Infectious mononucleosis after the age of 18 years carries a relative risk for MS of 7.9 (95% confidence interval 2–38).

□ MULTIPLE SCLEROSIS: AN EVOLUTIONARY HYPOTHESIS

MS did not begin with wandering Vikings distributing their genetic material throughout Europe and, through their descendants, to other parts of the globe. It evolved from a disease – neuromyelitis optica – already present in more ancient populations and leaving traces in the present day spectrum of disease. Th2 and humoral mechanisms acting against a particular genetic background targeted the disease process to the optic nerves and spinal cord, producing long necrotic lesions carrying a poor prognosis for functional recovery. The disease was never common but, by chance, the susceptibility factors were brought to Europe with the small founder group from Anatolia who contributed to the repopulation of northern Europe after the last Ice Age (ca 10,000 years BP).

Relapsing-remitting multiple sclerosis

This founder group from Anatolia is marked by the mitochondrial haplogroup J/T; traces of the association remain with MS in general and with the optico-spinal phenotype in particular. Thereafter, genetic drift and selection pressure from waves of epidemic disease favoured the emergence of high immune response genotypes clustered within the MHC. Those changes were sufficient to induce the Th1 to Th2 switch in immune response, triggering more frequent episodes and eventually breaking down the optico-spinal specificity – with checks and balances such that the lesions were smaller and more sharply defined but (individually) of less immediate functional significance. Thus arose relapsing-remitting MS. The triggers were infectious disease, with EBV playing a particular role, its impact emerging most floridly with cultural change consequent upon expansion of the population and industrialisation in the 19th century. Even now, the switch from optico-spinal to relapsing-remitting MS is seen on a smaller scale, as indicated by the shifting clinical phenotype of MS in Japan following cultural changes and industrialisation from the 1960s. Although still a much rarer disease than in the West, these social shifts exposed the innate vulnerability of those few individuals harbouring alleles that later underwent concentration and stratification amongst progeny of the Neolithic founders, leading to the sustained epidemic of MS that characterises northern Europeans.

□ CONCLUSIONS

This formulation makes many assumptions. An evolutionary approach to the origins of MS is novel but risky, leaving many issues unexplained. It is testable using the matrix of informative populations, mitochondrial and nuclear genetic markers, and discrete clinical phenotypes. The zoological record is in the spectrum of pathological changes, dubbed heterogeneity, and the transitional clinical cases. The archaeological record is in the global epidemiology of demyelinating disease.

REFERENCES

1 Sutherland JM. Observations on the prevalence of multiple sclerosis in northern Scotland. *Brain* 1956;**79**:635–54.

2 Poser CM. The dissemination of multiple sclerosis: a Viking saga? A historical essay. *Ann Neurol* 1994;**36**(Suppl 2):S231–43.

3 Wingerchuk DM, Hogancamp WF, O'Brien PC, Weinshenker BG. The clinical course of neuromyelitis optica (Devic's syndrome). *Neurology* 1999;**53**:1107–14.

4 Lucchinetti CF, Mandler RN, McGavern D, Bruck W *et al.* A role for humoral mechanisms in the pathogenesis of Devic's neuromyelitis optica. *Brain* 2002;**125**(Pt 7):1450–61.

5 Osuntokun BO. Neurological disorders in Nigeria. In: Spillane JD (ed). *Tropical Neurology.* London: Oxford University Press, 1973:161–90.

6 Sykes B. The molecular genetics of European ancestry. *Philos Trans R Soc Lond B Biol Sci* 1999;**354**:131-8; discussion 138–9.

7 Renfrew C. Genetics and language in contemporary archaeology. In: Cunliffe B, Davies W, Renfrew C. *Archaeology: the Widening Debate.* Oxford: Oxford University Press, The British Academy, 2002:43–76.

8 Reynier P, Penisson-Besnier I, Moreau C, Savagner F *et al.* mtDNA haplogroup J: a contributing factor of optic neuritis. *Eur J Hum Genet* 1999;**7**:404–6.

9 Harding AE, Sweeney MG, Miller DH, Mumford CJ *et al.* Occurrence of a multiple sclerosis-like illness in women who have a Leber's hereditary optic neuropathy mitochondrial DNA mutation. *Brain* 1992;**115**(Pt 4):979–89.

10 GAMES: Transatlantic Multiple Sclerosis Genetics Cooperative. A meta-analysis of whole genome linkage screens in multiple sclerosis. *J Neuroimmunol* 2003;**143**:39–46.

11 Lang HL, Jacobsen H, Ikemizu S, Andersson C *et al.* A functional and structural basis for TCR cross-reactivity in multiple sclerosis. *Nat Immunol* 2002;**3**:940–3.

12 Martyn CN, Cruddas M, Compston DA. Symptomatic Epstein-Barr virus infection and multiple sclerosis. *J Neurol Neurosurg Psychiatry* 1993;**56**:167–8.

Answers to self assessment questions

☐ ONCOLOGY

Should we be more aggressive in managing lung cancer?

1a True	2a True	3a False	4a True
b True	b False	b True	b False
c False	c True	c False	c False
d False	d True	d False	d True
e False	e False	e False	e False

Who should be screened for colorectal cancer?

1a True	2a True	3a False
b False	b False	b True
c False	c False	c True
d True	d False	d True
e True	e False	e True

☐ CARDIOLOGY

Contemporary treatment for atrial fibrillation

1a True	2a False	3a True
b True	b False	b False
c False	c False	c False
d False	d True	d True
e True	e False	e False

Risk stratification post-myocardial infarction

1a True	2a True	3a False	4a True
b True	b True	b False	b False
c True	c False	c False	c False
d False	d False	d True	d True
e True	e True	e True	e False

Cardiovascular funny turns

1a False	2a False	3a False	4a False	5a True
b False	b True	b True	b False	b False
c True	c False	c False	c False	c True
d False	d False	d True	d True	d True
e False	e True	e True	e True	e False

☐ ENDOCRINOLOGY

What to do with thyroid nodules and goitres

1a True	2a False	3a True
b False	b True	b False
c False	c True	c True
d False	d False	d False
e True	e False	e False

New management strategies for osteoporosis

1a True	2a True	3a True
b False	b False	b False
c True	c False	c False
d False	d False	d True

How to manage hypercalcaemia

1a True	2a False	3a False	4a False
b False	b True	b False	b True
c False	c False	c False	c False
d True	d True	d True	d False
e False	e False	e False	e False

☐ NEUROLOGY

Should transient ischaemic attack and minor stroke be managed as a medical emergency?

1a False	2a False	3a True
b True	b True	b True
c False	c False	c True
d True	d False	d False
e False	e False	e False

Epilepsy: update on new therapies

1a False	2a True	3a False
b True	b True	b True
c True	c False	c True
d False	d False	d False

Diagnosis and management of motor neurone disease

1a False	2a False	3a True
b False	b True	b True

c True	c False	c True
d False	d True	d False
e False	e False	e True

☐ RENAL

Uraemia and cardiovascular risk

1a True	2a True	3a False
b False	b False	b True
c True	c False	c True
d True	d True	d True
e True	e False	e True

Is proteinuria bad for the kidney?

1a False	2a True	3a True
b False	b True	b True
c True	c True	c True
d True	d True	d False
e False	e True	e False

Primary small vessel vasculitis

1a False	2a False	3a True	4a True	5a True
b False	b False	b False	b True	b False
c True	c True	c True	c False	c True
d False	d False	d False	d False	d False

Anaaemia in renal failure

1a False	2a True	3a False	4a False	5a False
b False	b False	b False	b True	b True
c False	c True	c False	c False	c False
d False	d False	d True	d True	d False
e True	e False	e False	e True	e False

☐ RESPIRATORY

Asthma or chronic obstructive pulmonary disease? Managing the acute exacerbation

1a False	2a True	3a False
b False	b False	b True
c False	c True	c True
d False	d True	d True
e False	e False	e False

Pulmonary embolism: the difficult diagnosis

1a True	2a False	3a False	4a False	5a True
b False	b False	b False	b False	b True
c True	c False	c True	c False	c True
d False	d True	d False	d False	d False

Community-acquired pneumonia

1a True	2a False	3a False	4a True
b False	b False	b False	b True
c True	c True	c False	c False
d False	d True	d False	d True
e False	e False	e False	e True

☐ GASTROENTEROLOGY

Management of dyspepsia

1a False	2a True	3a True	4a True	5a False
b True	b False	b True	b True	b True
c False	c True	c True	c False	c True
d True	d True	d True	d False	d False
e False	e True	e True	e False	e False

Advances in gastrointestinal bleed management

1a False	2a False	3a False	4a True
b False	b True	b True	b True
c False	c False	c True	c False
d False	d False	d True	d True
e True	e True	e False	e True

☐ HEPATOLOGY

Viral hepatitis and medical risks

1a False	2a False	3a False
b True	b True	b True
c False	c False	c False
d False	d False	d False
e True	e True	e True

Management of ascites

1a True	2a False	3a True
b True	b False	b False

c True	c False	c False
d False	d False	d False
e False	e False	e False

Non-alcoholic steatohepatitis and fatty liver disease

1a False	2a False	3a True
b False	b False	b True
c True	c True	c True
d False	d True	d False
e True	e False	e False

☐ TRANSPLANTATION

Bone marrow stem cells: from development to therapy

1a False	2a True	3a True
b False	b True	b True
c False	c True	c False
d True	d True	d True
e False	e False	e False

☐ MEDICINE IN PREGNANCY

How to manage renal disease in pregnancy

1a True	2a False	3a True	4a False
b True	b False	b True	b False
c True	c False	c False	c True
d True	d True	d False	d False
e True	e True	e True	e False

Congenital heart disease in pregnancy

1a True	2a False	3a True	4a True	5a True
b False	b True	b False	b False	b False
c True	c True	c True	c True	c True
d True	d False	d False	d False	d True
e True	e False	e True	e False	e False

☐ MANAGING RISK FACTORS

The epidemic of obesity: genes versus environment

1a True	2a False	3a True
b False	b True	b False
c True	c True	c True

d False	d False	d False
e False	e True	e True

The management of hypertension: what the trials have taught us

1a False	2a True	3a False
b True	b True	b False
c False	c False	c True
d False	d False	d False
e True	e False	e True

What to do about hormone replacement therapy

1a True	2a True	3a True
b False	b True	b True
c True	c True	c True
d True	d True	d False
e False	e True	e False

☐ INSTITUTE OF PHYSICS AND ENGINEERING IN MEDICINE

The clinical use of functional electrical stimulation in neurological rehabilitation

1a False	2a False	3a True	4a True	5a True
b True	b True	b True	b False	b False
c False	c True	c False	c False	c False
d False	d False	d False	d False	d False
e True	e True		e False	

Advances in renal dialysis technology: recent developments and future prospects

1a False	2a False	3a False	4a False
b True	b True	b True	b True
c False	c False	c True	c True
	d True	d True	

Advances in ultrasonic imaging

1a False	2a False	3a True	4a False	5a False
b True	b True	b False	b True	b True
c True	c True	c False	c True	c True
d False	d False	d True	d True	d True
e True	e False	e False	e False	e False